Oxford Handbook of
Perioperative Practice

Edited by

Suzanne J Hughes

Lecturer/Project Manager Learning & Teaching
Cardiff School of Nursing & Midwifery Studies
Cardiff University
Cardiff, UK

and

Andy Mardell

Practice Educator, Main Theatres
University Hospital of Wales
Cardiff, UK

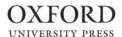

OXFORD
UNIVERSITY PRESS

OXFORD
UNIVERSITY PRESS

Great Clarendon Street, Oxford OX2 6DP

Oxford University Press is a department of the University of Oxford.
It furthers the University's objective of excellence in research, scholarship,
and education by publishing worldwide in

Oxford New York

Auckland Cape Town Dar es Salaam Hong Kong Karachi
Kuala Lumpur Madrid Melbourne Mexico City Nairobi
New Delhi Shanghai Taipei Toronto

With offices in

Argentina Austria Brazil Chile Czech Republic France Greece
Guatemala Hungary Italy Japan Poland Portugal Singapore
South Korea Switzerland Thailand Turkey Ukraine Vietnam

Oxford is a registered trade mark of Oxford University Press
in the UK and in certain other countries

Published in the United States
by Oxford University Press Inc., New York

© Oxford University Press, 2009

British Library Cataloguing in Publication Data
Data available

Library of Congress Cataloging in Publication Data
Data available

Typeset by Cepha Imaging Private Ltd., Bangalore, India
Printed in China
on acid-free paper by
Asia Pacific Offset Limited

ISBN 978-0-19-923964-1

10 9 8 7 6 5 4 3 2 1

Dedication

To Oliver, 'another story for you', love Mummy x

S.J.H

Dedication

Foreword

Supporting patients through their surgical experience is hugely rewarding but demands a wide range of skills from the professionals who choose to work in this field. Dealing with the complexities of procedures, range of equipment and drugs, and challenges encountered in the various stages of care can be daunting. The patient is wholly dependent on the expertise and knowledge of the multidisciplinary surgical team, with every member playing a vital role in securing a positive outcome. While procedures can vary in their technicality, for every patient undergoing a surgical treatment it is a 'big deal' and care must be tailored to meet their individual needs.

The advances we are enjoying in surgery and anaesthesia come at a time where the developed world is seeing a change in the demographics of its population, with increasing numbers of people living into old and very old age. As the saying goes, 'old age doesn't come alone' and many people are living into old age with one or more long-term or chronic conditions. This changing profile of surgical patients is adding complexity to an already complex area of care. The 'ageing' trend in the population is expected to continue during this century and practices need to evolve to meet the demands this brings.

The advent of the Internet has afforded easy access to information, resulting in a better informed populace. What this often means in practice is that patients are more likely to ask questions about their care and be knowledgeable about their conditions. Gone are the days of paternalistic care arrangements, patients expect and deserve to be partners in determining what treatments and care they receive. This can be uncomfortable for some practitioners, especially if patients choose not to consent to certain treatments. Resources such as this book provide a much needed overview of the patient journey, so that no matter where the practitioner is based they are able to answer patient queries about the likely pathway they will follow.

UK health regulators, such as the Nursing and Midwifery Council, all require that their registrants maintain their competence in practice and keep up to date. What this means is that every practitioner needs to be able to access reliable sources of information, based on the best available evidence, to inform their practice. This can be quite difficult in an area such as perioperative practice due to the diversity of patient conditions and procedures available. A book such as this clearly fits the bill, as its practical approach across a range of subjects, set out in 'bite size' sections, should prove useful to students, practitioners, and educators alike.

The contributors to this handbook have been able to highlight the importance of perioperative practice by setting out the key interventions and responsibilities of practitioners at each stage of the patient's journey. I applaud the aims of this book, as I firmly believe that an increased understanding of perioperative practice will increase the ability to deliver high quality patient-centred care.

Dr Jean White
Nursing Officer
Welsh Assembly Government

Preface

The subject of this book relates to practice within the perioperative environment. It addresses many key issues and outlines a thorough introduction to the principles and practice of anaesthetic practice, intraoperative care, recovery practice, and emergency care, including a comprehensive account of clinically-focused aspects of this highly specialised discipline.

The aim of the *Oxford Handbook of Perioperative Practice* is to provide practical, easily accessible, concise, and up-to-date evidence-based guidelines relating to all the essential elements of perioperative practice. This book has taken an inter-disciplinary and inter-professional approach to perioperative practice with contributors comprising of educationalists and clinicians from the fields of nursing, operating department practice, and pharmacy throughout the United Kingdom and from as far away as Australia.

This book is a sound introduction to perioperative practice for newly qualified practitioners, all those studying the subject, or those who are considering embarking on a career in this highly specialised environment. It is also intended to provide relevant and useful information at the fingertips of practitioners faced with managing difficult patient cases.

It is by no means exhaustive of all arenas of perioperative practice but serves to assist perioperative practitioners to meet the needs of surgical patients to ensure safe and efficient care delivery and management of this clientele. We hope that you will find it useful and that it contributes to your transition from novice to expert perioperative practitioner.

Suzanne J. Hughes
Andy Mardell

Acknowledgements

The increasing scope and complexity of perioperative care makes it more challenging for a sole author to encompass. Therefore, this text adopts an inter-disciplinary and inter-professional approach and I am very grateful to all of the contributors for their commitment to this project.

Special thanks to Jamie Hartmann-Boyce, Development Editor at Oxford University Press, whose endless support, encouragement, and motivation has been exemplary and very much appreciated, and whose administrative skills have brought the project to fruition.

I would like to thank my mum and dad, Anne and Brian Griffiths, who have been a consistent source of support and encouragement, throughout my life; love you!

Finally, special thanks to my husband, Charlie, my son, Oliver, and Mitzi, for their unconditional support and patience. I love you all.

Suzanne J. Hughes

I would like to acknowledge all the contributors who so willingly provided their expert knowledge to help make the publication of this book a reality. Gratitude is also due to those companies and organisations that allowed us to reproduce material to illustrate the work.

I would also like to thank our development editor Jamie Hartmann-Boyce at Oxford University Press for her constant support, encouragement, and enthusiasm.

Andy Mardell

Contents

Contributors

Kim Bennett
Cardiff University
Cardiff UK

- *The admission process*
- *Assessment of care*
- *Postoperative ward assessment*
- *Orthopaedic trauma surgery*
- *Management of fractures*

Nisha Bhudia
Royal Brompton &
Harefield NHS Trust
Harefield, Middlesex UK

- *Principles of drug action*
- *Absorption and distribution*
- *Metabolism and elimination*
- *Pharmacodynamics*
- *Medicine response relationships*
- *Medicine compatibility*
- *Common medicine problems*
- *Suspected adverse reactions*

Rachel Brent
University Hospital of Wales
Cardiff UK

- *Wound dehiscence*
- *Wound dehiscence: images*
- *Pain in recovery*
- *Hypothermia*
- *Patient discharge to ITU*
- *Overnight intensive recovery*

Olwen E Cooper
University Hospital
Llandough Cardiff UK

- **Chapter 10: Airway management**
- *Role of the anaesthetic practitioner*
- *Anaesthesia*
- *Triad of anaesthesia*
- *Inhalational anaesthesia*
- *Total intravenous anaesthesia*

Felicia Cox
Royal Brompton &
Harefield NHS Trust
Harefield, Middlesex UK

- **Chapter 23: Pain management**
- *Principles of drug action*
- *Absorption and distribution*
- *Metabolism and elimination*
- *Pharmacodynamics*
- *Medicine response relationships*
- *Medicine compatibility*
- *Common medicine problems*
- *Suspected adverse reactions*
- *Medicines administration: enteral*
- *Medicines administration: transmucosal (buccal and sublingual)*
- *Parenteral drug administration: 1*
- *Parenteral drug administration: 2*
- *Neuraxial analgesia*
- *Respiratory medicines administration*
- *Topical analgesia*
- *Patient-controlled analgesia*

Peggy Edwards
National Patient Safety Agency
London UK

- *Correct site surgery*

Hannah Grainger
Welsh Blood Service,
Cardiff UK

- *Intraoperative cell salvage*
- *Postoperative cell salvage*

Lois Hamlin
University of Technology
Sydney, Australia

- *Maintaining a sterile field*
- *Scrubbing up*
- *Draping of the patient*
- *Role of circulating practitioner*
- *Opening of sterile packs*
- *Movement within the theatre*
- *Communication with the surgical team*
- *Specimens*

Gaynor Hamlington
Wrexham Maelor Hospital
Wrexham UK

- *Ear, nose, and throat anaesthesia*
- *Transport to recovery*
- *Patient handover in recovery*
- *Patient assessment in recovery*

Jayne Hancock
Cardiff University
Cardiff UK

- *The admission process*
- *Assessment of care*
- *Postoperative ward assessment*
- *Management of fractures*
- *Orthopaedic trauma surgery*

Michelle Harding
University Hospital of Wales
Cardiff UK

- *Preoperative assessment*
- *Physical assessment*
- *Short stay surgery*

Paul Hennessy
Cardiff University
Cardiff UK

- *Medical gas cylinders*
- *Attaching cylinders to pin index system on an anaesthetic machine*
- *Oxygen therapy*
- *Local anaesthetic drugs*
- *Fluid therapy*
- *Crystalloids*
- *Colloids*
- *Blood*

Gillian Howell
Eastleigh, Hampshire UK

- *Minimal access surgery*
- *Arthroscopy*
- *Laparoscopy*
- *Endoscopy*
- *Use of lasers in surgery*

Charles W Hughes
Cardiff UK

- *Managing visitors in the perioperative environment*

Suzanne J Hughes
Cardiff University
Cardiff UK

- **Chapter 4: Pre-assessment of surgical patients**
- **Chapter 5: Patients with pre-existing disease**
- *Team working*
- *Interprofessional team working*
- *Theatre conduct*
- *Patients with special healthcare needs*
- *Physical disabilities*
- *Learning disabilities*
- *Mental illness*
- *Anxiety*
- *Children, parents, and carers*
- *Language barriers*
- *Prisoners in theatre*
- *Preoperative preparation*
- *Jewellery and body piercing*
- *Preoperative fasting*
- *Patient safety: surgical safety checklist*
- *Make-up, nail polish, and other considerations*
- *Venous thromboembolism*
- *Preoperative checklist*
- *Anaesthetic checklist*
- *Role of the anaesthetic practitioner*
- *Anaesthesia*
- *Triad of anaesthesia*
- *Inhalational anaesthesia*
- *Total intravenous anaesthesia*
- *The importance of airway management*
- *Laryngeal mask airway*
- *Additional supraglottic devices*
- *Paediatric and neonatal anaesthesia*
- *Neurosurgical anaesthesia*
- *Anaesthesia for burns surgery*
- *Anaesthesia for plastic surgery*
- *Cardiac anaesthesia*
- *Thoracic anaesthesia*
- *Principles of day surgery*
- *Management of a patient with an infection*
- *Intubated/ventilated patients in recovery*
- *Post-dural headache*
- *Extravasation*
- *Inadvertent intra-arterial injection*
- *Metabolism and elimination*
- *Medicine response relationships*
- *Routes of medicine administration [diagram]*
- *Anti-coagulant drugs*
- *Obstetric drugs*
- *Anti-muscarinic drugs*

- *Anti-cholinesterase drugs*
- *Anxiolytic benzodiazepine drugs*
- *Antagonists for central and respiratory depression and respiratory stimulants*
- *Anti-emetic drugs*
- *Anti-bacterial drugs*
- *Local anaesthetic drugs*
- *Bronchodilating drugs*
- *Nitrates*
- *Calcium channel blockers*
- *Intropic sympathomimetics*
- *Vasoconstrictor sympathomimetic drugs*
- *Professional, ethical, and legal and considerations of emergency care*
- *Death in the operating theatre*
- *Levels of consciousness*
- *Assessing levels of consciousness*
- *Ruptured abdominal aortic aneurysm repair*
- *Appendicectomy*
- *Gastrointestinal bleed*
- *Obstetrics surgery*
- *Gynaecology surgery*
- *Ophthalmology surgery*
- *Orthopaedic trauma surgery*
- *Common surgical abbreviations*

Ciarán Hurley
Sheffield Hallam University
Sheffield UK

- *Tourniquets*

Alister Jones
University Hospital Llandough
Cardiff UK

- *Preparing the anaesthetic room*
- *Stocking of essential items*
- *Perioperative drugs – overview*
- *Opiate analgesic drugs*
- *Non-opiate analgesic drugs and NSAIDs*

Arwel Jones
Ysbyty Gwynedd NHS Trust
Bangor UK

- *Monitoring obese patients*
- *Anaesthetic induction agents*
- *Depolarising muscle relaxants and non-depolarising muscle relaxants*
- *Inhalational drugs*

Barbara Jones
University Hospital Llandough
Cardiff UK

- *Malignant hyperpyrexia*
- *Suxamethonium apnoea*

Keith Jones
Cardiff University
Cardiff UK

- *Anaesthetic machines*
- *Ventilators*
- *Vaporisers*
- *Breathing systems*
- *Humidifiers*
- *Fluid/blood warmers*
- *Awareness under general anaesthesia*

Moyra Journeaux
Jersey General Hospital
St Hellier, Jersey UK

- *Infection control and prevention*
- *Common infection control terms*
- *Handwashing*
- *Management of a patient with an infection*
- *Accountability of swabs, sharps, and instruments*
- *Clinical waste*
- *Instrument trays*
- *Decontamination of equipment*
- *Protective clothing and eye protection*

Tim Lewis
Cardiff University
Cardiff UK

- *Anaphylaxis*
- *Respiratory arrest*
- *Causes of respiratory arrest*
- *Principles of emergency care*
- *A: airway*
- *B: breathing*
- *C: circulation*
- *Types of shock*
- *D: disability and E: exposure*
- *Professional, ethical, and legal considerations of emergency care*
- *Principles of resuscitation in adults*
- *Defibrillation in adults*
- *Principles of resuscitation in children*
- *Choking in children*

Andy Mardell
University Hospital of Wales
Cardiff UK

- **Chapter 13: Decontamination and sterilisation**
- **Chapter 14: Thermoregulation**
- **Chapter 17: Patient positioning for surgery**
- *Team working*
- *Interprofessional team working*
- *Theatre conduct*
- *Communication*
- *Dignity, anxiety, and promoting equality when preparing the patient for theatre*
- *Children and parents*
- *Theatre preparation: heating, lighting, and humidity*
- *Cleaning of the operating theatre*
- *The management of surgical equipment*
- *Surgical needles*
- *Wound dressings*
- *Operating microscopes*
- *Death in the operating theatre*
- *Ruptured abdominal aortic aneurysm repair*
- *Appendicectomy*
- *Splenectomy*
- *Bowel obstruction*
- *Gastrointestinal bleed*
- *Neurosurgery*
- *Ear, nose, and throat*
- *Common surgical abbreviations*

Paul Mathews
Royal College of Nursing
Glasgow, Scotland UK

- **Chapter 20: Preparation of the recovery room**

Rosanne MacQueen
Stracathro Hospital
NHS Tayside, Dundee UK

- *Role of the scrub practitioner*
- *Setting up of the surgical instrument tray*
- *Accountability of swabs, sharps, and instruments*
- *Administration of drugs during surgery*
- *Handling of surgical instruments*

Sherran Milton
The Association for
Perioperative Practice
Cardiff UK

- *Role of the anaesthetic practitioner*
- *Local anaesthesia*
- *Intravenous conscious sedation*
- *Epidural anaesthesia*
- *Caudal anaesthesia*
- *Spinal anaesthesia*
- *Patient positioning for regional anaesthesia*
- *Contraindications for spinal, epidural and caudal anaesthesia*
- *Patient monitoring*
- *Non-invasive monitoring*
- *Pulse oximetry*
- *Invasive monitoring*
- *Central venous pressure*
- *Acid aspiration syndrome*
- *High spinal*

Alun Morgan
Cardiff University
Cardiff UK

- **Chapter 9: Scientific principles**

Kevin Mulcock
Cardiff UK

- *Ophthalmic anaesthesia*
- *Electro-surgical equipment*

Anthony Pritchard
Cardiff University
Cardiff UK

- *Arterial blood gases*
- *Acid-base balance*
- *Neuromuscular junction blockade*

Tracey Radcliffe
Wrexham Maelor Hospital
Wrexham UK

- *Obstetric anaesthesia*
- *Caring for patients following spinal and epidural anaesthesia*
- *Caring for children and parents in the recovery room*
- *Postoperative documentation*

Hazel Smith
Spire Healthcare
London UK

- *Surgical incisions*
- *Haemostasis*
- *Wound closure*
- *Wound drains*
- *Prosthesis*

Ben Stanfield-Davies
Cardiff University & University
Hospital of Wales
Cardiff UK

- *Patients with special healthcare needs*
- *Patients with pre-existing disease - overview*
- *Lifestyle factors and induced disease*
- *Postoperative emergencies and management*
- *Respiratory disorders*
- *Cardiovascular disorders*
- *Neurological disorders*
- *Seizure/convulsion management*

Paula J Strong
Cardiff University
Cardiff UK

- *Postoperative problems*
- *Respiratory distress*
- *Postoperative nausea & vomiting*
- *Sore throat*
- *Delayed emergence from anaesthesia*
- *Post-anaesthetic shivering*
- *Sweating*
- *Hypotension*
- *Confusion and the violent patient*
- *Hypoglycaemia*

Judith Tanner
De Montfort University &
University Hospitals
Leicester UK

- **Chapter 15: Patient skin preparation**

Julie D Young
Cardiff University
Cardiff UK

- **Chapter 2: Professional issues in perioperative practice**

Sue Williams
Cardiff University
Cardiff UK

- *Clinical governance*
- *Applying principles of clinical governance*

Surgical terms

-OSCOPY: examination of a body cavity or deep structure using an instrument specifically designed for the purpose, e.g., gastroscopy, laparoscopy, arthroscopy and bronchoscopy.

-ECTOMY: removal of an organ, e.g., mastectomy, gastrectomy, orchidectomy, colectomy,

-ORRHAPHY: repair of tissues, e.g., herniorrhaphy

-OSTOMY: fashioning of an artificial communication between a hollow viscus and the skin, e.g., tracheostomy, colostomy, and ileostomy. The term may also apply to artificial openings between different viscera, e.g., gastro-jujunostomy, choledocho-duodenostomy.

-OTOMY: cutting open, e.g.. laparotomy, arteriotomy, fasciotomy, thoracotomy.

-PLASTY: reconstruction, e.g., pyloroplasty, mammoplasty, arthroplasty.

-PEXY: relocation and securing in position, e.g., orchidopexy, rectopexy.

-ITIS: inflammation of an organ or cavity, e.g., appendicitis, peritonitis.

Symbols and abbreviations

🕮	cross reference
>	greater than
<	less than
↑	increased
↓	decreased
🖫	downloadable document
🖰	website
AAA	abdominal aortic aneurysm
AADR	anaesthetic adverse drug reaction
AAGBI	Association of Anaesthetists of Great Britain and Ireland
ABC	airway, breathing, circulation
ABG	arterial blood gas
ACE	angiotensin-converting enzyme
ACh	acetylcholine
AChE	acetylcholinesterase
ACL	anterior cruciate ligament
ACORN	Australian College of Operating Room Nurses
ACT	activated clotting time
ADH	antidiuretic hormone
ADP	adenosine diphosphate
AED	automated external defibrillator
AF	atrial fibrillation
AFOI	awake fibreoptic intubation
AfPP	Association for Perioperative Practice
AICD	automatic implantable cardioverter defibrillator
AIDS	acquired immunodeficiency syndrome
AKA	above knee amputation
ALI	acute lung injury
ALL	anterior cruciate ligament
ALS	advanced life support
ANH	acute normovolaemic haemodilution
AORN	Association of periOperative Registered Nurses
AP	anteroposterior
APL	adjustable pressure-limiting
AR	aortic regurgitation

EEG	electroencephalogram
EMD	electromechanical dissociation
EMG	electromyography
EMLA	eutectic mixture of local anaesthetic
ENT	ear nose and throat
ePTFE	expanded polytetrafluoroethylene
EPO	erythropoietin
ERCP	endoscopic retrograde cholangiopancreatography
ERPC	evacuation of retained products of conception
ESR	erythrocyte sedimentation rate
$ETCO_2$	end-tidal carbon dioxide
ETT	endotracheal tube
EUA	examination under anaesthetic
FB	foreign body
FBC	full blood count
FES	fat embolism syndrome
FEV_1	forced expiratory volume in 1 second
FFP	fresh frozen plasma
FiO_2	fraction of oxygen in inspired air
Fg	French gauge (also FG or Ch)
FVC	forced vital capacity
G	gauge
G&S	group and save
G-6-PD	glucose -6- phosphate dehydrogenase
GA	general anaesthetic
GCS	Glasgow coma scale
GFR	glomerular filtration rate
GI(T)	gastrointestinal (tract)
	glyceryl trinitrate
	human albumin solution
	haemoglobin
	hepatitis B virus
	hepato carcinoma
	human chorionic gonadotrophin
	haematocrit
	hepatitis C virus
	high dependency unit
	haemolysis, elevated liver enzymes, low platelets
	high efficiency particulate air
	hydroxyethyl starches
	haemophilus influenzae B

ARDS	acute respiratory distress syndrome
AS	aortic stenosis
ASA	American Society of Anesthesiologists
ASD	atrial septal defect
ATLS	advanced trauma life support
AUR	acute urinary retention
AV	atrioventricular
AXR	abdominal x-ray
BBV	blood borne virus
BCC	basal cell carcinoma
BCG	Bacille Calmette-Guérin
bd	twice daily (bis diem)
BDZ	benzodiazepine
BiPAP	biphasic positive airway pressure
BKA	below knee amputation
BLS	basic life support
BMI	body mass index
BNF	British National Formulary
BP	blood pressure
bpm	beats per minute
BS	blood sugar
BSA	body surface area
BSE	bovine spongiform encephalopathy
BSL	British Sign Language
C&S	culture and sensitivity
CABG	coronary artery bypass graft
CAD	coronary artery disease
CAPD	continuous ambulatory peritoneal dialysis
CBD	common bile duct
CCF	congestive cardiac failure
CCU	critical care unit
CEA	carotid endarterectomy
CHD	coronary heart disease
CI	cardiac index
CJD	Creutzfeldt–Jakob disease
CKD	chronic kidney disease
CMV	cytomegalovirus or controlled mechanical ventilation
CNS	central nervous system
CO	cardiac output
CO_2	carbon dioxide
COAD	chronic obstructive airway disease

COPD	chronic obstructive pulmonary disease
CPAP	continuous positive airway pressure
CPB	cardiopulmonary bypass
CPP	cerebral perfusion pressure
CPR	cardiopulmonary resuscitation
CPX	cardiopulmonary exercise testing
CRF	chronic renal failure
CSE	combined spinal epidural
CSF	cerebrospinal fluid
C-spine	cervical spine
CSSD	central sterile supply department
CT	computerised tomography
CTZ	chemoreceptor trigger zone
CV	cardiovascular
CVA	cardiovascular accident
CVE	cardiovascular event
CVL	central venous line
CVS	cardiovascular system
CVP	central venous pressure
CWD	chronic wasting disease
CXR	chest X-ray
DHS	dynamic hip screw
DIC	disseminated intravascular coagulation
DLT	double-lumen tube
DM	diabetes mellitus
DMARD	disease modifying anti-rheumatoid drug
DMV	difficult mask ventilation
DNA	did not attend
DNR	do not resuscitate
DoH	Department of Health (UK)
DOPES	displaced ET tube, obstructed [...] equipment malfunction, stom[...]
DVT	deep venous thrombosis
Dx	diagnosis
EBV	Epstein–Barr virus
ECG	electrocardiogra[...]
ECF	extracellular fl[...]
ECM	external ca[...]
ECT	electroconvu[...]
ED	emergency depar[...]
EDD	estimated date of deli[...]

HIT	heparin-induced thrombocytopenia
HITT	heparin-induced thrombocytopenia and thrombosis
HIV	human immunodeficiency virus
HME	heat and moisture exchange
HPC	Health Professions Council
HR	heart rate
HRA	Human Rights Act
HRT	hormone replacement therapy
HSV	herpes simplex virus
Hx	history
IABP	intra-aortic balloon pump
IC	intermittent claudication
ICD	intracardiac defibrillator
ICU	intensive care unit
ICP	intra-cranial pressure
ID	internal diameter
IDDM	insulin-dependent diabetes mellitus
I:E ratio	inspired:expired ratio
IABP	intra-aortic balloon pump
IHD	ischaemic heart disease
ILMA	intubating laryngeal mask airway
IM	intramuscular
INPV	intermittent negative pressure ventilation
INR	international normalized ratio
IO	intra-osseous
IOP	intra-occular pressure
IPPV	intermittent positive pressure ventilation
IT	intrathecal
ITU	intensive treatment unit
IU	international units
IV	intravenous
IVC	inferior vena cava
JCAHO	Joint Commission on Accreditation of Healthcare Organizations
JVP	jugular venous pressure
L	litre(s)
LA	local anaesthetic
LAP	left atrial pressure
LAVH	laparoscopically assisted vaginal hysterectomy
LDL	low density lipid
LFT	liver function test

LH	luteinizing hormone
LIF	left iliac fossa
LMA	laryngeal mask airway
LMP	last menstrual period
LMWH	low molecular weight heparin
LOR	loss of resistance
LP	lumbar puncture
LSCS	lower segment Caesarean section
LSD	lysergic acid diethylamide
LT	laryngeal tube
LV	left ventricle
LVF	left ventricular failure
MAC	minimum alveolar concentration
MAO	monoamine oxidase
MAOI	monoamine oxidase inhibitor
MAP	mean arterial pressure
mcg	microgram(s)
MCV	mean corpuscular volume
MCRP	magnetic resonance cholangiopancreatography
MCV	mean cell volume
MEAC	minimum effective analgesic concentration
mg	milligram(s)
MH	malignant hyperthermia
MHRA	Medicines and Healthcare products Regulatory Agency
MI	myocardial infarction
ml	millilitre(s)
MLT	microlaryngoscopy tube
MMV	mandatory minute ventilation
MODS	multiple organ dysfunction syndrome
MR	mitral regurgitation
MRA	magnetic resonance angiography
MRI	magnetic resonance imaging
MRSA	meticillin (or multiple) resistant *Staphylococcus aureus*
NBM	nil by mouth
NCA	nurse-controlled analgesia
NG(T)	nasogastric (tube)
NIBP	non-invasive blood pressure
NIDDM	non-insulin-dependent diabetes mellitus
NICE	National Institute for Health and Clinical Excellence
NIPPV	non-invasive intermittent positive pressure ventilation
nocte	at night

NMB	neuromuscular blockade
NMC	Nursing and Midwifery Council
NSAID	non-steroidal anti-inflammatory drug
NSF	National Service Framework
O_2	oxygen
od	once daily
ODP	operating theatre practitioner
OGD	oesophago-gastro-duodenoscopy
OIR	overnight intensive recovery
PA	pulmonary artery or per axilla
$PaCO_2$	arterial carbon dioxide tension
PAD	preoperative autologous donation
PaO_2	arterial oxygen tension
PAP	pulmonary artery pressure
PAWP	pulmonary artery wedge pressure
PCA	patient-controlled analgesia
PCEA	patient-controlled epidural analgesia
PCNL	percutaneous nephrolithotomy
PCO_2	carbon dioxide tension
PCV	packed cell volume or pressure control ventilation
PDA	patent ductus arteriosus
PE	pulmonary embolism
PEEP	positive end-expiratory presure
PEFR	peak expiratory flow rate
PEG	percutaneous endoscopic gastrostomy
PICU	paediatric intensive care unit
PID	pelvic inflammatory disease
PMS	pain management service
PND	paroxysmal nocturnal dyspnoea
PO	orally (per os)
PONV	postoperative nausea and vomiting
POP	plaster of Paris
PO_2	oxygen tension
PPE	personal protective equipment
PPI	proton pump inhibitor
PPN	peripheral parenteral nutrition
PR	per rectum
prn	pro re nata (as required)
PSA	prostate specific antigen
PT	prothrombin time
PTE	pulmonary thromboembolism

PTT	partial prothrombin time
PU	polyurethane
PV	per vagina
PVD	peripheral vascular disease
qds	four times a day
RA	right atrial or rheumatoid arthritis
RAE	Ring, Adair, and Elwyn (tube)
RBC	red blood cell
RCN	Royal College of Nursing
RCoA	Royal College of Anaesthetists
RCS	Royal College of Surgeons
RCT	randomised controlled trial
RIF	right iliac fossa
RLMA	reinforced laryngeal mask airway
RS	respiratory system
RSI	rapid sequence induction
RTA	road traffic accident
SAH	subarachnoid haemorrhage
SaO_2	arterial oxygen saturation
SBE	subacute bacterial endocarditis
SC	subcutaneous
SCBU	special care baby unit
SCC	squamous cell carcinoma
SCD	sequential calf compression device
SEA	spinal epidural abscess
SHOT	serious hazards of transfusion
SIC	surgical intensive care
SIMV	synchronised intermittent mandatory ventilation
SIRS	systemic inflammatory response syndrome
SL	sublingual
SLE	systemic lupus erythematosus
SMA	superior mesenteric artery
SOB	shortness of breath
SOP	standing operating procedure
SPC	summary of product characteristics
SpO_2	peripheral oxygen saturation
SSAR	suspected serious adverse reaction
SSG	split skin graft
SSI	surgical site infection
SSRI	selective serotonin reuptake inhibitor
STEMI	ST elevation myocardial infarction

STI	sexually transmitted infection
(S)TOP	(suction) termination of pregnancy
SUSAR	suspected unexpected serious adverse reaction
SV	stroke volume or spontaneous ventilation
SVC	superior vena cava
SVI	stroke volume index
SvO_2	percentage oxygen saturation of mixed venous haemoglobin
SVR	systemic vascular resistance
SVT	supraventricular tachycardia
TB	tuberculosis
TBSA	total body surface area
TCA	tricyclic antidepressant
TCI	target-controlled infusion/to come in
TCRE	transcervical resection of endometrium
tds	three times a day
TEDS	thromboembolic deterrent stockings
TENS	transcutaneous electric nerve stimulation
THR	total hip replacement
TIA	transient ischaemic attack
TIVA	total intravenous anaesthesia
TMJ	temporomandibular joint
TNF	tumour necrosis factor
TNM	tumour nodes metastasis
TOE	transoesophageal echocardiography
TOF	tracheo-oesophyageal fistula
TPN	total parenteral nutrition
TRAM	transverse rectus abdominis myocutaneous
TSE	transmissible spongiform encephalopathy
TSSU	theatre sterile supply unit
TTE	transthoracic echocardiogram
TTI	transfusion transmitted infection
TUIP	transurethral incision in the prostate
TURP	transurethral resection of the prostate
U&E	urea and electrolytes
UFH	unfractionated heparin
UHMWPE	ultra-high molecular weight polyethylene
UPPP	uvulopalatopharyngoplasty
URTI	upper respiratory tract infection
UTI	urinary tract infection
vCJD	variant Creutzfeldt–Jakob disease

VF	ventricular fibrillation
VP	venous pressure or ventriculopertoneal
VQ	ventilation/perfusion scan
VR	ventricular rate
VRE	vancomycin-resistant *Enterococcus*
VSD	ventricular septal defect
VT	ventricular tachycardia
Vt or VT	tidal volume
VTE	venous thromboembolic disease
WCC	white cell count

Detailed contents

Section 1 **Principles of perioperative care**

Section 5 **Postoperative care**

Section 6 **Management principles of emergency care**

Principles of perioperative care

Perioperative practice

Team working

Surgery is a complex field that requires a coordinated, well directed, inter-disciplinary approach. There are three basic objectives of safe, surgical, patient-care delivery and management and all team members play a vital role in achieving these objectives:

- The delivery of a physiologically and psychologically prepared patient for the planned surgical journey.
- The safe, efficient, and therapeutic alleviation of the patient's problem is based on a sound evidence-based knowledge and a proficient technique.
- The careful guidance of the patient's immediate postoperative care in order to minimise the possibility of complications.

Teams often work across functional divides in that they are drawn from many disciplines with each member encompassing a distinct role and failure to develop a collaborative approach will often result in a fragmented service for patients.

The understanding of each team member's role is an important aspect of ensuring a coordinated and collaborative approach; no individual alone can deliver a high-quality service, therefore teamwork is vital in ensuring a first-class service.

Strategies pivotal to clinical governance include patient satisfaction, personal and professional growth, risk management, and team building. Effective teamwork can have a direct impact on health and well-being of team members and the mortality and morbidity of patients.

There is also a need to recognise that should errors occur, they cannot be eradicated completely, but they should be prevented in the future by systematically learning from them. This would encourage individual practitioners to share both error prevention and the actual errors with their team members without a fear of unfair treatment and to make error reduction in the future possible.

The focus of error prevention needs to be widened from individual to team responsibility and includes the underlying organisational factors as well. Therefore, fostering shared responsibility to minimise error making and to learn from mistakes should be intimately connected.

All healthcare practitioners have a duty to use evidence-based practice which encompasses research utilisation and highlights the impact that effective teamwork has on staff and patients.

In the modern NHS, with medicine and healthcare increasing in complexity, high quality care for patients will increasingly depend on high quality teamwork, so the quality of clinical teams is an important clinical governance issue.

References and further reading

Aritzeta A, Swailes S, and Senior B (2007) Belbin's team role model: development, validity and applications for team building. *Journal of Management Studies* **44**, 96–118.

Fairchild SS (1996). *Perioperative nursing: principles and practice* (2nd edn). Lippincott, Williams and Wilkins: Boston.

Masterson A (2002). Cross-boundary working: a macro-political analysis of the impact on professional roles. *Journal of Clinical Nursing* **11**(3), 331–9.

National Assembly for Wales (2001). *Clinical Governance: a tool kit for Clinical Teams*. NAfW: Cardiff.

Scholes J, Vaughan B (2001). Cross-boundary working: implications for the multiprofessional team. *Journal of Clinical Nursing* **11**(3), 399–408.

Silén-Lipponen M, Tossavainen K, Turunen H, *et al.* (2005). Potential errors and their prevention in operating room teamwork as experienced by Finnish, British and American nurses. *International Journal of Nursing Practice* **11**, 21–32.

Interprofessional team working

Defining the term *interprofessional* has proved problematic for almost a decade and there still does not appear to be a sound consensus of definition.

- The terms *interprofessional*, *multiprofessional*, *multidisciplinary*, and *interdisciplinary* are regularly used interchangeably without careful consideration to their underpinning meanings.
- Interprofessional working can be considered as interactions between team members; or a willingness to share and give up exclusive claims to specialised knowledge and authority if other professional groups can meet patient needs more efficiently and appropriately.
- Multiprofessional is seen as a group of people who come from different healthcare and social care professions but do not necessarily interact; or as a cooperative enterprise in which traditional forms and divisions of professional knowledge and authority are retained.
- Multi-disciplinary working is often viewed as describing practitioners who share the same professional background but who practice within different specialties.

The UK National Health Service (NHS) promotes and emphasises the importance of interprofessional teamwork as the way to providing seamless patient-centred care (Fig. 1.1).

Successful implementation of clinical governance within the NHS organisation depends upon leaders who are able to inspire and motivate others. Leaders are present throughout an organisation and are not necessarily the people at the top of the hierarchy or just managers. However, the running of the operating theatre should be undertaken by a theatre manager who is responsible for coordinating the operating lists and ensuring that effective communication systems are in place.

References and further reading

Masterson A (2002). Cross-boundary working: a macro-political analysis of the impact on professional roles. *Journal of Clinical Nursing* **11**(3), 331–9.

Scholes J and Vaughan B (2001). Cross-boundary working: implications for the multiprofessional team. *Journal of Clinical Nursing* **11**(3), 399–408.

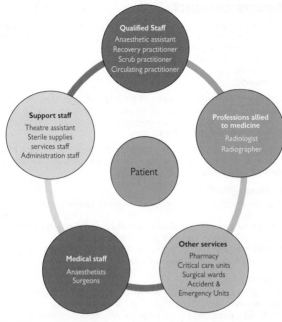

Fig. 1.1 Immediate interdisciplinary team for surgical patients.

Theatre conduct

The operating theatre has a unique atmosphere that can prove quite deceptive. However, there are certain conventions that the novice theatre practitioner ought to be aware of. These include:
- Minimising distraction of the surgical team.
- Noise levels.
- Teamwork.

There should be no direct contact of the surgeons when they are operating. Any communication must go through the scrub practitioner who will pass on any message at a convenient moment or invite the circulating member of staff to speak to the surgeon.

Similarly, the noise levels in the operating theatre must be kept to a minimum while surgery is taking place. Care should be taken to keep the volume of conversations as a low as possible.

Movement (traffic)
- The number of staff in the operating theatre should be kept to a minimum.
- All operating theatre staff should enter and leave the operating theatre via a clearly identified door so as not disturb airflow.
- Consideration should be given to the layout of the operating theatre to minimise flow of staff through the area.

Footwear
- Appropriate protective footwear with enclosed toes and heels should be worn and cleaned frequently.
- There is no evidence to suggest that the wearing of outside shoes in the operating theatre is a source of infection but they should be limited to contaminated cases only.
- The wearing of overshoes has been shown not only to be ineffective in reducing the bacterial load on the floor but also causes hands to become more easily contaminated when they are applied and removed.
- Local policy in respect of footwear should be adhered to.

Surgical masks
- These were originally designed to protect the patient from the bacteria contained in the breath of theatre staff.
- However, paper masks have been shown to be effective in reduction of contamination of the surgical field when worn by the surgical team but it is questionable whether they contribute to the overall reduction of wound infections.
- There would appear to be little rationale for the wearing of masks by circulating and anaesthetic staff.
- Hands should be washed after removing and discarding the mask.
- Protective face shields should be worn where there is the possibility of splashes.
- Local policy in respect of surgical masks should be adhered to.

Hats

- These should be donned prior to theatre clothing to reduce the amount of shedding of particles from the head onto the suit.
- All hair is to be covered and staff with long hair should wear a surgical hood or an elasticated hat for female members of staff.
- Men should wear a hood if they have facial hair.
- Most theatre departments purchase disposable hats, which are discarded at the end of the working day.
- Cloth caps should be laundered daily at a temperature of at least 60°C and changed if they become soiled.
- Hands should be washed after the removal of hats.
- Local policy in respect of theatre hats should be adhered to.

Theatre apparel

- All staff must wear a clean theatre suit upon entering the operating theatre area.
- Consideration should also be given to the donning of a fresh suit prior to each operating session.

References and further reading

Fairchild SS (1996). *Perioperative nursing: principles and practice* (2nd edn). Lippincott, Williams and Wilkins: Boston.

Hospital Infection Society Working Party (2001). *Behaviours and Rituals in the Operating Theatre*. Available from: ☐ www.his.org.uk/_db/_documents/Rituals-02.doc

Lipp A, Edwards P (2002). Disposable surgical facemasks for preventing surgical infection in clean surgery. *Cochrane Database of Systematic Reviews*. Issue 1.

Clinical governance

While practitioners may have been conscious of a decline in standards of care, or had concerns about individual practitioners, it took a number of publicised 'incidents' to draw public attention to the shortfalls in standards of service provision.[1] The lack of action by healthcare professionals could be attributed to the absence of an infrastructure for addressing deficits in clinical practice. Clinical governance has since emerged as the solution for resolving problems and regaining public confidence in health service provision.

Since its advent in the late 1990s, the term 'clinical governance' has become a regular feature of the health practitioner's vocabulary.

> 'Clinical governance is a framework through which NHS organisations are accountable for continuously improving the quality of their services and safeguarding high standards of care by creating an environment in which excellence in clinical care can flourish.'[1]

Very often, there is confusion regarding this definition, and this may exist from attempts to narrow the definition into something more tangible.

The overall aim of clinical governance is to 'ensure quality of care',[2] although to realise this vision, healthcare practitioners must embrace several components (see Fig. 1.2).

Engaging with clinical governance: role and responsibility of the nurse

Within any healthcare organisation, such as a hospital trust, overall responsibility for quality and safety lies with the chief executive. However, all NHS employers are responsible for delivering the clinical governance agenda, and working knowledge of the clinical governance themes is fundamental to its success. Endorsement of these principles is implicit within the code of conduct of the Nursing & Midwifery Council (NMC) and the Health Professions Council (HPC)—*provide a high standard of practice and care at all times.*[3,4]

Further guidance on how clinical governance principles should be implemented, are outlined by the Royal College of Nursing (RCN):[5]

- Applies to all healthcare; between all professional groups, between clinical staff and managers, and between patients and clinical staff.
- Clinicians must be patient-focused at all times and focused on improving the quality of patient care, whilst regarding public and patient involvement as essential.
- Individual practitioners are responsible and accountable for the quality of the care provided.
- Nurses have a key role to play in its implementation.
- It requires a safe, open, enabling culture which celebrates success and learns from mistakes.

Clinical governance is not a replacement for individual clinical judgement or professional self-regulation.

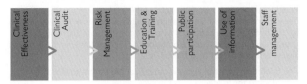

Fig. 1.2 Seven pillars of clinical governance.

References and further reading

1. NHS Executive (1999). *Performance assessment framework*. Available at: 🖥 www.dh.gov.uk/en/Publicationsandstatistics/Publications/PublicationsPolicyAndGuidance/DH_4009190

2. Department of Health (1997). *The new NHS: modern, dependable*. The Stationery Office: London.

3. Nursing & Midwifery Council (2008). *The code: standards for conduct, performance and ethics*. NMC: London.

4. Health Professions Council (2004). *Standards of conduct, performance and ethics*. HPC: London.

5. Royal College of Nursing (2003). *Clinical governance: an RCN resource guide*. RCN: London.

Department of Health (1998). *A first-class service: quality in the new NHS*. The Stationery Office: London.

Applying principles of clinical governance

Practitioners regularly work alongside other clinicians within the operating department and these partnerships should always work in collaboration for the benefit of the patient. However, recognising and addressing deficits in practice, particularly where omissions or mistakes are identified, should always reflect a proactive approach.

The operating department team can reflect the clinical governance ethos, by endorsing the following key principles:

Leadership
- This is key to ensuring the team is effective in meeting the outcomes of clinical governance.
- However, it is the responsibility of this person to ensure they have the knowledge and skills to undertake this role effectively, seeking appropriate development opportunities.

Communication
- Collectively meet and discuss the issues and disseminate relevant information to trust colleagues and patient user groups.

Staff management and performance
- Undertaking appraisals, identifying and addressing educational needs of self and staff.

Audit
- Formally reviewing service delivery, implementing recognised national standards, ensuring evidence-based practice.

Risk management
- Performing risk assessment and identifying risk profiles are essential to risk management.
- Clinical incidents reporting will also ensure potential 'at risk' situations are identified, and acted upon, before becoming a serious risk to patient/staff safety.
- Failure to acknowledge and address such situations reflects a breach of clinical governance principles.
- Departments will generate a risk profile that outlines the five or ten most common risks to the department and the actions that are taken to avoid these.
- Critical incident reports feed into this process and should be centrally managed within a department.
- This enables the manager to detect trends and deal with these appropriately. It is important that actions taken as a result of an incident form are fed back to departmental staff.

The National Patient Safety Agency (NPSA)[1] suggests we share safety lessons and encourage staff to use root cause analysis to learn how and why incidents happen. Failure to acknowledge and address such situations reflects a breach of clinical governance principles, and puts patients at risk. Furthermore, the NPSA provides a useful resource for preventing and managing patient safety incidents.[1]

Operating departments will generate a risk profile, outlining five out of ten most common risks to the department, and actions taken to avoid them. Areas of risk associated with the operating theatre department are identified by Kumar[2] in Box 1.1.

Box 1.1 Areas of risk in the operating theatre[2]

- Wrong patient
- Wrong surgical procedure, site or side
- Extension of surgery not covered by consent
- Retained swabs, needles, instruments
- Lack of written consent
- Drug error
- Patient injury
- Faulty equipment

References and further reading

1. National Patient Safety Agency (2004). *Seven steps to patient safety: An overview guide for NHS staff.* Available at: www.npsa.nhs.uk/nrls/improvingpatientsafety/

2. Kumar B (1998) *Working in the operating department* (2nd edn). Churchill Livingstone: London.

Royal College of Nursing (2003). *Clinical governance: an RCN resource guide.* RCN: London.

Professional issues in perioperative practice

Accountability and responsibility

Definitions
Accountable: to be held responsible or liable for an action.
Responsible: to be answerable or accountable.

Although the two words have very similar meaning, it is possible to identify differences in the meaning. Since the NMC[1] uses the term accountable, (but in 2004 noted that accountable means responsible[2]) and the HPC[3] uses only the term responsible it appears that for perioperative practitioners there is no need to differentiate between these two words.

Practitioners obviously have a moral accountability to themselves and to their families but, as professional accountability is the focus, this moral accountability is not discussed here.

When are perioperative practitioners accountable?
In their professional capacity, perioperative practitioners must comply with standards of conduct, performance, and ethics as stipulated by their professional regulatory body (HPC or NMC). Each practitioner is accountable for his/her own:
• Actions.
• Omissions.

A practitioner is therefore accountable for anything that he/she does, or fails to do, that does not meet the profession's required standard.

To whom are perioperative practitioners professionally accountable?
It is recognised that practitioners are accountable to:
• The patient.
• The public.
• The employer.
• The profession.

Accountability to the patient
• Each patient has a right to receive the standard of care required of the perioperative practitioner by his/her profession.
• Where the actions (or omissions) of the practitioner are not of the required standard the patient may seek redress.
• Where harm has been caused to the patient by the practitioner's action/omission the patient may choose to sue the practitioner for his/her negligence in the civil courts (📚 see Negligence, p.18).

Accountability to the public
• All perioperative practitioners must act within the law.
• In extreme cases where the practitioner's actions/omissions have led to the death of a patient, a criminal charge of manslaughter or murder may be brought.

Accountability to the employer

- Perioperative practitioners, by nature of their employment contracts, are required to undertake reasonable instructions of the employer.
- The employer may commence a disciplinary procedure against a practitioner whose actions/omissions are in breach of his/her employment contract (i.e. not the standard expected).
- Where the disciplinary procedure finds that the practitioner is in breach of contract, a range of sanctions, from a warning to dismissal, are available to the employer.

Accountability to the profession

- Regulatory bodies (e.g. the HPC and NMC) function to safeguard the health and well-being of the public.
- This function is discharged (in part) by considering any allegations of misconduct against registrants.
- Alleged misconduct is investigated in terms of the registrant's 'fitness to practise'.
- If the practitioner's actions/omissions are found to have affected his/her fitness to practise, the regulatory body has a range of sanctions it can apply.
- Sanctions include a caution, a Conditions of Practice Order, suspension, and ultimately a striking off order (removal of the registrant's name from the register).
- It should be noted that accountability to the patient, the public, or the employer may also result in the involvement of the regulatory body since any findings in any of these arenas may be reported to the regulatory body if 'fitness to practise' has been considered.

An example

A perioperative practitioner administers a massive overdose of a prescribed analgesic drug, without following the local policy of checking that drug dose, and the patient dies.

Although there are many aspects of this scenario that would be considered, it is possible (as a worse case scenario) that the patient's relatives sue for negligence (accountability to the patient), the practitioner is charged with manslaughter (accountability to the public), the employer commences disciplinary action (accountability to the employer), and the regulatory body reviews the practitioner's fitness to practise (accountability to the profession).

References

1. Nursing & Midwifery Council (2008). *The Code: standards of conduct, performance and ethics.* NMC: London.

2. Nursing & Midwifery Council (2004). *NMC code of professional conduct: standards for conduct, performance and ethics.* NMC: London.

3. Health Professions Council (2004). *Standards of conduct, performance and ethics.* HPC: London.

Negligence

Negligence claims can relate to any event where one party feels that he/she has been harmed by the negligent act or omission of another.

In most legal cases of clinical negligence, a claim for compensation is heard in the civil court. (Please note that other options, e.g. via the NHS complaints procedure, are not discussed in this chapter.)

The legal framework for clinical negligence claims

To succeed the claimant must prove that:

- He/she was owed a legal duty of care by the defendant health carer (perioperative practitioner) and/or health provider (NHS Trust).
- That the defendant was in breach of that duty of care (by failing to achieve the standard of care).
- The harm to the claimant (for which compensation is sought) was caused by, or materially contributed to, by the breach in the duty of care.

Duty of care

- It is an accepted legal principle that a practitioner who takes on the responsibility of caring for a patient owes a duty of care to that patient.
- There is no legal duty, in the UK, to act as a 'Good Samaritan' e.g. at the scene of an accident. However, if a practitioner does become involved then a duty of care will exist.
- Applies equally to all health professionals and to support staff.
- The NHS Trust (or other healthcare provider) may also have a duty of care and either be liable in negligence claims for its own actions (primary liability) or be vicariously liable for negligence actions of its employees.
- In most clinical negligence claims the duty of care is not disputed by the defendant(s).

Breach of duty

To identify whether a breach in duty occurred, a three-stage process is followed:

- There is a usual and normal practice for conducting the procedure/treatment in question.
  - 'Normal' practice is identified by examining the practice undertaken in relation to any existing national guidelines (e.g. National Institute for Health and Clinical Excellence [NICE] clinical guidelines) and evidence-based local policy.
  - If there is no 'normal' practice the practitioner is expected to assess and take precautions against known risks before acting in a reasonable manner.
- The practitioner responsible did not adopt that practice.
- The practice adopted is one that no practitioner in that profession with ordinary skill would have used if they had been acting with ordinary care.

It should be noted that if a practitioner undertakes expanded role practices or is learning new practices he/she will be judged by the standard of the profession that normally undertakes that role e.g. if acting as the first assistant to the surgeon, the practitioner's practice will be measured against the standard of the junior doctor, the person who normally undertakes this function.

Causation

Establishing that the breach of duty has caused the harm is notoriously difficult to prove in clinical negligence claims. There may be a number of reasons for the harm (that the patient claims) including pre-existing disease/trauma and recognised side effects of treatments. The following tests may be applied:

- The 'but for' test—used in straightforward cases. Would the harm have been caused *but for* the actions of the defendant? If not, the causal link is made.
- The 'chain of causation'—when there is an unbroken chain of events from the original act to the harm then the causal link is made.
- 'Reasonable forseeability'—is the harm which was caused not too remote from the act or omission?

The onus is always on the claimant to prove that the cause of the harm was the action or omission of the defendant(s). Where more than one possible cause may be presented, the decision by the court will be made using the civil standard of the 'balance of probabilities'—i.e. only if there is more than a 50% chance that the harm was caused by the negligence can the claim succeed.

Gross negligence

On rare occasions where the negligence is considered to be extreme (e.g. when a patient dies) a claim of gross negligence may take the form of a charge of manslaughter. Gross negligence is therefore seen in a prosecution through the criminal courts.

Further reading

Brazier M and Cave E (2007). *Medicine, Patients and the Law*. Penguin Books: London.

Conscientious objection

Perioperative practitioners, as registered health professionals, are required by their respective regulatory bodies to provide care for patients without discrimination and with respect for the patient's rights. Whilst few would disagree with these standards, difficulties do arise when practitioners find themselves in situations where participation in a patient's care is contrary to their own religious and personal beliefs.

This conscientious objection (to participation in care) can be considered in two ways:
- Legislation.
- Rights of the perioperative practitioner.

Legislation
- There are currently two Acts of Parliament that give health professionals the right to refuse to participate in procedures on the grounds of conscientious objection:
- Abortion Act 1967.
- The Human Fertilisation and Embryology Act 1990.

Requirements under the Acts
- In the event of an emergency, the practitioner is required to participate in the patient's care (i.e. cannot claim conscientious objection).
- Practitioners will be responsible for proving their conscientious objection should it be required in legal proceedings.

It has been established, through the courts, that conscientious objection to participation in either an abortion or procedures for assisted conception (under these Acts) only applies to those directly involved in the technical procedure (i.e. conscientious objection may be claimed by a practitioner in the operating theatre during a termination but not by a practitioner checking the patient into the department).

Rights of the perioperative practitioner
Where specific legislation does not address issues of conscientious objection the position is less clear. Perioperative practitioners cannot simply be selective about patients in their care as the regulatory bodies require practitioners to practice in a non-discriminatory way. There are, however, some situations where a practitioner may have real concerns about specific practices.

The Human Rights Act (HRA) 1998[1] identifies that:
- It is unlawful for any public authority (e.g. NHS Trusts) to act in a way that is incompatible with the HRA.
- Under Article 9, an individual (e.g. perioperative practitioner) has the right to freedom of thought, conscience, and religion, and the right to practice that religion.
- Rights under Article 9 are not absolute—there are a number of limitations including public order and the protection of the rights and freedoms of others.

If a perioperative practitioner objects to undertaking a specific practice, because it is contrary to the practice of his/her religion, the NHS Trust will need to consider the objection.

To date, this scenario has not been tested in the courts so no definitive guidance is available. Until such guidance is available perioperative practitioners must, whilst making their objections known, ensure that they adhere to the current standards of performance, conduct, and ethics as stipulated by their professional body by:

- Considering not accepting employment where practices are contrary to their beliefs.
- Informing the employer of the conscientious objection at the earliest opportunity—to allow other arrangements to be made to ensure that the patient's care does not suffer.
- Acknowledging that each patient has the right to make his/her own care decisions.
- Making no attempts to impose their beliefs on the patient.
- Treating all patients with respect and dignity.
- Accepting that in an emergency situation they cannot refuse to participate in the patient's care.

In light of the HRA 1998 it is evident that a balance between the rights of the patient to undergo a planned lawful surgical procedure and the rights of the practitioner to practice his/her religion has to be met.

Reference
1. Department of Constitutional Affairs (2006). *A Guide to the Human Rights Act 1998: Third Edition.* Available from 🖳 www.dca.gov.uk/peoples-rights/human-rights/index.htm

Chapter 3

Admission of surgical patients

The admission process

Surgery consists of emergency or elective admissions and the admission process will vary to accommodate the needs of the individual. Facilitating admission process is essential to quality care and communication within the surgical team. The surgical journey for patients who have a planned admission can be facilitated through:

- Pre-admission programmes.
- The provision of written information.
- Preoperative assessment clinics.
- Ward visits.

For urgent surgical admissions time is of the essence and preoperative care needs to be provided far more quickly to facilitate a comprehensive preoperative assessment and a safe patient journey. An essential element is effective communication between the patient and the team.

Patients' surgical journey

Patient group directives (PGDs) (Fig. 3.1)

- Formerly known as group protocols.
- They provide a framework for the supply and administration of medications without an individualised prescription.
- PGDs allow identified, responsible, trained healthcare professionals to supply and administer medication to a group of patients that fit specific PGD criteria.
- Trust-wide policy.
- Underpinned by best possible evidence base.
- Must be signed by a doctor, pharmacist, and organising authority before it can be used.

Integrated care pathways

- A guide to good practice.
- A multidisciplinary document that incorporates local and national policies/guidelines to plan safe/high quality, personalised care.
- Forms all or part of the clinical record and details essential steps in the care of the patient with a specific surgical condition.
- Patient progress can be monitored and audited.
- Known to reduce postoperative morbidity.

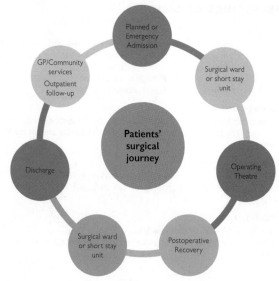

Fig. 3.1 Patient group directives (PGDs).

Assessment of care

Assessment

The aim of preoperative assessment is to minimise risk and ensure that the patient is prepared physically and psychologically for the procedure they are to undergo. Table 3.1 identifies some procedures to be undertaken during the assessment of surgical patients, although it should be noted that not all patients will require all investigations.

Planning care

The aim of planning care is to identify, reduce, or eliminate any individual risk factors that could potentially increase the risk to the patient during surgery.

Implementing care

Table 3.2 identifies procedures to be undertaken in the preparation of surgical patients. Additional procedures can be found in 📖 Chapter 4, pp.49–56.

Evaluating care

- Completion of preoperative checklist.
- Patient is safely prepared and transferred to the operating theatre team.

Table 3.1 Assessment of surgical patients

Baseline observations	Electrocardiogram (ECG)
Chest X-ray	Pulmonary function tests
Past medical history	Allergies
Medication	Haematological investigations
Health education—smoking, obesity, alcohol consumption	Height, weight, body mass index (BMI)
Screening for infection control e.g. methicillin-resistant *Staphylococcus aureus* (MRSA)—as per local policy	Complete local policy risk assessment tools e.g. Waterlow
Latex screen	Manual handling
Nutrition	Autar deep venous thrombosis (DVT)
Record last menstrual period (LMP)	Blood glucose

Table 3.2 Preparation of surgical patients

Confirm biographical data	Informed consent
Correlate results of investigations, scans, radiographic images	Record baseline observations of temperature, pulse, and respiration (TPR), blood pressure (BP), oxygen saturation.
Urinalysis	12-lead ECG
Anaesthetic assessment	Identify fasting regimen
Oral care	Hygiene needs
Identification of operation site	Record results of risk assessments
Document time pre-medication is given and ensure patient consent for rectal medication	Apply appropriate venous thromboembolism prevention, as per local protocol

Patients with special healthcare needs

- Patients with special health needs present complexities for staff and require specialist knowledge and skills in order to effectively manage their care. Special healthcare needs can be broadly categorised as physical disabilities, psychological disabilities, learning disabilities, and children and parents as identified in Fig. 3.2.
- Perioperative practitioners need a wide range of knowledge and skills to support the care of surgical patients with special healthcare needs.
- Patients with particular healthcare needs should be identified on the operating theatre list in order to ensure seamless care.
- By identifying and anticipating the needs of patients with complex problems, healthcare practitioners are able to quantify the nursing actions necessary to prevent problems occurring during the perioperative period.

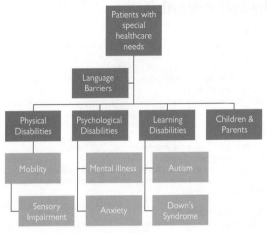

Fig. 3.2 Patients with special healthcare needs.

References

Graham D (2000). Perspectives on intraoperative care. In Manley K and Bellman L (eds). *Surgical Nursing: Advancing practice*. Churchill Livingstone: London.

Pudner R (2005). *Nursing the surgical patient* (2nd edn). Bailliere Tindall: London.

Physical disabilities

Mobility

- All patients with physical disabilities require care and consideration during the perioperative period.
- Patients with mobility difficulties caused by arthritis, or those with previous limb amputation, should be taken to theatre on a bed to avoid unnecessary transfers.
- Some procedures such as an epidural or spinal anaesthesia require positioning of the patient in the anaesthetic room.
- If a patient has restricted movement, the anaesthetic practitioner should identify:
  - How restricted is the movement?
  - Is the range of movement limited?
- Considerable care should also be taken when patients are anaesthetised in order to avoid nerve damage or excessive pressure on certain joints or limbs.

Sensory impairment

Healthcare practitioners need a special understanding of patients with auditory, visual, speech, and cognitive impairment. Patients with these impairments are vulnerable and often feel quite anxious and isolated regarding their prospective surgical procedures. Assistance or specialist aids can be provided to patients with hearing, visual, or speech impairment, enabling them to receive and respond to information.

- Assistance or specialist aids are provided to patients with speaking, sight, or hearing difficulties, special needs, or learning disabilities, enabling them to receive and respond to information.
- If necessary, people are provided with access to a translator or a member of staff with appropriate language skills.
- Some people may have a limited capacity to understand e.g. people with learning disabilities or mental illness. In such cases, every effort is made to help them comprehend what is being said and to involve them in the decision-making process with their carer or next of kin.

Hearing impairment

- Hearing aids and sound amplification technology can be of significant benefit to patients in the operating theatre.
- It is not necessary to remove a patient's hearing aid until he/she has been anaesthetised; it should then be replaced during reversal of anaesthesia.
- Ensure that any hearing aid is switched on and working and avoid the temptation to speak too loudly to the patient.
- Some patients can lip read so it is essential to face the patient and speak slowly and clearly.
- Some patients with a hearing impairment might prefer to communicate by writing; in this situation, handwriting should be clear, concise, and legible.
- British Sign Language (BSL) interpretation can be used for patients who request it, but adequate notice is generally required for interpreters— a family member can be involved with the patients' consent.

Visual impairment
- There are many conditions that can impair a patients' vision including cataract, glaucoma, diabetic retinopathy, age-related macular degeneration, acute closed-angle glaucoma, and primary open-angle glaucoma.
- In the perioperative environment, healthcare practitioners should stand or sit reasonably close to blind or partially sighted patients as they can often recognise outlines of individual faces.
- Sudden appearances at the theatre trolley or bedside should be avoided as this can startle patients.

Speech impairment
- Communication can be very difficult for patients, especially following a stroke; contact speech and language therapists for advice.

Cognitive impairment
- Some patients may have a limited capacity to understand e.g. patients with mental illness or learning disabilities.
- Every effort must be made to help them comprehend what is being said and to involve them in the decision-making process with a family member, friend, carer, or next of kin.
- Information already given may need to be repeated.
- Written information can be left to remind the patient.

References

Arnold E and Underman-Boggs K (2007). *Interpersonal relationships: professional communication skills for nurses* (5th edn). Saunders: Missouri.

Department of Health (2001). *The essence of care: patient-focused benchmarking for healthcare professionals.* The Stationery Office: London.

Welsh Assembly Government (2003). *Fundamentals of care: guidance for health and social care staff.* WAG: Cardiff.

Learning disabilities

Autism

- Autistic spectrum disorder refers to the whole range of 'autistic style' symptoms with varying ranges of symptoms and degrees of severity.
- Autism is a subgroup of autistic spectrum disorder.
- Autism is a brain development disorder that affects communication and social interaction (Box 3.1).
- Problems with language and communication are common and speech usually develops later than usual.
- No two autistic children are alike.

Box 3.1 Problems associated with autism

- Unable to express themselves well.
- Unable to understand gestures, facial expressions, or tone of voice.
- Saying odd things.
- Make up their own words.
- Anger or aggression if routines are changed.
- Children with autism often hurt themselves when they are angry— they might bang their head or hit their face to get attention.

In the perioperative environment

- Changes in routine can be frightening and disorientating.
- A preoperative visit by the anaesthesia team is vital to ensure a smooth experience for everyone involved.
- Parents should be encouraged to discuss their child's particular needs, fears, communication level, and ability to cooperate and understand.
- Children should be prepared for theatre as they would for any unusual activity.
- Explain the sequence of events to the parents.
- Both parents/carers should be allowed in the anaesthetic room until anaesthesia has been induced.
- Preoperative sedation may assist to ease the transition from the parents to the anaesthetic room.
- It should not be used in place of preparing the child ahead of time and instead of talking to the child in the preoperative area.
- Just because a child with autism has communication difficulties, **never** assume that the child does not understand what is happening.
- Listen to the parents/carers as they know the child best.

Down syndrome

Down syndrome is a common genetic disorder characterised by mental retardation, dysmorphic facial features, and a host of structural abnormalities. Individuals with Down syndrome tend to have a lower than average cognitive ability, often with mild-to-moderate learning disabilities. The life expectancy for people with Down syndrome is about 50–60 years. See Table 3.3 for associated medical conditions.

In the perioperative environment
- Patients may become belligerent when frightened.
- A preoperative visit by the anaesthesia team is vital to ensure a smooth experience for everyone involved.
- Encourage parents/carers to discuss the patient's particular needs, fears, communication level, and ability to cooperate and understand.
- Explain the sequence of events to the patient, parents, and/or carer.
- Parents/carers should be allowed in the anaesthetic room until anaesthesia has been induced.
- **Never** talk over the patient and never assume that the patient does not understand what is happening.

Table 3.3 Medical conditions associated with Down syndrome

Cardiac	Atrioventricular canal defects Ventricular septal defect, tetralogy of Fallot
ENT	Conductive, sensorineural, mixed hearing loss, otitis media, sinusitis, pharyngitis, obstructive sleep apnoea
Ophthalmic disorders	Cataracts, strabismus, nystagmus, congenital glaucoma, keratoconus
Gastrointestinal disorders	Oesophageal atresia, duodenal atresia, pyloric stenosis, Meckel's diverticulum, Hirschsprung's disease, imperforate anus, gastro-oesophageal reflux
Orthopaedic disorders	Hyperflexibility, scoliosis, hip dislocation, patellar subluxation/dislocation, foot deformity
Neurological disorders	Mental retardation, behavioural problems, Alzheimer's in older patients
Haematological disorders	Risk of infections Acute myeloblastic leukaemia Acute lymphoblastic leukaemia
Endocrine disorders	Hypothyroidism

References and further reading

Royal College of Nursing (2007). *Mental health nursing of adults with learning disabilities*. RCN: London.

Down's Syndrome Association: 🖥 www.downs-syndrome.org.uk

The National Autistic Society: 🖥 www.nas.org.uk

Mental illness

- Some surgical patients with mental illness will require considerable support in terms of explanation and understanding.
- Confused patients will require repeated explanations and reassurance.
- Establishing a relationship with mental health patients is sometimes a formidable challenge.
- Relatives/carers often play a vital role in helping to care for a patient with mental illness. They should be encouraged, with the patient's consent, to escort the patient to theatre, and stay if necessary, until anaesthesia has been induced.

Box 3.2 Types of mental health illnesses

- Depression
- Ante-natal and post-natal depression
- Antisocial personality disorders
- Obsessive compulsive disorders
- Bipolar disease
- Psychosis
- Self-harm
- Schizophrenia
- Drug misuse
- Dementia

Communication

- Effective communication with mental health patients is paramount in ensuring care and respect for patients' rights.
- The language used must be clear and concise.
- Check that information given has been communicated and understood.
- The presence of a registered mental health nurse is advantageous in the perioperative environment.
- The Mental Health Act 1983 clearly states that 'patients should be engaged in the process of reaching decisions which affect their care and treatment'.

References and further reading

Arnold E and Undermann-Boggs K (2007). *Interpersonal relationships: professional communication skills for nurses* (5th edn). Saunders: Missouri.

Department of Health (2008). *Code of Practice: Mental Health Act 1983.* The Stationery Office: London.

Mental Capacity Act 2005: 🖳 www.opsi.gov.uk/acts/acts2005/ukpga_20050009_en_1

Mental Health Act 2007: 🖳 www.opsi.gov.uk/acts/acts2007/ukpga_20070012_en_1

Royal College of Nursing (2007). *Mental health nursing of adults with learning disabilities.* RCN: London.

Anxiety

- Anxiety can be seen as a product of helplessness.
- Admission to hospital can accentuate this anxiety by disturbing the patient's integrity outside the context of their normal lives.
- During the perioperative period, the patient can be subjected to a variety of stresses associated with anxiety including:
  - Fear of pain.
  - Disfigurement.
  - Dependence.
  - Loss of life.
- Many patients enter hospitals and operating theatres with unnecessary fears and anxieties—this can stem from a lack of knowledge concerning their illness and the impending operative procedure.

Preoperative information giving

- Prolonged anxiety can lead to increased protein breakdown, decreased wound healing, decreased immune response, increased risk of infection, and fluid and electrolyte imbalances.
- Such physiological imbalances could delay recovery for surgical patients.
- Nurses should therefore, use interventions that reduce patients' anxiety levels (Fig. 3.3).
- Good psychological preparation preoperatively can contribute greatly to reduced analgesia requirements in the postoperative period.
- Psychological preparation can also reduce postoperative anxiety, pain levels, and episodes of nausea, thus leading to a shorter hospital stay.
- Explanation and information giving on admission to hospital before diagnostic tests and surgical operations have measurable benefits in terms of reducing anxiety, pain, and side effects in the majority of patients.
- The prospect of surgery can generate emotions such as fear of pain and death.
- To offer patients the best in perioperative care, practitioners need to create an environment in which patients are free to identify their fears.
- Practitioners also need to rethink how they assess for anxiety—they can then help patients to make the best out of an essentially unpleasant experience.

Within the perioperative environment

- Ensure a calm environment.
- Clearly and concisely explain procedures and events as they unfold.
- Provide constant support and reassurance using both verbal and non-verbal methods (listening, touch, eye contact).
- Answer questions honestly.
- Background music in the anaesthetic room and operating theatre can act as a distraction, particularly if a patient has regional anaesthesia.
- Hypnosis has been advocated for use to alleviate perioperative anxiety.

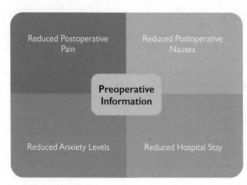

Reduced Postoperative Pain

Reduced Postoperative Nausea

Preoperative Information

Reduced Anxiety Levels

Reduced Hospital Stay

Fig. 3.3 Benefits of preoperative information.

References

Arnold E and Undermann-Boggs K (2007). *Interpersonal relationships: professional communication skills for nurses* (5th edn). Saunders: Missouri.

Hayward J (1975). *Information: a prescription against pain.* RCN: London.

Hughes SJ (2002). The effects of giving patients preoperative information. *Nursing Standard* **16**(28) 33–7.

Wilson-Barnett J (1979). *Stress in hospital: patients' psychological reactions to illness and healthcare.* Churchill Livingstone: Edinburgh.

Children and parents

The special needs of children and young people must be considered during all stages of perioperative care as they differ physiologically, emotionally, and socially from adults.

Operating theatres and operating lists specifically allocated for children are not always feasible. In these circumstances, children should be put to the start of the list with appropriately trained staff in the reception, anaesthetic room, theatre, and recovery areas.[1]

- Parents (and others in *loco parentis*) should, wherever possible, be involved in all aspects of care and decisions regarding the management of their children.
- Communication must be at a level which can be easily understood and it must also be culturally appropriate.
- Parents and children should be given the opportunity to ask questions during each stage of the perioperative journey.
- Provision should be made for parents to accompany children to the anaesthetic and recovery room.
- Provision should also be made for parents to stay in the anaesthetic room until the child has been anaesthetised; exceptions to this can include anticipated difficult intubation and rapid sequence intubation.
- When a parent accompanies a child into the anaesthetic room, a ward nurse or another suitable practitioner should also be present to escort the parent back to the ward.
- A registered children's nurse should be directly involved with children and young people within the perioperative environment.
- Healthcare practitioners caring for children and young people should be competent to practice advanced paediatric life support.
- Parents should be kept informed of their child's progress, especially if there is an unexpected delay in theatre.
- Many departments offer bleeps to parents so that they can be contacted in the event that anything needs to be discussed with them during surgery.

'Staff have a duty to understand and meet their legal responsibilities towards the children and young people they are caring for; including legal and ethical issues or potential conflicts between the interests of the child or young person and those of the parents.'[2]

Play and recreation

Children in hospital—either as a day case or inpatient—have a basic need for play and recreation; this should be met routinely in all hospital departments providing a service to children and young people.

- Play techniques should be encouraged across the interdisciplinary team, involving play-specialists, who can assist in the preparation for anaesthesia and surgery in children and young people.
- The team should be able to offer a variety of play interventions to support the child at each stage in his or her journey through the hospital system.

- Play may also be used to help the child gain control over a potentially frightening environment and prepare to cope with procedures and interventions.
- A pre-admission tour of the operating theatre department can allay some fears and anxiety for children and parents.

References and further reading

1. Department of Health and Department for Education and Skills (2004). *National Service Framework for children, young people and maternity services*. The Stationery Office: London.

2. *Children Act 1989*. HMSO: London.

Royal College of Anaesthetists (2004). *Guidelines for the provision of anaesthetic services*. Chapter 8, Paediatric services. RCoA: London.

Language barriers

- In a rapidly-growing multi-cultural society, it is inevitable that all healthcare practitioners will care for patients and relatives with language barriers at some point.
- To accommodate the vast range of ethnicities, the need for various forms of translation and interpreting in the health sector is great.
- Healthcare providers employ the use of translators, who should be available at any time during the day or night.
- Lists of named interpreters should be available within all departments of the hospital.
- Standards of care delivery and management can become compromised if healthcare providers are unable to communicate with patients who do not speak the home language.

'If a translator is needed, they must be thoroughly briefed on the context of the information they convey and on the requirement for confidentiality.'[1]

Language barriers in the perioperative environment

- Patients with language barriers within the perioperative environment are extremely vulnerable.
- Such language barriers can isolate patients.
- When patients cannot communicate with health professionals, they can become distressed and this can make their treatment stressful and confusing.
- Every effort should be made to contact a translator.
- Relatives and friends can be used as a temporary measure in cases such as emergency surgical treatment.
- Effective interpersonal skills are essential when caring for patients with language barriers.
- Attention should be paid to specific communication skills such as posture, eye contact, touch, and other non-verbal cues.

At no time should a child be expected to act as sole interpreter for another family member or patient.

References and further reading

1. Welsh Assembly Government (2003). *Fundamentals of care: guidance for health and social care staff.* WAG: Cardiff.

Department of Health (2001). *The essence of care: patient-focused benchmarking for healthcare professionals.* The Stationery Office: London.

Managing visitors in the perioperative environment

The continuing and often rapid development of products and techniques to provide improved treatment and more cost-effective practice, whilst maintaining the most beneficial outcomes for both patient and practitioner, realises the need for programmes of hands-on training and education, provided by the healthcare industries that specialise in the relative areas.

Historically, specialist representatives from industry, who have developed mutually beneficial partnerships with their colleagues within the critical care areas of the NHS, are often regarded as integral assets to the function of the department.

In a large number of cases, the specialist representative will have once worked within the operating theatre department. This is of course dependent on the ability of the representative to forge a long-term relationship and acquire a considerable degree of trust, which does not happen overnight.

With the appropriate training and guidelines, industry representatives have been welcomed into the operating theatres to provide support, education, and unbiased assessment of the needs and requirements of the department and its staff. This should, and no doubt will continue, with consideration to the following:

- The visitor should provide and constantly display, when practical, current identification relating to their role and their organisation.
- The theatre management team must assess the risks of the visit and admission of the representative to the department as required by the Health and Safety at Work Act 1974.[1]
- The visit, involving entry into the clinical area, must be agreed and pre-arranged by the senior nursing and medical staff involved in the project or activity.
  - It must be the equal responsibility of the representative and the operating theatre staff when confirming these arrangements to ensure that all parties have approved it and have communicated appropriately.
- Whether a former practitioner in the relative field or not, the representative should have successfully completed a registered and respected theatre access/operating theatre etiquette course.
  - This provides the theatre staff with the assurance and confidence that the visitor has been educated appropriately in regard to behaviour and protocols.
- It is necessary for the visitor to record their entry and exit times in the appropriate register and is prohibited from visiting areas of the department that are irrelevant to the procedures, without authorisation.
- Medical representatives must be suitably attired in accordance with the local operating theatre recommendations and must not, at any time, engage in assisting with patient care.

- Representatives must be provided with all the health and safety information in relation to the specific department e.g. fire exits, eye-wash and spill-stations, and the member of staff with first aid responsibilities.
- The respect, well being and integrity of the patient and their privacy are paramount; the visitor must be provided with boundaries that accentuate this.
- The patient must be consulted as to whether they wish to comply with the request that a representative be present during their procedure; this can be assisted in its presentation to the patient by the theatre staff member highlighting the relevant qualifications and experience of the visitor and the benefit that it will provide to the procedure being performed.
- Only with the consent of the medical staff can the representative assist in reassuring the patient directly of the relevance of their attendance during the procedure.
- When possible, demonstration and evaluation of the device in a non-clinical setting (i.e. a 'dry run') to the relevant nursing and medical staff is highly recommended, prior to the actual procedure itself.

Medical representatives 'are merely promoting technology that the healthcare industry, through its need to provide better and more economical patient care, has demanded'.[2]

References

1. Health and Safety at Work Act 1974. Available at: ⊞ www.hse.gov.uk/legislation/hswa.htm

2. Hughes CW (2003). A day in the life of a medical salesman. *British Journal of Perioperative Nursing* **13**(9) 346–8.

Prisoners in theatre

Prisons can be very challenging environments where friction between the interests of the prisoner and the health and social care of society are often magnified.[1] All prisons are served by a Medical Officer on a full or part time basis and although healthcare facilities are provided in prisons, occasionally a prisoner may require specialist surgical or medical treatment at an outside hospital.

General principles

According to the BMA 'hospitals are sometimes seen as the weak link in the chain of secure custody where detainees may try to give a false impression of their medical condition in order to attempt to escape'.[2]

- Prior to admittance to hospital the Medical Officer and the Governor would meet to discuss:
  - If the transfer to a community hospital was necessary as many prisons have their own operating theatres and minor ops are carried out on a regular basis.
  - Prior to discharge to a normal hospital the level of security would have been decided and the escorting officer briefed by the Security Department.
  - The escorting officers are solely responsible for the security of the person in their charge.
- Prisoner officers are accountable to the Governor, have jurisdiction over the prisoner, are required to maintain a secure environment at all times, and must be given appropriate respect and consideration.
- Each prisoner should be individually risk assessed and close communications is mandatory between healthcare practitioners and prison officers to discuss and observe security measures.
- The main risks associated with prisoners in hospital are violence and an attempt to escape.

Communication between surgical and prison staff is paramount—it helps to break down barriers, with both parties appreciating the role of each other.

The BMA advise that prisoners should be assessed and treated without restraints and without the presence of prison officers.[2] In an ideal world it would be of benefit to all concerned if 'all' medical procedures could be carried out without the presence of restraints. Unfortunately, it is often unrealistic to remove both the presence of prison staff and restraints from the consulting room

Prisoners in the perioperative environment

- All prisoners must be cared for confidentially, objectively, humanely, and with dignity.[3,4]
- Operating theatres should be warned in advance regarding the arrival of a prisoner, levels of escort, and possible use of restraints.
- At least two prison officers would escort the 'patient' to the operating theatre.

- They would be expected to change into appropriate theatre attire and remain with the 'patient' until he/she has been anaesthetised.
- They would at this point retire until the procedure has been completed and remain in the recovery room until medical and nursing staff have completed their postoperative observations.
- Returning to the ward may prove to be a high-risk excursion from the security angle, and prison staff would be extra vigilant during this short journey. They may even feel that restraints would be appropriate.
- Restraints, such as handcuffs, should be removed if it is likely to interfere with treatment or if the prisoner is incapacitated and is unlikely to abscond to cause harm to others.
- Caring for prisoners should be no different to caring for non-prisoners.
- Prisoners may also feel anxious regarding the forthcoming anaesthetic and surgical procedure and their presence in the perioperative environment can accentuate this anxiety.
- Ensure a calm environment and clearly and concisely explain procedures and events as they unfold and answer questions honestly.

Communication explaining normal medical/security procedures between both parties will help prevent tension and anxiety, and create as 'normal' an atmosphere during the hospital stay as possible under abnormal circumstances.

References and further reading

1. Dale C and Woods P (2002). Caring for prisoners: Their professional, educational and occupational needs. *Nursing Management* **9**(6) 16–21.

2. British Medical Association (2004). *Providing medical care and treatment to people who are detained.* BMA: London.

3. Health Professions Council (2008). *Standards of conduct, performance and ethics.* HPC: London.

4. Nursing & Midwifery Council (2008). *The Code: standards of conduct, performance and ethics.* NMC: London.

Section 2

Preoperative care

Chapter 4

Pre-assessment of surgical patients

Preoperative assessment

The primary aim of preoperative assessment is to identify the patient's health status and level of fitness and to optimise health in preparation for surgery and anaesthesia. It is also used to ascertain the functional ability/reserve of the patient and therefore quantify their operative risk.

Additional aims are:
- To identify possible undiagnosed conditions.
- To identify and instigate relevant investigations according to predetermined protocols.
- To increase the patient's understanding of pre- and postoperative care.
- To assess the patient's home situation, social circumstances, and availability of support.
- To reduce anaesthetic, surgical, and patient-specific risks of impending surgery.
- To establish that the patient is fully informed and wishes to undergo the planned procedure.
- To minimise the risk of late cancellations by ensuring that all essential resources and discharge requirements are identified.
- To provide information for the patient to decrease anxiety and fear.
- To provide an opportunity to discuss ways in which to improve their health and outcome of surgery such as weight loss and smoking cessation.
- To provide health education/promotion in order to reduce the potential for future co-morbidities.

Purpose of preoperative assessment

The purpose of preoperative assessment is to obtain a comprehensive review of the patient's presenting condition and past medical history, ensuring that no aspect is overlooked.

History taking

- Introduce yourself to the patient and explain the purpose of the visit.
- Confirm the patient's demographic details such as name, address, date of birth.
- Confirm the surgeon's findings with the patient i.e. the presenting condition.
- Establish the patient's symptoms and question whether they have resolved or deteriorated; establish the site and side involved, if applicable, such as an arthroscopy.
- Establish a rapport with the patient.
- Enquire about past surgical and anaesthetic history and document any difficulties or cause for concern. This might include major cardiovascular or respiratory events, rare inherited disorders such as malignant hyperthermia (MH), and pseudo cholinesterase deficiency.
- Establish any inherited blood disorders such as sickle cell disease and thalassaemia disorders.
- Ask questions about any allergies or sensitivities to medications, antibiotics, food, latex, or rubber; identify what reactions are experienced—these can include sneezing, wheezing, rash, nausea, vomiting, diarrhoea.

- Record details of any triggers to allergies such as asthma or eczema.
- Identify venous thromboembolism risk factors.
- Cardiopulmonary exercise testing may be necessary for some patients.

It is essential that patients provide a list of current medication name, dose, quantity per day/week; this should also include any alternative or over-the-counter medicines. Additionally, it is important to establish the patient's cardiorespiratory status and identify any instances of breathlessness, chest pain, palpitations, fatigue, and claudication or sleep apnoea.

Physical assessment

Preoperative assessment establishes if a patient is fit enough for anaesthesia, so the physical assessment and examination should focus primarily on the cardiorespiratory system. However, renal function, hepatobilary system, and the endocrine system is examined in some patients.

Vital signs should be monitored and documented. These include:
- Non-invasive BP.
- Pulse rate.
- Oxygen saturation.
- Height.
- Weight.
- BMI.

The following systematic approach is recommended for a physical examination:
- Observation.
- Palpation.
- Percussion.
- Auscultation.

Anaesthetic assessment

It is extremely important that a detailed medical, anaesthetic, and surgical history is taken and documented as this may indicate potential airway management difficulties.
- An airway assessment should always be undertaken following analysis of the medical history.
- Patients who have marked neck restrictions, anatomical abnormalities, a small mouth, or ill-fitting dentures could potentially be difficult to intubate.
- Congenital abnormalities such as Down syndrome, Marfan syndrome, and Treacher syndrome should be documented and brought to the attention of the anaesthetist.
- A history of snoring or obstructive sleep apnoea may be associated with airway difficulties and its presence should also be documented.

Mallampati classification

The Mallampati classification is used to determine a potentially difficult airway. The patient is required to protrude the tongue as far as possible, while the anaesthetist inspects the pharyngeal structures from patient eye-level.

Short stay surgery

The Association of Anaesthetists of Great Britain and Ireland (AAGBI) outline the fundamental principles of day care:[1]
- Patients should be selected according to their physiological status not their age.
- Fitness for a procedure should relate to the patient's health as found at pre-assessment and not limited by American Society of Anesthesiologists (ASA) status.
- Obesity is not an absolute contraindication for day care in expert hands and with appropriate resources.

Patient selection for short stay surgery will depend on:
- The procedure required.
- The general health of the patient.
- The patient's social circumstances.

Medical criteria for short stay surgery
- Free from disease.
- Disease controlled.
- Asthma—not on steroids.
- ↑BP—on treatment.
- Diastolic <100mmHg.
- Diabetes—diet controlled.
- No glycosuria.

The medical criteria and patients who are excluded from short stay surgery differ according to locally agreed protocols.

Patients excluded from short stay surgery
- Chest disease.
- Epilepsy.
- Renal failure.
- Uncontrolled hypertension.
- BMI >40—although some units will accept patients with a high BMI providing there is no other presenting co-morbidity.
- Insulin-dependent diabetes.
- Severe rheumatoid arthritis.
- Symptomatic hiatus hernia.
- Chronic neurological disease.
- Severe psychiatric illness.
- Previous adverse anaesthetic reactions (or relatives).

Social circumstances
- Patients should have adequate home circumstances with the presence of a responsible adult for 24 hours postoperatively.
- The patient's home situation should be compatible with postoperative care, with satisfactory standards of heating and lighting, together with adequate kitchen, bathroom and toilet facilities.[1]
- Patients should have telephone access.

- Patients should live within 15 miles (~24 kilometres)/1 hour from the hospital.
- Patients should have car transport home following surgery.
- If there is any doubt, medical referral is essential.

Patient investigations

- BP/pulse.
- Blood tests—FBC/LFT.
- FBC—menstruating age.
- Weight.
- ECG—patient >60 years.
- Assessed by anaesthetist.

Box 4.1 Patient discharge criteria for short stay surgery[2]

- Stable vital signs—1 hour.
- No sign of respiratory depression.
- Orientated to person, time, and place.
- Retain oral fluids.
- Void urine.
- Dress and walk without assistance.
- No excessive pain, bleeding, postoperative nausea or vomiting.
- Understands how to use oral analgesia supplied.
- Has a responsible adult to take them home.
- Has a carer at home for the next 24 hours.
- Written and verbal postoperative instructions have been received.
- Emergency contact number has been supplied.

Benefits of anaesthetic assessment

- Identifies potential anaesthetic difficulties.
- Identifies medical conditions.
- Allows careful planning of care.
- Improves safety—minimises risk.
- Provides preoperative information.
- Allays fear and anxiety.

Pre-assessment of in-patients

- Vital part of anaesthetic care.
- Available for elective and emergency surgery.
- Usually includes assessment by anaesthetist who is responsible for their anaesthetic.
- Ensures continuity and rapport for anaesthetist and patient.

Table 4.1 Advantages of short stay surgery

For the provider	For the patient
↓ cost of treatment	Less time in hospital
↓ recovery time	Fewer cancellations
↓ waiting lists	↓ infection
No emergencies	↓ anxiety
↑ efficiency/££££	
Develop services	

References and further reading

1. Association of Anaesthetists of Great Britain and Ireland (2005). *Day surgery (revised edition).* AAGBI: London.

2. British Association of Day Surgery (2002). Guidelines about the discharge process and the assessment of fitness for discharge. Available from: ▣ http://www.nodelaysscotland.scot.nhs.uk

Association of Anaesthetists of Great Britain and Ireland (2001). *Preoperative assessment: the role of the anaesthetist.* AAGBI: London.

Association of Anaesthetists of Great Britain and Ireland (2002). *Immediate post-anaesthetic recovery.* AAGBI: London.

Association of Anaesthetists of Great Britain and Ireland (2007). *Recommendations for standards of monitoring during anaesthesia and recovery* (4th edn). AAGBI: London.

National Institute of Clinical Excellence (2003). *Preoperative tests – The use of routine preoperative tests for elective surgery.* NICE: London.

Royal College of Anaesthetists. (2004). *Guidelines for the Provision of Anaesthetic Services.* RCoA: London.

Patients with pre-existing disease

Overview

- Pre-existing disease and illness impact greatly upon the provision of nursing care during the perioperative phase.
- Pre-existing disease can be classified as:
  - Lifestyle-induced disease.
  - Inherited disease/illness.
  - Acquired disease.
- Unfit patients frequently undergo surgery.
- Their illness/condition may be a result of smoking, excessive drinking, overeating, or an acquired or inherited disease.
- Assessment tools such as the ASA physical status (PS) grading serve to diagnose and classify illness.
- The results of such assessments can inform medical/nursing staff and be used to appraise the urgency for surgical intervention.

ASA grading of PS

The ASA grading system:
- Serves as a tool from which anaesthetists can classify patients, avoid unnecessary surgical procedures, and manage risk effectively.
- Aims to evaluate the severity of systemic diseases, physiological dysfunction, and anatomic abnormalities.

The tool is used to grade patient risk based on their medical history, appearance, and condition (Fig. 4.1).

ASA PS 1: a normal healthy patient
- No physiological, psychological, psychiatric, biochemical, or organic disturbances.
- Healthy individual with good exercise tolerance.
- Excludes the elderly and neonates.

ASA PS 2: patients with mild systemic disease
- No functional limitations; has a well-controlled disease of one body system.
- Examples: controlled diabetes mellitus, hypertension, asthma, chronic bronchitis.
- Mild lifestyle issues—tobacco abuse, obesity.

ASA PS 3: patients with severe systemic disease that restricts activity but is not incapacitating
- Some functional limitation; has a controlled disease of more than one body system or one major system.
- No immediate danger of death.
- Examples: stable angina, congestive cardiac failure, previous history of infarct, chronic renal failure (CRF).
- Lifestyle-affecting factors—morbid obesity.

ASA PS 4: patients with severe systemic disease that is a constant threat to life
- Has at least one severe disease that is poorly controlled or at end-stage.
- Possible risk of death as a result of disease.
- Examples: symptomatic chronic obstructive pulmonary disease (COPD), unstable angina, hepatorenal and/or endocrine failure.

ASA PS 5: moribund patients who are not expected to survive 24 hours without the operation
- Imminent risk of death.
- Surgery performed as a last resort or resuscitative effort.
- Multi-organ failure.
- Cerebral trauma.
- Examples: sepsis with haemodynamic instability, poorly controlled coagulopathy, ruptured aneurysm, large pulmonary embolism (PE)

ASA PS 6: a declared brain-dead patient whose organs are being harvested for donor purposes

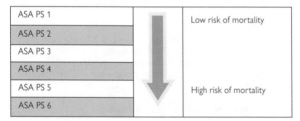

Fig. 5.1 ASA PS grading.

References and further reading

Hatfield A and Tronson M (2006). *The Complete Recovery Room Book* (3rd edn). Oxford University Press: Oxford.

Hoffer JL (1999). Anaesthesia. In Heeker MH and Rothrock JC (eds). *Alexander's Care of the Patient in Surgery* (11th edn). Mosby: St Louis.

Mason R (2001). *Anaesthesia Databook: A Perioperative and Peripartum Manual* (3rd edn). GMM: London.

Lifestyle factors and induced disease

Alcoholism

- Patients who are alcoholics and regular drinkers are tolerant to some sedatives (benzodiazepines) and anaesthetic agents (propofol) and will require higher dosages.
- Patients with alcoholism often emerge from anaesthesia in an aggressive and restless manner. They can thrash and move about in a semi-purposeful manner before they fully awake, e.g. they may try to sit up before rejecting their airway.
- They might appear dazed and will not respond to speech; this is a distinct feature.
- Thin/emaciated patients with alcoholism (usually in the latter stages of the disease) are prone to hypothermia.
- Postoperatively, some patients with alcoholism are susceptible to spontaneous hypoglycaemia.

Always monitor patients' blood glucose levels.

Drug addiction

- Patients who are street addicts and intravenous (IV) drug users are often malnourished and in poor physical health.
- They are most likely to attend for emergency surgery.
- They have a very high risk of containing blood-borne viruses (BBVs) and parasitic infections.

Standard precautions should be taken at all times.

Amphetamines and cocaine

- Stimulate the activity of the sympathetic nervous system, causing a state of 'hyper-alertness'.
- Displace endogenous noradrenaline from nerve endings; addicts are prone to noradrenaline depletion particularly after drug use.
- Patients can become profoundly hypotensive postoperatively in recovery due to noradrenaline depletion. They may even require noradrenaline infusion to restore and maintain their arterial pressure.

Opiate addiction

- Ideally, patients with opiate addiction will receive local/regional anaesthesia.
- Patients who are recovering from addiction may refuse opiates.
- In some cases, patients with drug addiction may overstate the intensity of their pain to obtain opiate analgesia.
- In general, patients with drug addiction will require higher doses than the average population due to opioid tolerance.
- Use caution if giving high doses and check the patient's drug history as he/she may be on a methadone regimen.
- ***Do not withold opiates.*** If the patient is in pain, administer analgesic.

Benzodiazepines (BDZ)

- Many elderly patients or those with anxiety disorders might be considered as 'drug addicts' as they have been taking BDZ such as nitrazepam or diazepam for many years.
- Withdrawal of these drugs can cause acute agitation, aggression, violence, and even convulsions.
- If the patient is BDZ dependent, administer their dose (if they have not already received it).

Caution is advised when caring for severely dependant patients who are experiencing withdrawal as they can become very violent.

Obesity

- Obese patients will require higher O_2 concentrations due to increased consumption as there is more tissue to be perfused.
- Positioning is very important, if possible, sit the patient up.
- BP readings cannot be relied on due to excess of body fat.
- If possible, monitor BP invasively via arterial access.
- IV access can be difficult to obtain due to body fat; this should therefore be well secured.

References and further reading

Hatfield A and Tronson M (2008). *The Complete Recovery Room Book* (4th edn). Oxford University Press: Oxford.

Hoffer JL (1999). Anaesthesia. In Heeker MH and Rothrock JC (eds). *Alexander's Care of the Patient in Surgery* (11th edn). Mosby: St Louis.

Mason R (2001). Anaesthesia Databook: A Perioperative and Peripartum Manual (3rd edn). GMM: London.

National Obesity Forum. Available from: 🖳 www.nationalobesityforum.org.uk

National Obesity Forum (2005). National Obesity Care Pathway.
Available from: 🖳 http://nationalobesityforum.org.uk/images/stories/Obesity_Care_Path.pdf

Respiratory disorders

Asthma

- Asthma is defined as reversible airflow obstruction due to constriction of smooth muscles in the airways.[1]
- Symptoms can include breathlessness, wheeze, cough, and sputum production.
- Patients with mild or well-controlled asthma rarely require additional treatment pre- and post-anaesthesia and surgery.
- Patients with more severe asthma may require additional medication and/or steroid therapy perioperatively if additional problems develop e.g., chest infection.

Chronic obstructive pulmonary disease (COPD)

- COPD involves chronic bronchitis and emphysema and symptoms can include breathlessness, wheeze, cough, and sputum production.
- Nebulized bronchodilators are recommended prior to anaesthesia and surgery and continued for up to 48 hours.
- Intubation should be avoided but spontaneous breathing may be unsuitable for some patients.
- Patients should be monitored and observed closely perioperatively for potential pneumothorax.
- Deciding whether or not to proceed with surgery should rest with a consultant anaesthetist and consultant surgeon, taking account of the presence of co-morbidities, the functional status of the patient, and the necessity of the surgery.[2]
- The medical management of the patient should be optimised prior to surgery and might involve pulmonary rehabilitation.

Preoperative management

- Patients with respiratory disease are at risk of developing problems postoperatively.
- It is advisable that elective surgery occurs only when respiratory function is optimal.
- Preoperative assessment of patients with respiratory disease requiring surgery should include:
  - Drug history; peak flow rates.
  - Smoking history; cough and sputum production.
  - Exercise tolerance test, as this can provide a reliable test of respiratory function.
  - FBC to identify anaemia or polycythaemia.
  - BMI calculated.
- Patients may benefit from preoperative chest physiotherapy.
- McCormick[3] identifies that perioperative pulmonary problems may occur when the following factors are present:
  - Patients over 60 year of age.
  - Smoking history.
  - History of malignancy.
  - Abdominal and thoracic surgery.
  - Abnormal chest x-ray.

Anaesthesia management
- Regional anaesthesia may be beneficial for patients with pulmonary impairment.

Postoperative management
- Ensure patient is sitting in an upright position.
- Chest physiotherapy in recovery and on the ward as prescribed.
- Early mobilisation.
- Bronchodilator therapy as prescribed.
- Effective analgesia to aid respiratory function.
- Accurate monitoring of fluid balance as patients with respiratory disease are at increased risk of pulmonary oedema.

Table 5.1 Respiratory definitions[4]

Tidal volume	The amount of air that is moved in and out of the lungs during each breath
Minute volume	The volume of air that is moved in and out of the lungs in 1 minute
Hypercarbia	Excess carbon dioxide (CO_2) in the body
Hypoxia	Lack of O_2 that affects the normal function of cells
Hypoxaemia	PaO_2 falls below 60mmHg
Hypoventilation	Failure of the lungs to eliminate CO_2 and measured by a rise in the partial pressure of CO_2 in arterial blood

References and further reading

1. Sheldon C and Wilson I (2000). Respiratory disorders. In Nicholls A, Wilson I (eds). *Perioperative medicine: managing surgical patients with medical problems.* Oxford University Press: Oxford.

2. National Institute for Health and Clinical Excellence (2004). *Chronic obstructive pulmonary disease: Management of chronic obstructive pulmonary disease in adults in primary and secondary care.* NICE: London.

3. McCormick B (2006). Respiratory disease. In Allman KG and Wilson IH (eds). *Oxford Handbook of Anaesthesia* (2nd edn). Oxford University Press: Oxford.

4. Hatfield A and Tronson M (2008). *The Complete Recovery Room Book* (4th edn). Oxford University Press: Oxford.

National Institute for Health and Clinical Excellence respiratory guidelines. Available from: www.nice.org.uk/guidance/index.jsp?action=byTopic&o=7308&set=true

Royal College of Anaesthetists (2004). *Guidelines for the Provision of Anaesthetic Services.* RCoA: London.

Cardiac disorders

- Cardiac disease is one of the commonest causes of morbidity and mortality in surgical patients.[1]
- Patients with coronary heart disease (CHD) are at risk of a myocardial infarction (MI) and this risk increases with age, hypertension, diabetes, and renal disease.
- Increased perioperative risks are associated with the following cardiac problems:
  - Ischaemic heart disease.
  - Heart failure.
  - Arrhythmia.
- Unstable ischaemic heart disease mandates optimisation prior to elective surgery to reduce operative risk as it is a main contributory factor to postoperative morbidity and mortality.

Preoperative management

- Comprehensive pre assessment by a consultant anaesthetist and pre-assessment nurse should include:
  - Past medical history including cardiac events.
  - Observe colour, signs of cyanosis, breathlessness.
  - Monitor vital signs including non-invasive BP.
  - 12-lead ECG.
  - Cardiopulmonary exercise testing may be necessary for some patients.
- Elective surgery should be postponed for up to 6 months following recent MI—refer to cardiologist if necessary.
- Assess renal function.
- Patients with pacemakers should have these identified and checked to ensure its good working order.
- Patients with pacemakers should also have an ECG preoperatively to assess function.
- Liaison with pacemaker clinics is sometimes necessary for cardiovascular evaluation for non-cardiac surgery.

Anaesthesia management

- Close patient monitoring during the perioperative period.
- Invasive monitoring including arterial BP, and central venous pressure (CVP) ± cardiac output if necessary for major surgery.
- Ensure availability of intensive care bed for emergency surgery, unstable disease, and recent MI.
- Close monitoring of fluid balance is essential.
- Short bursts of bipolar diathermy are recommended as electrocautery for patients with pacemakers.
- Regional analgesia is effective in reducing the risk of tachycardia.

Postoperative management

- Accurate fluid balance should be monitored frequently with recordings of hourly urine output.
- Monitoring of vital signs including TPR, BP, peripheral O_2 saturation (SpO_2).
- Invasive monitoring including arterial BP, CVP ± cardiac output may be required following emergency surgery, unstable disease and recent MI.
- O_2 as prescribed.
- Analgesia as prescribed to reduce the risk of tachycardia.

References and further reading

1. Dean J and Telford R (2000). Cardiovascular disorders. In Nicholls A and Wilson I (eds). *Perioperative medicine: managing surgical patients with medical problems*. Oxford University Press: Oxford.

Department of Health (2000) *National service framework for coronary heart disease*. The Stationery Office: London.

National Institute for Health and Clinical Excellence. Cardiovascular guidance. Available from: www.nice.org.uk/guidance/index.jsp?action=byTopic&o=7195&set=true

Sinclair M and Evans R (2006). Cardiac surgery. In Allman KG and Wilson IH (eds). *Oxford Handbook of Anaesthesia* (2nd edn). Oxford University Press: Oxford.

Telford R (2006). Cardiovascular disease. In Allman KG and Wilson IH (eds). *Oxford Handbook of Anaesthesia* (2nd edn). Oxford University Press: Oxford.

Neurological and muscular disorders: overview and multiple sclerosis

- Patients with neurological and muscular disorders should be cared for by practitioners with the appropriate neurological and resuscitation skills and facilities.[1]
- An inter-disciplinary approach to care delivery and management is essential to maximise the patient experience.
- Treatment must comply with national and local standards and guidelines.

Examples of neurological and muscular disorders

- Myasthenia gravis.
- Multiple sclerosis.
- Stroke.
- Parkinson's disease.
- Muscular dystrophy.
- Motor neurone disease.
- Myasthenic syndrome.
- Epilepsy.
- Dementia.
- Guillain–Barré syndrome.
- Dystrophia myotonica.
- Malignant hyperthermia.

Multiple sclerosis (MS)

- MS is a common disabling neurological disease and autoimmune condition, resulting from damage to the myelin sheath which interferes with transmission of messages between the brain and other parts of the body.
- Treatment can involve disease-modifying drugs, complementary and alternative therapy, analgesia for neuropathic pain, and stem cell treatment in some instances.

Problems associated with multiple sclerosis

- Balance.
- Constipation.
- Dysphagia.
- Memory.
- Mood swings.
- Pain.
- Tremor.
- Bladder and bowel incontinence.
- Chronic fatigue.
- Dysphasia.
- Muscle spasms and stiffness.
- Muscle spasticity.
- Sexual dysfunction.
- Visual disturbances.

Preoperative management
- Detailed neurological assessment.
- Assessment of respiratory function.
- Anti-embolic stockings should be applied to reduce the risk of DVT and PE.

Anaesthesia management
- General anaesthesia is usually advocated as it does not alter the course of MS.
- Caution should be applied to the use of non-depolarising drugs.
- Suxamethonium should be avoided.
- Regional anaesthesia may aggravate the condition.
- Local anaesthesia should be minimal.
- Cardiovascular monitoring is essential.

Postoperative management
- Monitor all vital signs, especially temperature as hypothermia can delay recovery.
- Patients may experience difficulty coughing up sputum, increasing the risk of chest infection; sputum clearance is essential to reduce the risk of respiratory compromise.
- Leg movement should be encouraged in recovery if appropriate to reduce spasticity.

Reference and further reading

1. Department of Health (2005). *National service framework for long term conditions*. The Stationery Office: London.

Hardie R and Day C (2000). Neurological disorders. In Nicholls A and Wilson I (eds). *Perioperative medicine: managing surgical patients with medical problems*. Oxford University Press: Oxford.

Multiple Sclerosis Society. Available at: 🖳 www.mssociety.org.uk

National Institute for Health and Clinical Excellence (2003). *Management of multiple sclerosis in primary and secondary care*. NICE: London.

Teasdale A (2006). Neurological and muscular disorders. In Allman KG and Wilson IH (eds). *Oxford Handbook of Anaesthesia* (2nd edn). Oxford University Press: Oxford.

Neurological disorders: epilepsy

- A neurological condition characterised by recurrent epileptic seizures unprovoked by any immediately identifiable cause.
- An epileptic seizure is the clinical manifestation of an abnormal and excessive discharge of a set of neurons in the brain (NICE 2004).
- A comprehensive care pathway utilising an inter-disciplinary approach to care delivery and management is essential.
- Epilepsy nurse specialists should be an integral part of the care of patients with epilepsy.

Preoperative management

- Short stay surgery and anaesthesia is suitable for patients with well-controlled disease.
- Comprehensive pre-assessment of patient to include drug history and frequency of seizures.
- Anti-epileptic therapy should be continued until the time of surgery.

Anaesthesia management

- Premedication can include the use of diazepam or lorazepam.
- Thiopental is the drug of choice for induction of general anaesthesia, due to its anti-convulsant properties.
- Atracurium or cisatracurium is recommended for muscle relaxation.
- Suxamethonium and vecuronium can increase the risk of dystonias.

Postoperative management

- Epilepsy drugs should be recommenced as soon as possible postoperatively.
- Ensure IV access.
- Ensure availability of ventilatory support if required.
- Monitoring of vital signs including TPR, BP, SpO_2.
- Anti-emetic therapy should include ondansetron or cyclizine to reduce the risk of dystonias.
- Monitor for postoperative convulsions.

Status epilepticus can be controlled with propofol or thiopentone.

- If seizure occurs, call for anaesthetist and:
  - Maintain airway.
  - Administer O_2.
  - Assess cardiorespiratory function.
  - Ensure safety of patient but do not restrain.
  - Constant reassurance is necessary as the patient may be confused and not fully aware of surroundings.
  - Monitor length of seizure.
  - Patients may feel tired and need to sleep following a seizure.

Reference and further reading

National Institute for Health and Clinical Excellence (2004). *The diagnosis and management of the epilepsies in adults and children in primary and secondary care*. NICE: London.

Department of Health (2005). *National service framework for long term conditions*. The Stationery Office: London.

Hardie R and Day C (2000). Neurological disorders. In Nicholls A and Wilson I (eds). *Perioperative medicine: managing surgical patients with medical problems*. Oxford University Press: Oxford.

Teasdale A (2006). Neurological and muscular disorders. In Allman KG and Wilson IH (eds). *Oxford Handbook of Anaesthesia* (2nd edn). Oxford University Press: Oxford.

The National Society for Epilepsy. Available at: 🖳 www.epilepsynse.org.uk

Neurological disorders: myasthenia gravis

- An autoimmune disease characterised by fluctuating muscle weakness that can sometimes be fatal.
- Symptoms usually include facial weakness, ptosis, diplopia, bulbar palsy, and respiratory insufficiency.
- Treatment involves the use of anticholinesterase drugs such as neostigmine and atropine to counteract the muscarinic side effects that can include abdominal cramps and bradycardia.
- Myasthenic crisis causes paralysis of the respiratory muscles necessitating ventilation.

Preoperative management

- Patients with stable disease can usually present for most surgical procedures.
- Postoperatively, patients with myasthenia gravis are at risk of respiratory difficulties due to inadequate cough reflex to clear their mucous due to intrinsic muscle weakness.
- Sputum can then block the bronchi causing collapse of the lung.
- Comprehensive pre-assessment of patient to include assessment of neurological and respiratory function.
- Anticholinesterase therapy should be continued until induction of anaesthesia.
- Pre-medication is not recommended.

Anaesthesia management

- Regional anaesthesia should be considered to avoid the use of opiate drugs and the possibility of respiratory depression.
- Rapid sequence induction may be employed with general anaesthesia utilising a minimal dose of suxamethonium.
- Neuromuscular blockade should be avoided as intubation and ventilation are achievable in the absence of muscle-relaxing drugs.
  - If non-depolarising muscle relaxants are used, the drugs of choice include atracurium, vecuronium, or mivacurium.
- Reversal agents are not recommended due to risk of overdose—if necessary, one dose of neostigmine is advocated.
- Nerve stimulators should be used to assess neuromuscular function prior to extubation.

Postoperative management

- Delayed emergence from anaesthesia may occur.
- Ventilatory support should be available postoperatively.
- Transfer to intensive treatment unit (ITU) for postoperative management may be necessary.
- Full patient monitoring—TPR, BP, ECG, SpO_2, level of consciousness, urinary output.
- Drug therapy should be recommenced immediately; enteral administration of medicines via a nasogastric tube may be necessary.
- Postoperative analgesia—epidural or patient-controlled analgesia (PCA).

- Respiratory problems may occur e.g. infection, sputum retention, respiratory failure.
- Intensive physiotherapy may be required pre- and postoperatively.

References and further reading

Department of Health (2005). *National service framework for long term conditions*. The Stationery Office: London.

Hardie R and Day C (2000). Neurological disorders. In Nicholls A and Wilson I (eds). *Perioperative medicine: managing surgical patients with medical problems*. Oxford University Press: Oxford.

Myasthenia Gravis Association. Available at: 🖳 www.mgauk.org

Teasdale A (2006). Neurological and muscular disorders. In Allman KG and Wilson IH (eds). *Oxford Handbook of Anaesthesia* (2nd edn). Oxford University Press: Oxford.

Haematology disorders

Haematology disorders can include anaemia, sickle cell disease, coagulation disorders, thrombocytopenia, haemophilia, and porphyria.

Anaemia

- Anaemia can be defined as a reduction in red cell mass leading to a lowered haemoglobin and haematocrit level in the blood.
- The most common form of anaemia is iron-deficiency anaemia and this occurs when the haemoglobin (Hb) levels falls below the following levels:
  - Females = <12g/dL.
  - Males = <13g/dL.
- The most common symptoms associated with iron deficiency anaemia include:
  - Tiredness.
  - Lethargy.
  - Dyspnoea.
  - Palpitations.
- Changes in physical appearance can also occur including dry, flaking nails, spoon-shaped nails, pale complexion, abnormally smooth tongue, painful ulcers on the corners of the mouth.
- One of the commonest causes of anaemia is gastrointestinal (GI) blood loss and this can occur with stomach ulcers, cancer, menstruation, pregnancy, diet, and non-steroidal anti-inflammatory drugs (NSAIDs).

Perioperative considerations

- Pre-assessment prior to surgery to include FBC and anaemia corrected by oral iron or vitamin B_{12} injections if necessary.
- Blood transfusion is only recommended if HB is <7g/dL.
- Transfusing a patient with pernicious anaemia may increase the risk of heart failure.
- Adequate patient monitoring is essential and should include:
  - SpO_2.
  - TPR.
  - BP.

Sickle cell disease

- Sickle cell anaemia is one of the most common genetic diseases in the United Kingdom (UK) and affects the ability to carry O_2 around the body
- The shape and texture of blood cells change, becoming hard and sticky and shaped like sickles. These cells then die prematurely, leading to a shortage of red blood cells.
- Sickle cell anaemia is more prevalent in Afro-Caribbean, black African, and black British people.
- The only cure for sickle cell anaemia is a bone marrow transplant.
- The symptoms of sickle cell anaemia usually commences from 3 months of age and can include:
  - Anaemia.
  - Hand–foot syndrome.

- Jaundice.
- Frequent infections.

Perioperative considerations
- Preoperative assessment should include antibody screening.
- Consideration should be given to the possibility of dehydration, hypoxia, infection, and pain and be avoided.
- The operating theatre should be warmed to avoid patient hypothermia.
- Adequate patient monitoring is essential and should include:
  - SpO_2.
  - TPR.
  - BP.
- Consider perioperative fluid regimen.
- Postoperative O_2 therapy as prescribed.

References and further reading

Lee R and Purday J (2000). Haematological disorders. In Nicholls A and Wilson I (eds). *Perioperative medicine: managing surgical patients with medical problems*. Oxford University Press: Oxford.

National Institute of Health and Clinical Excellence. Blood guidance. Available from: www.nice.org.uk/guidance/index.jsp?action=byTopic&o=7164&set=true

Purday J (2006). Haematological disorders. In Allman KG and Wilson IH (eds). *Oxford Handbook of Anaesthesia* (2nd edn). Oxford University Press: Oxford.

Sickle Cell Society. Available from: www.sicklecellsociety.org

Renal disorders

- Chronic kidney disease (CKD) can be defined as a gradual and eventual permanent loss of kidney function over time.
- CKD has been identified as a condition that is often under-diagnosed with no obvious symptoms.
- Common causes include hypertension, diabetes, and familial, and the damage usually occurs very gradually over years.
- Patients with kidney problems tend to be susceptible to heart attacks and strokes.
- Afro-Caribbean and South Asian patients are at significantly greater risk of renal failure than people from white ethnic backgrounds.
- For patients in established renal failure, the optimal choice is renal transplantation.
- It is recommended that the use of NICE[1] guidance on preoperative testing should be followed in all surgical units.

Preoperative management

- Pre-assessment should include drug history and drug allergies.
- Regular monitoring of vital signs.
- Consider anaemia or cardiovascular problems if reduced exercise tolerance is identified.[2]
- An intensive care bed should be available for major surgical procedures.

Anaesthesia management

- The use of non-invasive BP and cannulation should be avoided in an arm with an antrioventricular (AV) fistula.
- Cannulation of the dorsum of the dorsum of the hand is recommended.
- Cannulation of the forearm and antecubital fossa should be avoided.
- The majority of drugs used in anaesthesia can reduce glomerular filtration rate, urine output, and blood flow (Table 5.2).

Postoperative management

- Accurate fluid balance should be monitored frequently with recordings of hourly urine output.
- Avoid dehydration.
- NSAIDs should be avoided.

Renal failure

- Renal failure can occur perioperatively when oliguria and a rising serum creatinine develop. Patients at risk of acute renal failure include the following:
- Septic shock.
- Fluid depletion.
- Heart failure, hypertension, vascular disease.
- CRF.
- Elderly patients with hypertension and diabetes.
- Patients taking NSAIDs, ACE inhibitors, diuretics, and chemotherapy.

Table 5.2 Safe anaesthetic drugs in chronic renal failure[3]

Premedication drugs	Midazolam, temazepam
Induction agents	Propofol, thiopental, etomidate
Inhalational agents	Isoflurane, halothane, desflurane
Muscle relaxants	Suxamethonium, atracurium, cisatracurium
Opiate drugs	Remifentamil, alfentanil
Local anaesthetic drugs	Lidocaine, bupivacaine
Analgesic drugs	Paracetamol

References and further reading

1. National Institute for Health and Clinical Excellence (2003). *Preoperative Tests: The use of routine preoperative tests for elective surgery.* NICE: London.

2. Nicholls A (2000). Renal disorders. In Nicholls A and Wilson I (eds). *Perioperative medicine: managing surgical patients with medical problems.* Oxford University Press: Oxford.

3. Milner Q (2006). Renal disease. In Allman KG and Wilson IH (eds). *Oxford Handbook of Anaesthesia* (2nd edn). Oxford University Press: Oxford.

British Renal Society. Available at: 🖳 www.britishrenal.org/

Department of Health (2004). *National Service Framework for Renal Services - Part One: Dialysis and transplantation implementation toolkit for commissioners based on best practice.* The Stationery Office: London.

Department of Health (2005). *National Service Framework for Renal Services Part Two: Chronic kidney disease acute renal failure and end of life care.* The Stationery Office: London.

Department of Health (2007) *National Service Framework for Renal Services.* Available from: 🖳 www.dh.gov.uk/en/Healthcare/NationalServiceFrameworks/Renal/DH_4102636

Department of Health (2007). *National Service Framework for Renal Services: Second Progress Report.* The Stationery Office: London.

Harrison R and Daly L (2006). *Acute medical emergencies: a nursing guide* (2nd edn). Churchill Livingstone: Edinburgh.

National Institute of Clinical Health and Excellence. Urinary tract system surgery guidance. Available from: 🖳 www.nice.org.uk/guidance/index.jsp?action=byTopic&o=7610

National Institute of Clinical Health and Excellence. Urogenital guidance. Available from: 🖳 www.nice.org.uk/guidance/index.jsp?action=byTopic&o=7317&set=true

Nicholls A (2000). Oliguria and renal failure. In Nicholls A and Wilson I (eds). *Perioperative medicine: managing surgical patients with medical problems.* Oxford University Press: Oxford.

Bone and joint disorders

Rheumatology

- Rheumatoid arthritis is defined as a chronic, disabling autoimmune disease characterised by inflammation of the synovial tissue of the peripheral joints[1] and is more prevalent in women than in men.
- Symptoms can include stiffness, swelling pain, and progressive joint destruction.
- An inter-disciplinary approach to managing musculoskeletal conditions is multidisciplinary is recommended usually involving the following health disciplines:
  - Rheumatologists; orthopaedic surgeons; nursing; physiotherapy; occupational therapy
  - Orthotics, prosthetics, podiatry and dietetics usually support the above disciplines
- Rheumatology services provide specialist advice, treatment and support for considerable numbers of people affected by rheumatological conditions (Table 5.3).

Preoperative management

- Pre-assessment is essential by members of the nursing, anaesthetic, and medical team and should include the following investigations:
- Chest x-ray, ECG, FBC, urea and electrolytes (U&Es).
- Neck x-ray for cervical instability.
- Airway assessment to assess intubation risk.
- Assessment may also be undertaken by occupational therapists and physiotherapists to discuss the home environment and postoperative exercise regimens.
- Steroid cover should be implemented perioperatively and reduced to maintenance level postoperatively.[2]

Anaesthetic management

- Airway management with sedation can be problematic as patients are often in the supine position for orthopaedic surgery.
- Ensure anti-embolic prophylaxis.
- A protective neck collar is recommended prior to induction of anaesthesia for patients with cervical instability.[2]
- The use of spinal and epidural anaesthesia may prove difficult in some patients with joint deformities.
- Tracheal intubation might be problematic in patients with scoliosis and spondyloarthropies.
- Care should be taken when moving, handling, and transferring patients with bone and joint disorders.
- Patients should be positioned carefully with appropriate protection and padding of pressure areas.
- Patients should be actively warmed intraoperatively.
- General anaesthesia ± epidural is recommended for major orthopaedic procedures.

Postoperative management

- All patients with bone and joint disorders should be transferred onto beds following surgery.
- O_2 therapy as prescribed.
- Effective postoperative analgesia and NSAIDs should be prescribed.
- DVT prophylaxis until patient is mobilising.
- Accurate fluid balance should be monitored.
- For patients with rheumatoid disease, disease-modifying anti-rheumatoid drugs (DMARDs) should be resumed as soon as possible following surgery.
- Pressure area care for immobile and frail patients.

Table 5.3 Rheumatology conditions[3]

Inflammatory diseases	Ankylosing spondylitis Psoriatic arthritis Reactive arthritis
Auto-immune rheumatic diseases	Rheumatoid arthritis Systemic lupus erythematosus (SLE) Scleroderma Myositis Sjogren's syndrome Systemic vasculitis
Soft tissue/regional pain disorders	Generalised and non-articular pain syndromes Tendonitis Bursitis
Bone diseases	Osteoporosis Paget's disease
Osteoarthritis	
Back pain	

References and further reading

1. National Institute of Clinical health and Excellence (2007). *Rheumatoid arthritis in adults.* Available from: ▣ www.nice.org.uk/guidance/index.jsp?action=download&o=37807

2. Marshall P (2000). Bone and joint disorders. In Nicholls A and Wilson I (eds). *Perioperative medicine: managing surgical patients with medical problems.* Oxford University Press: Oxford.

3. Department of Health (2006). *Musculoskeletal Services Framework. A joint responsibility: doing it differently.* The Stationery Office: London.

Marshall P (2006). Bone, joint, and connective tissue disorders. In Allman KG and Wilson IH (eds). *Oxford Handbook of Anaesthesia* (2nd edn). Oxford University Press: Oxford.

National Institute of Health and Clinical Excellence. Musculoskeletal guidance. Available from: ▣ www.nice.org.uk/guidance/index.jsp?action=byTopic&o=7299&set=true

Worms R and Griffiths R (2006). Orthopaedic surgery. In Allman KG and Wilson IH (eds). *Oxford Handbook of Anaesthesia* (2nd edn). Oxford University Press: Oxford.

Endocrine and metabolic disorders: overview and diabetes

Examples of endocrine and metabolic disorders

- Acromegaly.
- Diabetes mellitus.
- Hypernatraemia.
- Hyponatraemia.
- Parathyroid disease.
- Cushing's syndrome.
- Hyperkalaemia.
- Hypokalaemia.
- Obesity.
- Thyroid disease.

Diabetes

There are two main types of diabetes:

- *Type 1 diabetes*: occurs when the body is unable to produce insulin; onset is usually before the age of 40 and is the least common of the two types.
- *Type 2 diabetes*: is the most common of the two types and develops when the body doesn't make enough insulin; onset is usually after the age of 40 and is linked to obesity.

The main problem experienced by diabetic patients is blood glucose control. Complications of this can include:

- Ischaemic heart disease.
- Retinopathy.
- Peripheral vascular disease.
- Cerebrovascular disease.
- Neuropathy.
- Nephropathy.
- Hypoglycaemia:
  - Blood glucose <3.5mmol/L.
  - Symptoms include sweating, tachycardia, confusion, unconsciousness, convulsions.
- Hyperglycaemia:
  - Blood glucose up to 20–25mmol/L.
  - Symptoms include thirst, dehydration.

Preoperative management

- Diabetes is the most common endocrine disease encountered before surgery.
- Fasting times, the surgical stress response, and inactivity can all have a negative impact on blood sugar control.
- Preoperative fasting times for patients with diabetes should be minimal.
- Diabetic patients should be first on the operating theatre list.
- Short stay surgery and anaesthesia is suitable for patients with well-controlled disease.

- Comprehensive pre-assessment of patient to include monitoring of blood glucose levels, urine analysis, creatinine and electrolytes, and ECG if the patient is over 30 years old.
- Regular monitoring of blood sugar levels is essential.
- Locally agreed regimens for blood sugar control of diabetic patients should be in place.
- Risks associated with complications of diabetes should be minimised.

Anaesthetic management
- If blood glucose level >10mmol/L, consider insulin/glucose regimen.
- Rapid sequence induction of general anaesthesia may be required as diabetic patients are prone to gastric reflux.
- Hypoglycaemia may not be evident during anaesthesia so blood glucose levels should be monitored regularly.
- Regional anaesthesia should be considered for surgery to the extremities.

Postoperative management
- Monitoring of blood glucose levels.
- Monitoring of vital signs including TPR, BP, SpO_2.

References and further reading

Blanshard H (2006). Endocrine and metabolic disease. In Allman KG and Wilson IH (eds). *Oxford Handbook of Anaesthesia* (2nd edn). Oxford University Press: Oxford.

Diabetes UK. Available at: ⬚ www.diabetes.org.uk

Department of Health (2005). *National service framework for long term conditions*. The Stationery Office: London.

Hattersley A and Saddler J (2000). Endocrine and metabolic disorders. In Nicholls A and Wilson I (eds). *Perioperative medicine: managing surgical patients with medical problems*. Oxford University Press: Oxford.

National Institute for Health and Clinical Excellence (2008). *Type 2 diabetes: The management of type 2 diabetes*. NICE: London.

Royal College of Anaesthetists (2004). *Guidelines for the Provision of Anaesthetic Services*. RCoA: London.

Endocrine and metabolic disorders: obesity

Body weight and weight gain are influenced by many factors, including life-style and genetic make-up. Patients who are classed as obese increase the risk of developing:

- Osteoarthritis.
- Coronary heart disease.
- Type 2 diabetes.
- Certain types of cancer.

The degree of overweight or obesity in adults should be defined as per NICE guidelines, shown in Table 5.4.

Preoperative management

- Bariatric surgery for adults with a BMI >50kg/m^2 is recommended where surgery is considered appropriate and the patient is fit and meets the criteria for anaesthesia and surgery.
- Weight management programmes can be employed prior to elective surgery and identified during pre-assessment.
- One of the main problems for obese patients is respiratory compromise, which can be accentuated in the following positions:
  - Head-down.
  - Supine—aorto-caval compression may occur.
- Other problems that give rise for concern for both the anaesthetic and surgical team can include:
  - Venous access.
  - Airway management.
  - Regional anaesthesia—not usually recommended.
  - Hiatus hernia and the risk of aspiration.
  - BP monitoring—appropriate sized cuff should be used.
  - Wound dehiscence.
- Prophylactic anti-embolic therapy is advised with subcutaneous heparin and anti-embolic stockings to reduce the risk of DVT and PE.
- Premedication with medicines causing respiratory depression is not recommended.
- Anti-emetic therapy and prophylactic antacids are advised before surgery to reduce the risk of acid aspiration.

Anaesthetic management

- Airway management is often difficult in obese patients.
- Possible difficult airway should be assessed with consideration give to awake intubation.
- Rapid sequence induction with preoxygenation is required as obese patients are prone to gastric reflux.
- Antacids such as sodium citrate are advocated for use in the anaesthetic room prior to induction.
- Patients should be extubated awake in an upright position.

Postoperative management

- Patients should be nursed in the upright position to aid respiratory function.
- Airway should be constantly monitored.
- Nasopharyngeal airway can aid breathing and reduce obstruction.
- Supplemental O_2 should be given as prescribed.
- Postoperative analgesia via IV route and/or PCA is recommended as intramuscular (IM) injection is often administered subcutaneously (SC).
- Transport of patients may prove difficult so consideration should be given to transporting and transferring patients on a bed.
- Ensure there are enough staff for safe transfer and transport.
- Monitoring of vital signs including TPR, BP, SpO_2.
- Invasive monitoring is recommended following major surgery.

Also see Monitoring obese patients, p.158.

Table 5.4 NICE guidelines for classification of obesity[1]

Classification	BMI (kg/m²)
Healthy weight	18.5–24.9
Overweight	25–29.9
Obesity I	30–34.9
Obesity II	35–39.9
Obesity III	40 or more

References and further reading

1. National Institute for Health and Clinical Excellence (2006). *Obesity guidance on the prevention, identification, assessment and management of overweight and obesity in adults and children.* NICE: London.

Association of Anaesthetists of Great Britain and Ireland (2007). *Perioperative management of the morbidly obese patient.* AAGBI: London.

Blanshard H (2006). Endocrine and metabolic disease. In Allman KG and Wilson IH (eds). *Oxford Handbook of Anaesthesia* (2nd edn). Oxford University Press: Oxford.

Hatfield A and Tronson M (2008). *The Complete Recovery Room Book* (4th edn). Oxford University Press: Oxford.

Hattersley A and Saddler J (2000). Endocrine and metabolic disorders. In *National Obesity Forum.* Available from: www.nationalobesityforum.org.uk

National Obesity Care Pathway (2005). Available from: http://nationalobesityforum.org.uk/images/stories/Obesity_Care_Path.pdf

Nicholls A and Wilson I (eds) (2000). *Perioperative medicine: managing surgical patients with medical problems.* Oxford University Press: Oxford.

Gastrointestinal disorders

GI disorders encompass a wide range of diseases including liver disease, obstructive jaundice, inflammatory bowel disease, and gastric ulceration.

Gastro-oesophageal reflux

- Patients with oesophageal reflux are at risk of acid aspiration during general anaesthesia.
- An antacid prophylactic regimen is usually administered to patients a few days prior to surgery.
- Sodium citrate can be administered orally immediately prior to induction of anaesthesia.
- Consider rapid sequence induction for general anaesthesia.
- Extubate head-down in left lateral position.

Liver disease

- Causes of liver disease in adults can include alcohol, cirrhosis, hepatitis B and hepatitis C infection.
- Causes of liver disease in children can include congenital, biliary atresia, and viral hepatitis.
- Risks associated with liver disease include bleeding, acute renal failure, and decompensation of chronic liver disease.
- Complications of liver disease can include bleeding, hypoglycaemia, ascites, renal failure, infection, and encephalopathy.
- See Table 5.5 for a list of safe anaesthetic drugs for use in liver failure.

Perioperative considerations

- Pre-assessment of patient is essential prior to anaesthesia and surgery.
- Avoid use of halothane due to the possibility of postoperative liver dysfunction.
- Inform appropriate healthcare professionals if a patient has positive hepatitis viral serology.
- Postoperative monitoring of renal function is required.
- Assess levels of consciousness.
- Monitor blood glucose levels.

Table 5.5 Safe anaesthetic drugs in liver failure[1]

Premedication drugs	Lorazepam
Induction agents	Propofol, thiopental, etomidate
Inhalational agents	Isoflurane, sevoflurane, desflurane
Muscle relaxants	Atracurium, cisatracurium
Opiate drugs	Remifentanil
Analgesic drugs	Paracetamol

References and further reading

1. Purday J (2006) Hepatic disease. In Allman KG and Wilson IH (eds). *Oxford Handbook of Anaesthesia* (2nd edn). Oxford University Press: Oxford

Daneshmend T and Dow A (2000) Gastroenterological disorders. In Nicholls A and Wilson I (eds). *Perioperative medicine: managing surgical patients with medical problems.* Oxford University Press: Oxford.

NICE Gastrointestinal guidance. Available from: 🖳 www.nice.org.uk/guidance/index.jsp?action=byTopic&o=722

Preparing the patient for theatre

Preoperative preparation

A preoperative checklist (Box 6.1) must be completed prior to any surgical intervention and it is the responsibility of all surgical and perioperative practitioners to undertake this task. The ward nurse/nurse in charge must ensure that the patient is fully prepared for theatre. Patients should be assessed to ensure adequate preoperative education has been received and that they understand the nature and potential outcome of the surgery. The preoperative checklist should be checked prior to induction of anaesthesia on at least 4 or 5 occasions:

- At ward level when the patient is being prepared for surgery.
- Prior to the patient leaving the ward for the operating theatre.
- When the patient arrives at the operating theatre.
- When the patient arrives in the anaesthetic room.
- Immediately prior to induction of anaesthesia.

Box 6.1 Preoperative checklist

- Correct patient
- Nil by mouth (NBM)
- Informed consent
- Allergy status
- Dentures and crowns
- Caps and loose teeth
- Weight—children/elderly
- Make-up and nail polish

- Surgical site marking
- Skin preparation
- Prosthesis
- Jewellery and body piercing
- DVT prophylaxis
- Medical records
- Nursing records
- X-rays and blood results

Patient safety

- Ensure the patient is scheduled for surgery as per theatre list although some variance may occur between elective and emergency procedures.
- Identification band on wrist and ankle.
- Identification band has correct information.

Patient wristbands

Standardising the design of patient wristbands, the information on them, and the processes used to produce and check them will improve patient safety. Patients' ID wristbands must meet the NPSA design requirements. Clear guidelines from the NPSA outline how wristbands should be produced, applied, and checked as follows:

- Wristbands should be white with black text and applied to the dominant hand.
- They should be generated and printed from hospital information systems and must include surname, first name, date of birth, and ID/NHS number.
- A red wristband should be worn by patients with allergies and by those who do not wish to receive blood.
- In Wales, wristbands must include the first line of the patient's address.

Informed consent

- Must be written, verbal, or implied as all are equally valid in law.
- Consent in writing is infinitely superior as a form of evidence.
- Patients should receive an explanation of the surgery and the risks involved.
- If the patient has any doubt, call the surgical team back.
- 📖 Refer to Chapter 3, p. 23 for further information.

Allergy status

- *Hypersensitivity*—refers to a drug-induced antigen–antibody reaction.
- Type I —anaphylactic reaction.
- Type IV—delayed reaction.
- This must be identified to theatre staff by use of a prominent red band.
- Common allergies include antibiotics, iodine, sticky plasters, latex.

Teeth and dentures

- Dental crowns, caps, bridges, and loose teeth must be identified and recorded as these may be damaged, dislodged, or inhaled during intubation
- Some anaesthetists allow dentures that are securely fitted to remain in situ as this can improve the structure of the airway.
- Problems can occur with a oropharyngeal airway and may need to be replaced with nasal airway.

Patient's weight

- The patient's weight must be documented on the prescription chart.
- The weight of paediatric and elderly patients must be recorded anaesthetic drugs are calculated according to the weight of these patients.

References

Dimond B (2002). *Legal aspects of nursing* (3rd edn). Longman: London.

National Patient Safety Agency (2007) *Standardising hospital wristbands will improve patient safety.* Available from: 🖳 www.npsa.nhs.uk/display?contentId=6076

Jewellery and body piercing

All jewellery should be removed and kept on the ward or given to relatives, although wedding rings can remain but should be securely taped.

- All metal jewellery carries electrical conduction risks e.g. electrosurgical cautery.
- Care should be taken if a patient wishes to keep jewellery on for religious reasons; these should be securely taped to avoid injury to the patient and/or perioperative personnel.

Nursing and medical staff are constantly faced with various types of body piercing. Although each NHS Trust usually has its own set of guidelines, each case should be dealt with individually and sensitively according to the type of anaesthesia or surgical procedure.

There are four main types of jewellery used for body piercing:

- *Labret stud*—a straight bar with a fixed flat end and an unscrewable ball on the other end.
- *Barbell*—a straight bar with an unscrewable ball at one end.
- *Captive ring*—an open ring in which a ball with two small dimples is inserted and the ball is clicked into position and held in place.
- *Flesh tunnel*—a ring inserted through a hole, usually the ear, to enlarge the hole in the skin.

A general guide for body piercing is that if it is not in the way, and does not interfere with anaesthesia or the surgical site/procedure, leave it alone. However, it is important to ensure that piercings are secure and documented. If body jewellery is to be removed, the best person to undertake this task is the patient.

Risk assessment

Body piercings have the potential to be caught and/or ripped by ECG leads, drapes, surgical clips, or instruments. There is an increased risk of pressure to chin/lip causing soft tissue damage from anaesthetic masks or nipple-piercing pressure if the patient is to lie prone. This should be assessed and documented by the anaesthetic practitioner prior to commencement of anaesthesia.

Surgical procedures

Body piercings should generally be removed if they are in close proximity to the surgical site or any other associated procedure (Table 6.1). However, this is ultimately the decision of the anaesthetist and/or surgeon.

Tongue and lip piercing

All tongue and lip jewellery should be removed before a general anaesthetic but advice should be sought from the anaesthetist

- Barbells may cause obstruction to the airway during anaesthesia.
- Tongue labrets can contain a gemstone which is at risk of falling out and entering the airway as they are only glued in.

Nasal and naval piercing

- Nasal septum, nose, or ear piercing should be removed if the patient is to have ear, nose, and throat (ENT) surgery.

- Naval and breast piercing should be removed for laparoscopic or breast surgery.

Male genital piercing
- Penile piercing can be pulled to one side if the patient requires a urinary catheter.
- For urological surgery it should be removed.

Female genital piercing
- The site of piercing should be assessed for surgical access.
- It should be removed if it is likely to hinder the type of surgery to be performed.
- It does not have to be removed if the surgical procedure is elsewhere on the body.

Table 6.1 Area and position of body piercings

Body	Position
Ear lobes	Cartilage of ear
Nostril	Base of nostril; septum
Tongue	Inch from tip in centre
Lip	Bottom or top
Navel	Anywhere around navel
Chin	Centre of lower lip
Female nipple	Base of nipple
Male nipple	Placed well into areola
Female genitals	Labia majora, labia minora, clitoris
Male genitals	Foreskin, head of penis, underside of penis

Infection risk

If there are signs of infection around the piercing site, it must be removed. Treatment for the infection may precede the surgery.

If the body piercing remains for the surgical procedure
- The site and type of piercing should be documented on the preoperative checklist.
- A check should be made in the postoperative period to ensure it is still in situ, which should also be documented.

References and further reading

Marenzi B (2004). Body piercing: a patient safety issue. *Journal of Perianaesthesia Nursing* **19**(1), 4–10.

Meyer D (2000). Body piercing: old traditions creating new challenges. *Journal of Emergency Nursing* **26**(6), 612–14.

Preoperative fasting

The purpose of fasting patients preoperatively is to minimise the volume of gastric contents and reduce the risk of regurgitation and aspiration during anaesthesia. Recent fasting guidelines are:[1]

• Solid food (milk and milky drinks)—6 hours.
• Breastfed infants—4 hours.
• Clear fluids (water, black tea, and coffee)—2 hours.

The chewing of gum is controversial but the pragmatic approach is to treat it as if it were an oral fluid and prohibit for 2 hours preoperatively.[2] Many studies have emphasised the harmful effects of prolonged fasting but patients continue to be deprived of food and drink for excessively long periods (Table 6.2). There is evidence to suggest that patients who fast for long periods during the preoperative phase often recover slowly postoperatively. Prolonged fasting can have both physical and psychological implications postoperatively and is particularly harmful in small children and elderly, infirm patients. Altered digestion can occur with pain, injury, and opiate analgesia.

The benefits of implementing evidence-based preoperative fasting times are outlined by Oshodi[3] and include a decreased incidence of:

• Dehydration.
• Headache.
• Postoperative nausea and vomiting.
• Hunger and thirst.
• Anxiety and discomfort.

Table 6.2 Implications of prolonged fasting

Physical	Psychological
Dehydration	Anxiety
Catabolism	Discomfort
Nausea	Irritability
Vomiting	
Hypoglycaemia	
Ketosis	
Electrolyte imbalance	

Dehydration

Dehydration is an excessive loss of fluid and minerals from the body and it can be described as mild, moderate, or severe. Nurses must be cognisant of the risk of fluid imbalance and patients should be monitored for signs of dehydration. Postoperative fluid replacement is often prescribed to counteract fasting and blood loss. Patients who remain fasted following surgery will often be administered IV fluid to avoid dehydration. Water, as a means of hydration, can reduce confusion and headache[4] so it is therefore essential that patients are not fasted longer than the recommended timescale.

Stages and symptoms of dehydration
- Mild—headache, lack of energy, tiredness.
- Moderate—dry mouth, decreased alertness, sunken eyes, muscle cramps.
- Severe—confusion, disorientated, tachycardia, tachypnoea.

Nausea and vomiting

Prolonged fasting preoperatively can cause nausea and vomiting in the postoperative period, and reintroducing oral fluid postoperatively can sometimes be equally problematic. Smith *et al.*[5] claim that if patients are nauseous on induction of anaesthesia, this is likely to persist into the postoperative period. The RCN[1] recommend that postoperative patients should be encouraged to drink when they are ready, providing there are no medical or surgical contraindications.

Headache

Preoperative fasting can be associated with postoperative headache and the interruption of daily caffeine consumption can cause caffeine withdrawal headache. Dehydration, prolonged preoperative fasting, and caffeine withdrawal can cause headaches during the perioperative period.[6] Caffeine normally induces vasoconstriction, acute withdrawal in those with high daily intake will cause rebound vasodilatation and headache. Prophylactic administration of caffeine tablets might be considered for surgical patients who are accustomed to a high daily intake of caffeine.[7]

Hypoglycaemia

Hypoglycaemia occurs when the blood glucose falls to 2.7–3.3mmol/L and can be caused by too much insulin, excessive physical activity, or too little food.
- The clinical manifestations of mild-to-moderate hypoglycaemia can include sweating, tachycardia, nervousness, hunger, headache, confusion, light headedness, and drowsiness.
- Elderly patients are at an increased risk of dehydration.
- Patients who are prescribed insulin or insulin-secretion stimulating medication may experience hypoglycaemia as a result of perioperative fasting.

References

1. Royal College of Nursing (2005). *Perioperative fasting in adults and children: an RCN guideline for the multidisciplinary team.* RCN: London.

2. Association of Anaesthetists of Great Britain and Ireland (2001). *Preoperative assessment: the role of the anaesthetist.* AAGBI: London.

3. Oshodi TO (2004). Clinical skills: an evidence-based approach to preoperative fasting. *British Journal of Nursing* **13**(16), 958–62.

4. Royal College of Nursing, National Patient Safety Agency (2007). *Water for health: Hydration best practice toolkit for hospitals and healthcare.* Available at: 🖳 www2.rcn.org.uk/campaigns/nutritionnow/tools_and_resources/hydration

5. Smith AF, Vallance H, and Slater RM (1997). Shorter preoperative fluid fasts reduces postoperative emesis. *British Medical Journal* **314**, 1486.

6. Werrett G (2002) Perioperative headache. *Update in Anaestheisa* **15**, Article 14. Available from: 🖳 www.nda.ox.ac.uk/wfsa/html/u15/u1514_01.htm.

7. Hampl KF, Schneider MC, Ruttimann U, *et al.* (1995). Perioperative administration of caffeine tablets for prevention of postoperative headaches. *Canadian Journal of Anesthesia* **42**(9), 789–92.

Patient safety: surgical safety checklist

In 2008, the World Health Organization (WHO) launched its campaign, 'Safe Surgery Saves Lives', to reduce the number of errors occurring in surgery. The focus of the campaign is the *surgical safety checklist*.[1]

The checklist comprises three phases of a surgical procedure (Figure 6.1):
- *Sign in*: signifies prior to induction of anaesthesia.
- *Time out*: signifies prior to skin incision.
- *Sign out*: signifies prior to the patient leaving the operating theatre.

During each phase, the WHO emphasise that a checklist coordinator must confirm that the surgical team has completed the listed tasks before it proceeds with the procedure.

A surgical safety checklist and implementation manual provides suggestions for implementing the checklist, whilst recognizing that different practice settings will adapt it to their own circumstances.[1,2]

The implementation manual is designed to help ensure that surgical teams are able to implement the checklist consistently so that healthcare professionals can minimise the most common and avoidable risks endangering the lives and well-being of surgical patients.[2]

References and further reading

1. World Health Organization (2008). *WHO Surgery Safety Checklist (First Edition)*. Available from: ⬚ www.who.int/patientsafety/safesurgery/ss_checklist/en/index.html

2. World Health Organization (2008). *Implementation Manual WHO Surgical Safety Checklist (First Edition)*. Available from: ⬚ www.who.int/patientsafety/safesurgery/ss_checklist/en/index.html

Department of Health (2008). *Chief Medical Officer's Annual Report 2007*. DoH: London.

Figure 6.1 Surgical safety checklist*

Prior to induction of anaesthesia	Prior to skin incision	Prior to patient leaving theatre
SIGN IN	**TIME OUT**	**SIGN OUT**
Patient has confirmed: ☐ • Identity • Surgical site • Surgical procedure • Consent	Confirm all team members have introduced themselves by name and role ☐	**Nurse verbally confirms with the team:** • The name of the procedure recorded • All instruments, swabs and needle counts are correct if applicable ☐ • How the specimen is labelled ☐ • If any equipment problems need addressing ☐
Surgical site marked / not applicable ☐	Anaesthetist, surgeon and nursing staff verbally confirm: ☐ • Correct patient • Correct surgical site • Correct surgical procedure	Anaesthetist, surgeon and nursing team review the main concerns for recovery and management of the patient ☐
Anaesthetic safety check list completed ☐	**ANTICIPATED CRITICAL EVENTS** Anaesthesia team reviews: Identify concerns that are patient-specific ☐	
Pulse oximeter on patient and functioning ☐	Surgical team reviews: Identify the critical steps or unexpected steps, duration of surgery, anticipated blood loss ☐	
Does the patient have a:	Nursing team reviews: Confirm sterility (include indicator results); identify concerns with equipment or other issues ☐	
• Known allergy? YES ☐ NO ☐	Has prophylactic antibiotic therapy been administered during the last 60 minutes? YES ☐ N/A ☐	
• Difficult airway / aspiration risk? YES ☐ NO ☐	Is essential imaging displayed? YES ☐ N/A ☐	

• Risk of >500mL blood loss
  (7mL/kg for paediatric patients)
  YES ☐ NO ☐		

*Adapted with permission from WHO (2008). *Implementation Manual: Surgical Safety Checklist (First Edition)*, pp. 3–4, Document number: WHO/IER/PSP/2008.05. Copyright © World Health Organization, 2008.

Make-up, nail polish, and other considerations

All make-up and nail vanish should be removed prior to surgery.

Make-up

Foundation and lipstick may disguise changes in the patient's colour e.g. cyanosis. Coloured and clear nail vanish can distort or disguise changes in the patient's peripheral colour.

Nail polish

Nail polish is routinely removed prior to surgery as previous research suggested nail polish can reduce pulse oximeter reading by 2–6%. However, Rodden et al.[1] evaluated use of nail polish and effects and variances of SpO_2 reading. SpO_2 readings were taken and compared with baseline results and they found:
- Presence of nail polish, tattoos, or jaundice can distort SpO_2 reading.
- Blue and brown polish caused largest variances but no colours had variances greater than 1% (within 2% clinical threshold).

Acrylic nails

Artificial acrylic nails are fashionable and are usually used to strengthen and lengthen nails. Peters[2] investigated effects of unpolished acrylic nails on SpO_2 measurement using a sample of 30 women, aged 18–61 years.
- Baseline reading obtained on each subject's natural nail.
- Reading taken following application of acrylic nail.
- Mean SpO_2 reading at baseline = 97.33%
- Mean SpO_2 reading after acrylic nails = 97.58%
- No statistical difference existed between readings

Although current research suggests that patients may not need to remove acrylic nails before surgery, it is safer to err on the side of caution and remove the nails until further research has been undertaken.

Prosthetic devices

- Some prosthesis should normally be removed for safe keeping and retained on the ward.
- The removal of devices such as wigs, false eyes, glasses, contact lenses, and artificial limbs can cause distress to patients and it is not always necessary to remove these.
- Maintaining patients' dignity is essential so the necessity for removal should be discussed with the anaesthesia and/or surgical team and the patient; if removal is necessary, a prosthesis can be removed immediately prior to anaesthesia and replaced in the recovery room.
- It is often practical to allow patients to retain hearing aids for induction, reversal, and post-anaesthetic care.
- Some prosthetic devices such as orthopaedic implants should be documented appropriately and brought to the attention of perioperative personnel.

Surgical site marking

Although surgery performed at an incorrect site is rare, when it happens it can be devastating for patients and their families. The NPSA and the Royal

College of Surgeons (RCS) developed national guidelines for implementation across NHS, which are shown in Table 6.3.[3]

Table 6.3 NPSA/RCS guidelines for surgical site marking[3]

How to mark	Indelible marker pen
Where to mark	Mark at or near intended incision
Who marks	Operating surgeon/other present
With whom	Patient/carer involvement
Time and place	Mark on day of surgery
Verify	Documented by surgeon, check by nurse

Surgical skin preparation

- Shower or bath to prepare skin.
- Operation site marked correctly.
- Hair removal at the operative site is mostly carried out according to surgeon's preference.
- Research shows it is preferable to remove hair as near as possible to the time of surgery.

Shaving

- Close skin shaving can cause soft tissue abrasions and cuts which can encourage growth of bacteria.
- Depilatory creams are not widely used due to localised skin reactions.
- Electric shavers are preferred as they cause less trauma to skin.
- Razors can increase the risk of infection.

Premedication

Due to the difficulty of timing premedication to optimise effectiveness, there is a tendency to use them less frequently. However, they may be prescribed for the following reasons:
- Prophylactic antibiotic therapy.
- Prophylactic anti-emetic therapy.
- Postoperative analgesia e.g. diclofenac per rectum (PR).
- Sedative agents to reduce patient anxiety.

References

1. Rodden AM, Spicer L, Diaz VA, *et al.* (2007). Does fingernail polish affect pulse oximeter readings? *Intensive and Critical Care Nursing* **23**(1) 51-5.

2. Peters SM (1997). The effect of acrylic nails on the measurement of oxygen saturation as determined by pulse oximetry. *American Association of Nurse Anaesthetists Journal* **65**(4) 361–3.

3. National Patient Safety Agency (2005). *Patient safety alert: Correct site surgery.* NPSA: London.

Venous thromboembolism

Venous thromboembolism (VTE) is the formation of a blood clot in a vein, which on occasions, may dislodge and give cause to an embolism. A deep vein thrombosis (DVT) is a clot that forms mostly in the deep veins of the legs or pelvis; whereas a pulmonary embolus (PE) is the result of the DVT breaking off and travelling through the right side of the heart into the pulmonary circulation, leading to an infarct within the lung tissue.

The deep veins in the leg that are likely to be affected include:
• Great saphenous vein.
• Femoral vein.
• Popliteal vein.
• Deep veins of the knee.

If a VTE occurs, it is usually diagnosed 3–14 days postoperatively. There is an increased risk of developing VTE with middle-aged and elderly patients, patients on prolonged bed rest, and following major surgery of the lower abdomen pelvis or hip joints (see Box 6.2).

All patients should be individually assessed on admission to hospital to identify risk of developing a VTE. They should also be provided with written and oral information on the signs and symptoms of VTE.

> ### Box 6.2 Patient risk factors for VTE[1]
>
> • Cancer treatment.
> • Cardiac/respiratory failure.
> • Acute medical illness.
> • Age over 60 years.
> • Immobility.
> • Obesity—BMI of >30.
> • Pregnancy.
> • Familial.
> • Use of oral contraceptives.
> • Varicose veins.
> • Severe infection.
> • Continuous travel of >3 hours 4 weeks pre/post surgery.

Prophylactic treatment of VTE

There are two main forms of prophylactic treatment to reduce the risk of VTE:
• Mechanical treatment:
  • Graduated compression stockings, which work by promoting venous flow and reducing stasis.
  • Intermittent pneumatic compression.
• Pharmacological treatment:
  • Anticoagulant therapy with low-molecular weight heparin (LMWH) for immediate effect, followed by warfarin in the long term to reduce the risk of recurrence

- Anti-platelet drugs will decrease platelet aggregation and inhibit thrombus formation; they are usually effective in the arterial circulation, where anticoagulants have little effect.[2]
- Aspirin, an anti-platelet drug, provides some protection against VTE but is considered less effective than other pharmacological methods.[3]

NICE recommend that both methods of treatment (mechanical and pharmacological) should be considered for all patients to reduce the incidence of VTE.[1]

Early ambulation should be encouraged following surgery. Adequate analgesia postoperatively will encourage early mobilisation and will also decrease the risk of VTE.

Patients should be encouraged to continue the use of compression stockings until normal mobility has been restored.

Anaesthesia and VTE

In the perioperative environment the immobility of the patient during anaesthesia, can deprive the deep veins in the legs of the pumping action of the calf muscles, causing pooling of venous blood and venous dilation that can predispose the patient to thrombosis formation.

Regional anaesthesia can further reduce the risk of VTE in comparison to general anaesthesia.[1]

References and further reading

1. National Institute for Health and Clinical Excellence (2007). *Venous thromboembolism: reducing the risk of venous thromboembolism in inpatients undergoing surgery.* NICE: London.

2. British National Formulary. Available at: ▣ www.bnf.org

3. Campbell B (2006). Prophylaxis of venous thromboembolism. In: Allman KG and Wilson IH (eds). *Oxford Handbook of Anaesthesia* (2nd edn). Oxford University Press: Oxford.

Harrison R and Daly L (2006). *Acute medical emergencies: a nursing guide* (2nd edn). Churchill Livingstone: London.

Illingworth C and Timmons S (2007). An audit of intermittent pneumatic compression (IPC) in the prophylaxis of asymptomatic deep vein thrombosis (DVT). *Journal of Perioperative Practice* **17**(11), 522–8.

Preoperative checklist

Table 6.4 Preoperative checklist

Patient's name:
Patient's address:
Hospital number:
Consultant:
Ward:
Theatre no:

	Yes	No	Comments
Correct patient ID bands × 2			
Consent form signed/dated			
Patient's weight recorded			
Allergies recorded			
Last ate (use 24-hour clock)			
Last drank (use 24-hour clock)			
Dentures, caps, crowns, loose teeth, bridges			
Jewellery/body piercings removed/covered			
Surgical site prepared and marked			
Make-up/nail vanish removed			
Prosthesis removed Wigs, hair pieces			
Implants (state side)			
Spectacles/contact lenses			
Cardiac pacemaker Internal defibrillator			
Socially clean/shaved			
Last blood glucose level (time) if appropriate			
Pre-medication (time)			
Patient's documentation Medical/nursing notes			
Prescription chart			
Vital signs chart			
Fluid balance chart			
X-rays			
Blood results			
Voided urine			

Anaesthetic checklist

It is recommended that a final anaesthetic check (Table 6.5) is also performed immediately prior to induction of all methods of anaesthesia by an anaesthetic practitioner.

Remember—you cannot 'over check' a patient's details.

Table 6.5 Anaesthetic checklist

	Yes	No	Comments
Correct patient for correct surgery in correct theatre			
ID bands × 2			
Consent form signed/dated			
Allergies recorded as per NPSA guidelines			
Last ate (use 24-hour clock)			
Last drank (use 24-hour clock)			
Dentures, caps, crowns, loose teeth, bridges			
Surgical site prepared and marked			
Hearing aid with the patient			
Patient's documentation Medical/nursing records			
Prescription chart			
Vital signs chart			
Fluid balance chart			
X-rays			
Blood results			

Communication

Patients who are undergoing surgery may be anxious and feeling vulnerable. This can be the case if they are undergoing elective surgery, where the final outcome is unknown, such as surgery for cancer where the prognosis is not clear, or in an emergency when events may unfold very quickly and there is an equal amount of uncertainty as to what is going to happen.

For most practitioners, their interaction with patients will be prior to their anaesthetic and then in the recovery room. As the practitioner and patient are unlikely to have met previously, there is little time to establish a relationship in a manner that other professionals might. It is vital therefore that the perioperative practitioner is able to gain the trust of the patient and the family, should they be present. This is a skill that most practitioners will grow more confident in with more experience.

Surgery under local anaesthetic
- It is good practice to have a member of staff attend to the patient while the patient is undergoing the procedure.
- The member of staff should provide the information and reassurance as required.
- The member of staff should let the patient know what is going to happen and what is happening while it occurs.

Non-verbal communication
This is a large part of communication. Types include:
- Eye contact and gaze.
- Facial expression.
- Proximity.
- Touch.
- Paralanguage.

Patients who do not speak English
Under these circumstances an independent interpreter may need to accompany the patient into the anaesthetic room and be present in the recovery room to ensure that the patient can understand instructions and advice.

Use of family members
- It is considered poor practice to utilise a member of the patient's family. However, in urgent or emergency circumstances when it is not possible to use an official interpreter, it may prove necessary.
- Where possible, use an official interpreter. These are often available thorough the hospital or organisation's advocacy arrangements and need to be arranged prior to the patient's arrival at the theatre doors.

Other communication difficulties
Patients with hearing difficulties
- Patients who have regional/local anaesthesia should keep their hearing aids in throughout the surgical procedure.

- Patients with hearing difficulties who normally wear hearing aids should be allowed to wear these until the last possible moment, which is usually when the general anaesthetic has been commenced; in some instances a hearing aid can just be 'turned off' and 'turned on' again in the recovery room.
- If a hearing aid is removed, it should be safely stored until it can re-positioned to aid communication in the recovery period.
- The hearing aid can be repositioned as soon as a patient emerges from anaesthesia, either before the patient leaves theatre or as soon as the patient enters the recovery room.
- With patients that are hard of hearing:
  - Position yourself so that they can see you talking.
  - Ensure that speech is clear and at an appropriate volume.
  - Use touch where appropriate.

Patients with visual impairment

- Introduce yourself to the patient in the normal way by telling them your name and who you are so that they become familiar with your voice.
- Touch may be useful where appropriate.
- Allow spectacles to be worn until the last possible moment (usually when the general anaesthetic has been commenced) and allow them to be put on as soon as possible in the recovery stage.
- Children with visual impairment are generally accompanied to theatre with their parents or guardians and it is often best to be guided as to what works with the child by utilising the parents in the pre- and postoperative phase.

Dignity, anxiety, and promoting equality when preparing the patient for theatre

Dignity

Vulnerable perioperative patients have the right to be treated in a dignified manner whether conscious or anaesthetised. Practitioners should consider the way that they would want themselves or family members treated whilst undergoing perioperative care.

Introduction

- Greet the patient in a professional manner. Introduce yourself by name and a simple explanation of your title. Remember that members of the general public are unlikely to understand specialist titles.
- E.g. 'Hello Mr/Mrs/Ms/Miss (name) my name is (your name) and I am one of the team looking after you today'.
- Refer to patients by their title and last name unless invited to do otherwise. This is particularly true of older patients who may feel uncomfortable being called by their first name by a younger person.

Exposure

When the patient is being prepared for anaesthetic or surgery and access is required to their body, such as when skin preparation is being applied, the minimal area should be exposed and only when it is necessary to do so.

Postoperative phase

During this phase, the practitioner should, when appropriate, introduce themselves (this may be required more than once) and inform the patient what they do and what they will be doing. Care should be taken when looking under the patient's bedclothes for drains by explaining to the patient that this is being done and why since the patient may be drifting off to sleep and be startled by such an intervention.

Anxiety

Patients undergoing a surgical intervention are likely to have some anxiety even if they have undergone a procedure in the past. Anxiety may manifest itself in several different ways. Some people will want to talk or be spoken to, while others may be quiet. Some patients will want to know everything, while others may be so frightened that they would prefer to know nothing and simply place their trust in the healthcare professional looking after them. This is a professional call made by the staff member. Each patient should be treated in appropriate manner that is right for them.

Ways to reduce anxiety

- Providing information helps reduce anxiety and pain.
- Explanations should be given to the patient (and their carer or family member if present) as to what will be happening to them.
- Information should be given in a suitable way so that the patient understands.
- Patients should be given the opportunity to ask questions.

Promoting equality

All staff are required to treat patients without favour or discrimination. All patients are equal in terms of the care that is delivered, no matter how difficult a member of staff feels that a person or a group may be. This is enshrined in both the NMC code of professional conduct (*The Code: Standards of conduct, performance and ethics for nurses and midwives, 2008*) and the HPC's *Standards of conduct, performance and ethics* (2008).

References and further reading

1. Nursing & Midwifery Council (2008). *The Code: Standards of conduct, performance and ethics for nurses and midwives.* NMC: London.

2. Health Professions Council (2008). *Standards for conduct, performance and ethics.* HPC: London.

Department of Health (2008). *Code of Practice: Mental Health Act 1983.* The Stationery Office: London.

Department of Constitutional Affairs (2006). *A Guide to the Human Rights Act 1998: Third Edition.* Available at: www.dca.gov.uk/peoples-rights/human-rights/index.htm

Mental Capacity Act 2005 www.opsi.gov.uk/ACTS/acts2005/ukpga_20050009_en_1

Mental Health Act 2007 www.opsi.gov.uk/ACTS/acts2007/ukpga_20070012_en_1

Children, parents, and carers

It is now accepted practice to allow one or both parents of a baby or child into the anaesthetic room. This serves two main purposes:
- To help minimise the trauma to the child.
- To help the parents to be included in the child's care.

Parental involvement in the preoperative stage
- The child is accompanied to the theatre department by the parent(s).
- After the final preoperative checks are made, the receiving theatre practitioner should accompany the child and parent(s) to the anaesthetic room. Since the parent(s) will remain until the child is anaesthetised another member of staff will be required to escort them from the anaesthetic room.
- Where appropriate the parent(s) may be able to distract the child so the anaesthetist can undertake the IV cannulation.
- Once the child is anaesthetised, the parent(s) can be escorted from the anaesthetic room and then the department.
- Before the parent(s) leave, the practitioner should explain to them what the arrangements are for meeting up with their child in the recovery room following the operation.
- This can be an emotional time and parents may need a few moments to compose themselves.

Parental involvement in the postoperative stage
- Usually, the parent(s) come into in the recovery room as the child is awakening from the anaesthetic.
- It is advisable to have a short conversation with the parent(s) before they come into the recovery room to explain to them:
  - What to expect in the way of the child's condition, drains, drips, and items of monitoring equipment.
  - If the unit is not exclusively paediatrics, it is worth mentioning that there are adults present as well as other children.
- The parent(s) should be involved with as much of the child's care as possible as this can be of comfort to the child and parent(s).
- Throughout this process appropriate explanations should be provided of interventions such as the administration of medication.
- At the appropriate time the child will be allowed to leave the recovery room and to return to the ward area. The practitioner should accompany the child and parent(s) from the unit.

Communication
- Careful and appropriate explanations of what is to happen will be required for the parent(s) and the child.
- The age of the child will determine the manner and terms used to speak to the child.

Further reading

Argyle M (1983). *The Psychology of Interpersonal Behaviour*. Penguin: London.

Hayward J (1976). *Information: a prescription against pain*. RCN: London.

Health Professions Council (2008). *Standards for conduct, performance and ethics*. HPC: London.

Nursing & Midwifery Council (2008). *The Code: Standards of conduct, performance and ethics for nurses and midwives*. NMC: London.

Section 3
Principles of anaesthesia

Principles of anaesthesia

Role of the anaesthetic practitioner

An anaesthetic practitioner is a qualified nurse or an operating department practitioner (ODP) who provides continual assistance to the anaesthetist during the delivery, maintenance, and reversal of anaesthesia.

In order to maintain safe levels of patient care throughout any surgical or anaesthetic procedure, the anaesthetic practitioner must be clinically competent and have a current and sound knowledge base of:
- Relevant anatomy and physiology.
- The principles and practice of elective and emergency anaesthesia.
- Airway management and difficult airway management.
- Pharmacodynamics and pharmacokinetics of anaesthetic pharmacology.
- Principles and practice of resuscitation.

Priorities for the anaesthetic practitioner include:
- Ensuring best practice and the patients' best interests at all times in accordance with local, national, and legal frameworks.
- Contributing to all aspects of patient care, which includes the provision of emotional and physical support of the patient throughout the perioperative phase.
- Anticipating the patient's and anaesthetist's requirements.
- Patient management options.
- Airway management and difficult airway management and protocols and procedures for difficult and failed intubation.
- Monitoring of the patient during anaesthesia.
- Monitoring of the patient during transfer to the recovery unit or intensive treatment unit (ITU); ensuring that the patient's needs are met until care has been transferred to another healthcare professional.

Ensuring compliance with professional and mandatory training at all times, the anaesthetic practitioner must also engage with professional and educational development in the specialist area of perioperative care within regulatory requirements. Additionally, practitioners must contribute to the training and development of students and non-regulated personnel. Also see Box 7.1.

Box 7.1 Additional aspects of the anaesthetic practitioner role

Duties
- Excellent interpersonal skills including verbal and non-verbal communication skills.
- Preparation and checking of the anaesthetic room and operating theatre environment and equipment.
- Checking and stocking of all anaesthetic equipment to be used including any emergency equipment that may be required.
- Participating, if required, with the emergency response team to provide clinical assistance to all environments within the hospital e.g. cardiac arrest calls.
- Care of catheters, drains, CVP lines, epidural catheters, arterial lines, and peripheral lines.
- Caring for ventilated patients.
- Perioperative teaching and information giving.
- Ensuring and adhering to handling and moving policies when transferring patients to trolleys and beds; ensuring safe and correct positioning of patients.

Knowledge
- Principles and practice of cross-infection.
- Evidence-based practice and national guidelines.
- Risk management strategies in the clinical area.
- Post-anaesthesia care in a range of surgical specialties.

References

Allman KG and Wilson IH (eds) (2006). *Oxford Handbook of Anaesthesia* (2nd edn). Oxford University Press: Oxford.

Association of Anaesthetists of Great Britain and Ireland (2005). *The anaesthesia team.* AAGBI: London.

Difficult Airway Society. Available at: 🖳 http://www.das.uk.com

Royal College of Anaesthetists (2004). *Guidelines for the Provision of Anaesthetic Services.* RCoA: London.

Anaesthesia

The term 'anaesthesia' is derived from two Greek words, which together mean 'loss of feeling or sensation'. Today the term reflects modern day anaesthetic techniques and can also mean 'relaxation and pain relief for surgery'. Anaesthesia is one of the most significant developments of modern medicine as it allows once-unbearable surgical procedures to be performed while the patient is unconscious, pain free, and relaxed. There are predominantly four types of anaesthesia:

- General anaesthesia.
- Local anaesthesia.
- Regional anaesthesia.
- Combination of these three.

General anaesthesia

General anaesthesia is defined as:

- A state of total unconsciousness resulting from anaesthetic drugs within a controlled environment.
- The administration of an agent or agents to render the patient unconscious and insensitive to pain and non-reactive to any form of surgical stimulation.
- Induction of anaesthesia is achieved by IV or inhalational methods.

The development of new technology and safer anaesthetic pharmacology means that modern anaesthesia is now relatively safe, and is usually used for all surgical procedures that cannot be performed under a local or regional anaesthetic. General anaesthetic drugs produce anaesthesia by their effect on the brain. Anaesthetic gases are inhaled, and are then transferred from the lungs to the circulation, and finally to the brain to be effective.

IV induction

- Suitable for routine and emergency surgical procedures.
- In an emergency situation, patients are often pre-oxygenated with 100% O_2 using a face mask.
- All anaesthetic drugs necessary for the procedure should be prepared and appropriately labelled.
- The AAGBI recommend that all patients should be monitored in the anaesthetic room prior to induction of anaesthesia.[1] This should include:
  - Capnography.
  - ECG.
  - NIBP.
  - Respiratory rate.
  - SpO_2.
- The following must also be available:
  - A nerve stimulator whenever a muscle relaxant is used.
  - A means of measuring the patient's temperature.
- Anaesthesia induction agents include:
  - Propofol.
  - Thiopental.
  - Etomidate.

Complications of IV induction
- Cardiovascular and respiratory depression
- Arterial injection
- Injection into subcutaneous tissue
- Drug reaction

References and further reading

1. AAGBI (2007). *Recommendations for standards of monitoring during anaesthesia and recovery* (4th edn). Association of Anaesthetists of Great Britain and Ireland: London.

Allman KG and Wilson IH (eds) (2006). *Oxford Handbook of Anaesthesia* (2nd edn). Oxford University Press: Oxford.

Kumar B (1998). *Working in the operating department.* Churchill-Livingstone: London.

Morton NS (1997). *Assisting the anaesthetist.* Oxford University Press: Oxford.

Royal College of Anaesthetists (2004). *Guidelines for the Provision of Anaesthetic Services.* RCoA: London.

Simpson PJ and Popat M (2002). *Understanding anaesthesia* (4th edn). Butterworth-Heinemann: Oxford.

Triad of anaesthesia

The triad of anaesthesia was developed to describe the three basic requirements of an anaesthetic that must be achieved to ensure a successful outcome. The triad is associated with all anaesthetic techniques and these requirements provide a balanced combination of anaesthetic drugs and other agents that induce:

- Narcosis.
- Analgesia.
- Relaxation.

Narcosis

Narcosis means that the patient is rendered unconscious/unaware following the administration of:

- Narcotic drugs.
- Sedative drugs.
- IV anaesthetic induction agents.
- Inhalational gas induction agents.

Analgesia

- Analgesia means lack of pain and suppresses physiological reflexes that occur following surgical stimulation and is often achieved by powerful narcotics, local block, or local infiltration.
- A surgical incision induces a complex series of physiological responses if made in a conscious patient[1] and can cause:
  - Tachycardia.
  - Hypertension.
  - Hyperventilation.
  - Sweating.
  - Vomiting.
- The administration of narcotic analgesic drugs limits such physiological responses to surgical stimulation.

Relaxation

- Relaxation refers to the reduction or absence of muscle tone which can be retained even when the patient is deeply unconscious, and is achieved by the use of muscle relaxing drugs and local blockade.
- Following the administration of relaxation drugs, patients will then require assisted or controlled ventilation until the drug has been reversed.
- Patient relaxation is important for endotracheal intubation, abdominal and laparoscopic surgery.

Maintenance of anaesthesia can then be provided with O_2, nitrous oxide (N_2O), and either a volatile agent or continuous infusion with propofol, with additional increments of muscle relaxant as required. Modern anaesthetic agents allow the proportions of the three components of the triad to be more easily adjusted according to patients' individual requirements. The introduction of muscle relaxant drugs has meant that adequate relaxation may be obtained by an IV injection while the patient is only lightly anaesthetised.

Reference and further reading

1. Whelan E and Davies H (2000). The pharmacology of drugs used in general anaesthesia. In Davey A and Ince C (eds). *Fundamentals of operating department practice*. Greenwich Medical Media Ltd.: London.

Allman KG and Wilson IH (eds) (2006). *Oxford Handbook of Anaesthesia* (2nd edn). Oxford University Press: Oxford.

Morton NS (1997). *Assisting the anaesthetist*. Oxford University Press: Oxford.

Royal College of Anaesthetists (2004). *Guidelines for the Provision of Anaesthetic Services*. RCoA: London.

Simpson PJ and Popat M (2002). *Understanding anaesthesia* (4th edn). Butterworth-Heinemann: Oxford.

Inhalational anaesthesia

Inhalational anaesthesia is the delivery of a volatile agent from a vaporiser through a breathing circuit to a patient. Inhalational anaesthesia can be sub-divided into:
- Induction.
- Maintenance.

Induction

The potency of an inhaled anaesthetic is quantified by its minimum alveolar concentration (MAC). The alveolus is the area of the lung in which gas leaves the lung and enters the bloodstream. MAC is defined as the amount of gas in the lungs required to prevent 50% of humans from moving when given a painful stimulus like a surgical incision. IV medications can be characterised as to their 'equivalent MAC' so that their potencies can be compared to the inhaled medications.

During respiration, the patient inhales the volatile agent, the concentration of which builds in the alveoli which diffuses across the alveoli capillary membrane into the bloodstream, resulting in the gradual loss of consciousness.

Indications for use
- To avoid IV induction with children or patients with needle phobia.
- To maintain spontaneous respiration where difficult intubation is expected e.g. acute epiglottitis or anatomical anomalies.
- Bronchopleural fistula.
- Inhaled foreign body.

Management
- Explanation and emotional support for patients.
- Close-fitting facemask.
- Preparation for immediate IV access.
- Availability of full range airway management equipment.

Complications:
- Delay in induction due to breath holding or obstruction.
- Difficulties with cannulation.
- Staff exposure to the inhalational agent.

Unconsciousness in most cases may be reversed promptly by the withdrawal of the inhalational agent. The use of volatile agents is contraindicated for use in patients with any history or familial association with malignant hyperthermia.

Maintenance

Volatile agents are the choice for maintenance of anaesthesia, in conjunction with O_2, analgesia, and muscle relaxants. These agents include:
- Isoflurane.
- Sevoflurane.
- Desflurane.

Management
- Monitoring and maintaining the level of volatile agent within the vaporiser.
- Ensuring patency of breathing circuits.
- Minimise the risk of environmental pollution with the use of active scavenging.
- Ensure availability and use of a vapour analyser.
- Circle breathing systems with vapour and CO_2 analysers are indicated for use with volatile agents to minimise cost and environmental pollution.

Complications
- Disconnection of breathing circuits.
- Delayed recovery.

Stages of anaesthesia

All anaesthetic drugs produce anaesthesia by their effect on the brain and anaesthetic gases are inhaled and are then transferred from the lungs to the circulation and finally to the brain to be effective. By administering an anaesthetic gas alone the progress of each patient towards deep anaesthesia is divided into four stages[1] (Table 7.1).

Table 7.1 Stages of anaesthesia[1]

Stage	Progress of anaesthetic gas induction
1	The stage of analgesia; lasts from the beginning of administration of the gas until consciousness is lost
2	Refers to the stage of excitement, which lasts from loss of consciousness until regular breathing begins and settles. During this stage patients have been known to hold their breath, struggle, cough, or even vomit
3	Indicates that surgical anaesthesia has been achieved; once the patient's breathing has settled the procedure may begin
4	If additional anaesthetic is administered, the patient reaches the fourth stage, otherwise referred to as 'overdose' and breathing and circulation will cease

References
1. Morton NS (1997). *Assisting the anaesthetist*. Oxford University Press: Oxford.

Allman KG and Wilson IH (eds) (2006). *Oxford Handbook of Anaesthesia* (2nd edn). Oxford University Press: Oxford.

Association of Anaesthetists for Great Britain and Ireland (2007). *Recommendations for standards of monitoring during anaesthesia and recovery* (4th edn). Association of Anaesthetists for Great Britain and Ireland: London.

Simpson PJ and Popat M (2002). *Understanding anaesthesia* (4th edn). Butterworth-Heinemann: Oxford.

Total intravenous anaesthesia

Total intravenous anaesthesia (TIVA) is the delivery of anaesthesia with no inhalational agents. Delivery is via a microprocessor controlled syringe pump which delivers a prescribed target does of an anaesthetic agent which is calculated on the basis of weight, age and gender. TIVA may also be called target controlled anaesthesia (TCA) or target controlled infusion (TCI).

Indications for use
- Anaesthetist's choice.
- Availability of equipment.

Advantages
- Rapid induction of general anaesthesia.
- Rapid recovery with minimal 'hangover' effect.
- Can be used for sedation or as an adjunct to regional anaesthesia
- Reduced postoperative nausea and vomiting (PONV).
- Laryngoscopy/bronchoscope where inhalational agents may cause airway irritation.
- Safe for use with patients with malignant hyperthermia.
- Predictability for bariatric patients.
- Suitable for high risk patients e.g. the elderly and patients with relevant pre-existing disease (📖 see Chapter 5 pp. 57–84 for further details).
- Gentle gradual approach.
- Control over depth of anaesthesia.

Disadvantages
- Pain on induction.
- Contraindicated for patients with hypolypidaemia for long-term use i.e. ITU.
- Propofol TCI is not licensed for paediatric use.
- Potential interruption to delivery.

Clinical management
- IV access must be protected, visible, and accessible at all times. If the IV access becomes dislodged or detached this will interrupt delivery and therefore predispose the patient to awareness. This is an added concern with patients that are paralysed as part of their management.
- IV delivery systems must include an anti-reflux valve at the access site to ensure anti-siphon and prevent reflux. It is suggested that if TIVA is used in conjunction with IV fluids it should have separate and dedicated IV access point.
- Accurate assessment of depth of anaesthesia is difficult during TIVA, so care in preventing awareness is essential, especially if muscle relaxants are used.

References and further reading

Allman KG and Wilson IH (eds) (2006). *Oxford Handbook of Anaesthesia* (2nd edn). Oxford University Press: Oxford.

Royal College of Anaesthetists (2004). *Guidelines for the Provision of Anaesthetic Services*. RCoA: London.

The Virtual Anaesthesia Textbook: *Intravenous agents, TCI and TIVA*. Available at: 🖳 http://www.virtual-anaesthesia-textbook.com/vat/iva.htm

Local anaesthesia

Local anaesthetics are drugs that reversibly block the conduction of nerve impulses along nerve axons. Occasionally patients can be sedated throughout the local anaesthetic procedure if they are particularly anxious. There are many ways in which the local anaesthesia can be used; this will depend on potency, toxicity, duration of action, stability, solubility in water, and the ability to penetrate mucous membranes by the drug. Other variations which will determine the local anaesthetic which is used will be the type of procedure and the mode of delivery for the local anaesthetic.[1]

Administration

When administering local anaesthetics care should be taken in calculating safe drug dosage. Account should be given to:
- Patient's age.
- Weight.
- Physique and health.

Other factors include:
- Absorption.
- Excretion.
- Potency of the drug.
- Vascularity of the area in which the local anaesthesia is to be applied when injecting.[1]

Local anaesthetics will also cause some degree of vasodilatation; consequently, quite often vasoconstrictors will be added to the local anaesthetic which increase its potency and duration of action by ensuring the drug is localised in the tissue. The vasoconstrictors also increase the safety by decreasing the rate of absorption. Adrenaline-containing solutions should never be used for infiltration around end-arteries e.g., penis, ring block of fingers or other areas with a terminal vascular supply as the intense vasoconstriction may lead to severe ischemia and necrosis.[2]

Local anaesthetic often does not work when injected in and around infected tissue. This is due to the infected tissue having a more acidic environment, therefore delaying the action and reducing the effect of the local anaesthetic. Infected tissue often has an increased blood supply therefore the anaesthetic is removed from the injection area before it can affect the nerve axon and neuron.[3] Local anaesthesia can be administered in several ways:

Topical: topical anaesthetics are normally applied to both the skin or mucus membrane and its onset of action can range from 5–60 minutes. Topical anaesthetics are used typically prior to injection or cannulation and cutaneous contact (usually under an occlusive dressing) should be maintained for the maximum period directed by the drug data sheet prior to venepuncture to ensure maximum effect.[2]

Local infiltration: this technique is normally used for minor procedures such as dental extractions and suturing of skin wounds.

Regional (conductional anaesthesia): this can be divided into minor and major nerve blockade. Minor nerve blockade will include blocking ulnar, radial, or intercostal nerves; whilst major nerve blockade relates to the deeper nerves or trunks such as brachial plexus.[4]

Local anaesthesia can also be used in the treatment of acute and chronic pain. Acute pain can refer to labour pain, postoperative pain, and trauma. Chronic pain is complex and therefore require treatment by an expert in pain management. Often local anaesthetics are given in these cases with a combination of opioids, non-steroidal drugs, and anticonvulsants.

Toxicity[4]

Coma, circulatory collapse, cardiac arrest, and apnoea may occur in toxicity. Signs and symptoms of central nervous system (CNS) toxicity include:
- Light-headedness.
- Dizziness and circumoral paraesthesia which may precede visual and/or auditory disturbances which can include difficulty focusing and tinnitus.

Other symptoms of toxicity include:
- Disorientation and feelings of drowsiness.
- Respiratory depression.

Signs of CNS toxicity are usually excitatory and include:
- Shivering.
- Muscular twitching and tremors initially involving muscles of the face and distal parts of the extremities.
- Ultimately, convulsions of a tonic-clonic nature occur.

If a dose of local anaesthetic is given rapidly IV or the administered dose is too great for an individual, then the initial signs of excitation may progress very quickly to generalised CNS depression and coma.[1] The AAGBI have produces guidelines for management of patients with severe local anaesthetic toxicity.[5]

Respiratory depression may result in respiratory arrest. CNS toxicity is exacerbated by hypercarbia and acidosis. When injecting local anaesthesia into vascular areas, great care should be given to avoid intravascular injection; should accidental intravascular injection occur, signs and symptoms would be convulsions and cardiovascular collapse which can occur rapidly.

References and further reading

1. British National Formulary. Available from: http://www.bnf.org/bnf/bnf/current/6684.htm

2. Simpson PJ and Popart MT (2002). *Understanding anaesthesia* (4th edn). Butterworth-Heinemann: Oxford.

3. Illingworth KA and Simpson K H (1998). *Anaesthesia and analgesia in emergency medicine* (2nd edn). Oxford University Press: Oxford.

4. Salender D (2005). *The Illustrated guide to peripheral nerve blocks.* Available at: www.anaesthesia-az.com/sites/156/imagebank/typearticleparam509589/Page_02-09.pdf

5. Association of Anaesthetists of Great Britain and Ireland (2007). *Guidelines for the management of severe local anaesthetic toxicity.* AAGBI: London.

Adams AP and Cashman JN (1991). *Anaesthesia, analgesia and intensive care.* Edward Arnold: London.

Williams T (2007). Obstetric anaesthesia. In Smith B, Rawlings P, Wicker P, *et al. Core topics in operating department practice.* Cambridge University Press: Cambridge.

Intravenous conscious sedation

- Intravenous conscious sedation (IVCS) refers to mild-to-moderate depression of levels of consciousness allowing the patient to maintain their own airway.
- IVCS allows patients to respond to commands and/or physical stimulation.
- Patients are normally given sedatives to reduce anxiety and tolerate medical and nursing procedures.
- Sedation can also be used in intensive care for ventilated and spontaneous breathing patients.
- Sedation can be delivered either by continuous infusion or bolus doses through either a central line (for long-term sedation) or IV line.
- It is essential that the line is secured properly as any disruption of the infusion or delivery of the sedation will result in emergence.
- It must be ensured that the patient is monitored appropriately throughout.[1] This should include:
  - ECG.
  - NIBP.
  - Respiratory rate.
  - SpO_2.
- Some degree of respiratory depression may be observed along with fluctuation in BP, heart rate, and rhythm.

Drugs commonly used are:
- IV anaesthetic agents: propofol infusions are commonly used as propofol is controllable—produces rapid changes in consciousness e.g. can wake patients up to allow them to breath spontaneously and assess neurologically. Propofol however, can cause hypotension in some patients especially those who are hypovolaemic or dehydrated.
- Benzodiazepines: potent amnesiacs.
- Opioids: these are often used for pain relief, supported sometimes by sedatives.

Reference and further reading

1. Association of Anaesthetists of Great Britain and Ireland (2007). *Recommendations for standards of monitoring during anaesthesia and recovery* (4th edn). AAGBI: London.

Adams AP and Cashman JN (1991). *Anaesthesia, analgesia and intensive care.* Edward Arnold: London.

Allman KG and Wilson IH (eds) (2006). *Oxford Handbook of Anaesthesia* (2nd edn). Oxford University Press: Oxford.

Davey A and Ince CS (2000). *Fundamentals of operating department practice.* Greenwich Medical Media Ltd.: London.

Fortunato NH (2000). *Berry and Kohn's operating room technique* (9th edn). Mosby: London.

Hutton P and Prys-Roberts C (1994). *Monitoring in anaesthesia and intensive care.* Saunders: London.

Simpson PJ and Popart MT (2002). *Understanding anaesthesia* (4th edn). Butterworth-Heinemann: Oxford.

Epidural anaesthesia

- Epidural anaesthesia is achieved by the administration of a local anaesthetic drug into the epidural space via an epidural catheter.
- The advantages of an epidural over spinal anaesthesia are that the epidural catheter allows for the epidural to be 'toped-up' with a local anaesthetic, therefore prolonging the duration of action.
- Epidural has a slower onset than spinal anaesthesia and can take up to 45 minutes for surgical anaesthesia to be achieved.
- Local anaesthetic solutions can be delivered through the epidural catheter with a single shot, intermittent top-up, or continuous via a pump.
- Epidural anaesthesia can be used in obstetric, general, gynaecological, and orthopaedic surgery.
- Epidurals can also be used as an on-demand system such as PCEA for postoperative pain relief as per local policy.
- When epidurals are being sited and dressed, a sterile technique must be adhered to and the epidural site dressed according to local policy and practice.
- It must be ensured that the patient is monitored appropriately throughout.[1] This should include:
  - ECG.
  - NIBP.
  - Respiratory rate.
  - SpO_2.

Complications of epidural anaesthesia include:
- Hypotension.
- CSF/dural puncture.
- Respiratory depression.
- Failed block.
- Pruritus.
- Total spinal effect may occur from accidental dural puncture.

Reference and further reading

1. Association of Anaesthetists of Great Britain and Ireland (2007). *Recommendations for standards of monitoring during anaesthesia and recovery* (4th edn). AAGBI: London.

Adams AP and Cashman JN (1991). *Anaesthesia, analgesia and intensive care.* Edward Arnold: London.

Allman KG and Wilson IH (eds) (2006). *Oxford Handbook of Anaesthesia* (2nd edn). Oxford University Press: Oxford.

Anaesthesia UK (2008). Bromage Scale. Available at: 🖳 http://www.frca.co.uk/article.aspx?articleid=100316

Davey A and Ince CS (2000). *Fundamentals of operating department practice.* Greenwich Medical Media Ltd.: London.

Simpson PJ and Popart M T (2002). *Understanding anaesthesia* (4th edn). Butterworth-Heinemann: Oxford.

Smith B, Rawlings P, Wicker P, et al. (2007). Core topics in operating department practice: anaesthesia and critical care. Cambridge University Press: Cambridge.

Caudal anaesthesia

- This is described as a low approach to the epidural space through the sacral hiatus, which is an anatomical gap in the sacrum.
- The caudal anesthesia produces a block of the sacral and lumbar nerve roots.
- This procedure is prominently used in children as higher volumes of local anaesthetic are needed to produce an effective block in adults.
- As this can be unpleasant for children, caudal anaesthetics are normally performed once the general anaesthesia has been induced and before surgery.
- There are now caudal anaesthesia kits available with catheters similar to the epidural catheters which allow for the block to be prolonged during the course of surgery.

Complications of caudal anaesthesia are the same as epidural anaesthesia.

References and further reading

Adams AP and Cashman JN (1991). *Anaesthesia, analgesia and intensive care*. Edward Arnold: London.

Allman KG and Wilson IH (eds) (2006). *Oxford Handbook of Anaesthesia* (2nd edn). Oxford University Press: Oxford.

Association of Anaesthetists of Great Britain and Ireland (2007). *Recommendations for standards of monitoring during anaesthesia and recovery* (4th edn). AAGBI: London.

Davey A and Ince CS (2000). *Fundamentals of operating department practice*. Greenwich Medical Media Ltd.: London.

Simpson PJ and Popart MT (2002). *Understanding anaesthesia* (4th edn). Butterworth-Heinemann: Oxford.

Smith B, Rawlings P, Wicker P, et al. (2007). *Core topics in operating department practice: anaesthesia and critical care*. Cambridge University Press: Cambridge.

Spinal anaesthesia

Spinal anaesthesia is also known as a sub-arachnoid block or spinal analgesia and is the introduction of local anaesthetic solutions directly into the CSF which produces spinal anaesthesia.

- Spinals usually involve the lower part of the body, with a complete sensory and motor block of the affected area resulting in a total loss of sensation including pain, temperature, and position.
- Spinal anaesthesia can also have the effect of total or partial loss of power in the numb area for the duration of the block.
- Depending on the agent used, and the dose/volume given, the technique is fast onset with the duration of the block lasting anywhere between 1–4 hours.
- The area blocked can extend between the nipple levels (T10) to toes.
- It must be ensured that the patient is monitored appropriately throughout.[1] This should include:
  - ECG.
  - NIBP.
  - Respiratory rate.
  - SpO_2.
- Patients can become hypotensive because of sympathetic blockade and vasodilation so the circulation system may need supporting with IV fluids.
- Vasoconstrictors such as ephedrine need to be available when this procedure is taking place and patients should be monitored appropriately throughout.
- The level of the spinal anaesthetic is measured for spread and height of the block. This is normally done with ice and/or light touch. Ethyl chloride is no longer commonly used, due to it being an atmospheric pollutant which tests afferent function.
- Motor function is normally tested with the bromage scale (Table 7.2).
- Spinal anaesthesia is suitable for surgical anaesthesia and is sometimes supported with a combination of epidural anaesthesia. The epidural allows for prolonged block for surgery and/or pain relief post-surgery.
- When a spinal injection is being performed and dressed, a sterile technique must be adhered to and the spinal injection site dressed according to local policy and practice.
- Spinal anaesthesia is predominantly used in obstetric, orthopaedic, general, and gynaecological procedures.

Complications

See Box 7.2.

Contraindications include:

- Surgical procedures above the thorax.
- Hypovolaemia.
- Local/systemic infection.
- Raised intracranial pressure.
- Surgical procedures of long duration i.e. lasting >2 hours.

Table 7.2 Bromage scale[2]

Grade	Definition
1	Free movement of legs and feet
2	Just able to flex knees with free movement of feet
3	Unable to move knees but with free movement of feet
4	Unable to move legs or feet

Box 7.2 Complications of spinal anaesthesia

- Failure of spinal anaesthesia.
- Uncommon complication is neurologic disorder due to trauma.
- Localised bruising and back pain.
- Respiratory depression with opiates.
- PONV.
- High spinal block.
- Bladder distension.
- Bradycardia.
- Infection.
- Spinal headache.
- Hypotension: local anaesthetic drugs block the sympathetic nerves to the blood vessels therefore causing vasodilatation.

References

1. Association of Anaesthetists of Great Britain and Ireland (2007). *Recommendations for standards of monitoring during anaesthesia and recovery* (4th edn). AAGBI: London.

2. Anaesthesia UK (2008). Description of Bromage Scale. Available at: ▣ http://www.frca.co.uk/article.aspx?articleid=100316

Further reading

Allman KG and Wilson IH (eds) (2006). *Oxford Handbook of Anaesthesia* (2nd edn). Oxford University Press: Oxford.

Davey A, Ince CS (2000). *Fundamentals of operating department practice.* Greenwich Medical Media Ltd.: London.

Simpson PJ and Popart M T (2002). *Understanding anaesthesia* (4th edn). Butterworth-Heinemann: Oxford.

Smith B, Rawlings P, Wicker P, et al. (2007). *Core topics in operating department practice: anaesthesia and critical care.* Cambridge University Press: Cambridge.

Yentis S, May A, and Malhotra S (2007). *Analgesia, anaesthesia and pregnancy: a practical guide.* Cambridge University Press: Cambridge.

Continuous spinal anaesthesia

- Continuous spinal anaesthesia was first described by Edward Tuohy in 1944.
- Small-bore catheters for continuous spinal anaesthesia are available but 'they do not enjoy wide-spread popularity'.[1]
- Once a microspinal catheter has been inserted, it must be clearly labelled to avoid accidental injection of an epidural-style dose.

Advantages

- Good quality block with the ability to titrate the dose and avoiding the risk of inadvertent total spinal block.
- Allows repeated boluses (or infusion) of local anaesthetic.
- Acceptable for patients in labour and operative delivery.
- Decreases the possibility of cardiovascular instability during anaesthesia.
- Can be left in place for postoperative analgesia.
- Smaller decrease in BP and lower incidence of vasopressor use in elderly patients.
- Rapid onset of action, better quality of analgesia, and better muscle relaxation.

Disadvantages

- It is uncommon in the UK.
- Associated with the development of cauda equina syndrome.
- Handling of the microspinal catheters is difficult.
- Risk of post-dural puncture headache.
- Mistaking the microspinal catheter for an epidural catheter.
- Persistent parasthesia and lower back pain.
- Risk of infection.
- Expensive.

Reference and further reading

1. Simpson PJ and Popart M T (2002). *Understanding anaesthesia* (4th edn). Butterworth-Heinemann: Oxford.

Association of Anaesthetists of Great Britain and Ireland (2007). Recommendations for standards of monitoring during anaesthesia and recovery (4th edn). AAGBI: London.

Allman KG and Wilson IH (eds) (2006). *Oxford Handbook of Anaesthesia* (2nd edn). Oxford University Press: Oxford.

Davey A, Ince CS (2000). *Fundamentals of operating department practice*. Greenwich Medical Media Ltd.: London.

Smith B, Rawlings P, Wicker P, et al. (2007). *Core topics in operating department practice: anaesthesia and critical care*. Cambridge University Press: Cambridge.

Yentis S, May A, and Malhotra S (2007). *Analgesia, anaesthesia and pregnancy: a practical guide*. Cambridge University Press: Cambridge.

Patient positioning for regional anaesthesia

Spinal and epidural anaesthesia are often performed with the patient awake and in a sitting position.

- The sitting position allows for the patient to position themselves in the optimum position for the spinal/epidural anaesthesia to take place.
  - When possible, the patient rounds his/her back to open the gaps between vertebrae.
  - Place chin to chest.
  - The patient leans over a pillow on his/her lap and relaxes shoulders down.
  - Their feet should rest on a stool.
- The patient can also be placed on their side in a foetal position as is required for caudal anaesthesia if sitting is not possible. Lateral position however, distorts the midline anatomy.
- It is a matter of individual judgement whether the advantages of the sitting position outweigh the discomfort for the patient in cases such as trauma or obstetrics.
- It is essential that one member of the anaesthetic team is solely dedicated to helping the patient maintain their position through the course of the procedure and continually monitors the patient's comfort and safety at all times.

References

Allman KG and Wilson IH (eds) (2006). *Oxford Handbook of Anaesthesia* (2nd edn). Oxford University Press: Oxford.

Anaesthesia UK (2008). *Bromage Scale.* Available at: ▣ http://www.frca.co.uk/article.aspx?articleid=100316

Association of Anaesthetists of Great Britain and Ireland (2007). *Recommendations for standards of monitoring during anaesthesia and recovery* (4th edn). AAGBI: London.

Davey A and Ince CS (2000). *Fundamentals of operating department practice.* Greenwich Medical Media Ltd.: London.

Simpson PJ and Popart M T (2002). *Understanding anaesthesia* (4th edn). Butterworth-Heinemann: Oxford.

Smith B, Rawlings P, Wicker P, et al. (2007). *Core topics in operating department practice: anaesthesia and critical care.* Cambridge University Press: Cambridge.

Contraindications for spinal, epidural and caudal anaesthesia

- Technical/anatomical difficulties: If the spinal/epidural/caudal proves to be technically difficult, as a general rule after two or three unsuccessful attempts seek more experienced help or an alternative technique. The anaesthetic assistant must be aware how to contact additional support should this be required.
- Lack of patient cooperation or if patient refuses.
- Lack of full resuscitation equipment available.
- If the patient's coagulation means there is heightened risk of haemorrhagic complications.
  - Patient is receiving anticoagulants such as warfarin prior to the spinal/epidural anaesthesia.
  - Here the international normalised ratio (INR) results need to be within acceptable limits to avoid haemorrhagic complications
  - Normal INR = 1.
  - Acceptable INR = 0.8–1.2.
- Localised skin infection.
- Raised intracranial pressures.
- Patients with fixed cardiac output states.

References and further reading

Allman KG and Wilson IH (eds) (2006). *Oxford Handbook of Anaesthesia* (2nd edn). Oxford University Press: Oxford.

Davey A, Ince CS (2000). *Fundamentals of operating department practice*. Greenwich Medical Media Ltd.: London.

Simpson PJ and Popart M T (2002). *Understanding anaesthesia* (4th edn). Butterworth-Heinemann: Oxford.

Smith B, Rawlings P, Wicker P, et al. (2007). *Core topics in operating department practice: anaesthesia and critical care*. Cambridge University Press: Cambridge.

Essential anaesthetic equipment

Preparing the anaesthetic room

The checks and preparation detailed in this topic should be carried out before commencing each and every operating session and should be in accordance with the relevant AAGBI recommendations.[1]

Checking machines

- The anaesthetic machine should be clean and free from damage and debris.
- Check that the machine is directly connected to a mains electrical supply and has a well charged battery back-up (where appropriate).
- Connect gas pipelines to corresponding mains outlets and perform 'Tug test', ensuring each gas outlet exclusively supplies its corresponding flowmeter.
- The mains supply pressure for each gas should be 400–500kPa.

Check the following according to the AAGBI guidelines for checking anaesthetic equipment[1]

- An audible O_2 fail alarm sounds when O_2 supply is shut off.
- Anti-hypoxia guard present: you should not be able to deliver a gas mix of more than 75% N_2O:25% O_2, and N_2O flow should shut off if O_2 supply fails.
- All gas flowmeters move freely throughout ranges.
- Reserve O_2 cylinder fitted, functioning, and sufficiently full.
- Additional cylinders fitted and contents checked, as required.
- Emergency O_2 bypass control.
- Vaporiser(s) correctly mounted on back bar and locked in place (when one vaporiser is switched on it should lock off all other vaporisers from use).
- Calibrate O_2 and gas flow sensors and assess function.
- Circle breathing circuit, and ventilation limb and bag patent, intact, and in date (these are disposable items and have a defined period of use).
- Adjustable pressure-limiting (APL) valve and one-way flow valves function.
- Perform low pressure breathing circuit leak test.
- Ventilator function.
- Auxiliary/common gas outlet function.
- Soda lime (CO_2 absorber) intact.
- Anaesthetic gas scavenging system operational.

Don't forget to sign and date the anaesthetic machine log book.

Remember: if the anaesthetic machine fails any of these tests:

- It must be removed from service.
- Complete failure documentation.
- Inform anaesthetic service team and anaesthetic department.

Checking equipment

Check availability and function of:

- Operational head down (Trendelenberg) facility on bed/trolley.
- Essential minimal patient monitoring (ECG, NIBP, SpO_2, end-tidal carbon dioxide ($ETCO_2$)).
- Appropriate airway management equipment— see Chapter 10, p. 185.

- Mains suction with Yankaur sucker and a selection of suction catheter sizes (suction is incorporated into some anaesthetic machine design).
- Difficult/emergency airway equipment—McCoy laryngoscope blades, intubating laryngeal mask airway (LMA), fibreoptic laryngoscope, cricothyroidotomy kit.
- Alternative anaesthetic breathing circuit e.g. Bains, Waters.
- Self-inflating bag and alternative O_2 cylinder.
- Peripheral nerve stimulator—for assessing neuromuscular blockade.
- Infusion pressure cuff/rapid infusion devices.
- Temperature monitoring equipment.
- Patient/fluid warming devices.

Reference and further reading

1. Association of Anaesthetists of Great Britain and Ireland (2004). *Checking anaesthetic equipment.* AAGBI: London.

Association of Anaesthetists of Great Britain and Ireland (2007). *Recommendations for standards of monitoring during anaesthesia and recovery* (4th edn). AAGBI: London.

Royal College of Anaesthetists (2004). *Guidelines for the Provision of Anaesthetic Services.* RCoA: London.

Stocking of essential items

A sufficient stock level of the following consumable items should be kept in each anaesthetic room to cover not only the planned operating session but also any emergencies that may potentially arise.

- Facemasks.
- Oropharyngeal ('Guedel') and nasopharygeal airways.
- LMAs—sized by patient weight (see Table 8.1).
- Endotracheal (ET) tubes—selected by internal diameter (ID) (see Table 8.1); always have a tube one size below that selected immediately available.
- Laryngoscope handle and blades—Macintosh size 3 and 4 (always check the bulb of the laryngoscope is secure, bright, and focuses on the tip of the blade. Keep spare batteries and bulbs in the anaesthetic room).
- Bougie/introducer and stylet.
- Water based lubricant for LMA/ET tube.
- Tie/tape for securing LMA/ET tube.
- Gauze roll throat pack.
- Eye pads/protection.
- Gum guard and petroleum/paraffin jelly for teeth and lip protection.
- Heat and moisture exchange (HME) bacterial/viral filter.
- O_2 masks and other airway O_2 enrichment devices (e.g. T-piece, T-bag).
- Anaesthetic drugs, emergency drugs and fluids.
- Syringes and needles—various sizes.
- IV cannulae (various sizes) and giving sets/taps/extensions.

All of these items are now available as single-patient use products.

Preparing the anaesthetic tray

After securing the patient's airway the anaesthetic tray should hold everything you require for intra- and postoperative airway management. Most commonly:

- Laryngoscope.
- Magill's forceps.
- Syringe—for inflating cuffs on airway devices.
- Facemask.
- Oro-/naso-pharyngeal airway (for post-extubation).

Table 8.1 Guidelines for selection of LMAs and ET tubes*

LMA		ET tube	
Size	Patient weight	ID (in mm)	Patient group
3	30–50 kg	7.0/7.5/8.0	Female
4	50–70 kg	8.0/8.5/9.0	Male
5	70–100 kg		
6	>100kg		

* LMA sizes derived from Intavent Orthofix Ltd. guidelines. ET tube sizes for adults patients.

Anaesthetic machines

During general anaesthesia medical gases are delivered to the patient via the anaesthetic machine and anaesthesia breathing systems. In addition, the modern day anaesthetic machine has the facility to provide additional monitoring for physiological parameters and ventilation.

Modern anaesthetic machines incorporate a circle breathing system and possess the following features (adapted from Al-Shaikh and Stacey[1]):
- Pressure gauges—colour coded.
- Pressure regulators.
- Flowmeters—colour coded.
- Vaporisers.
- O_2 flow meter controlled by a single-touch coded control knob.
- O_2 concentration monitor or analyser.
- High-flow O_2 flush.
- N_2O cut-off device when O_2 pressure is low.
- O_2, N_2O ratio monitor and controller.
- Pin index safety system.
- O_2 failure warning alarm.
- Ventilator disconnection alarm.
- Reserve O_2 cylinder in case of pipeline failure.

The anaesthetic machine is checked by the anaesthetic practitioner according to the AAGBI checklist for anaesthetic equipment guidelines.[2] This helps to inform standardisation of practice. However all anaesthetists have the responsibility to carry out checks of the anaesthetic equipment prior to commencement of the operating list.

All modern anaesthetic machines have the ability to be connected to an external power supply which means they need to be switched on. When this occurs some anaesthetic workstations enter into a self-test programme and calibration exercise. These functions do not have to be retested.

Safety systems
- Piped gases are colour coded and connectors are specific to the gas being used so that for example an O_2 pipeline (white) cannot be connected to a N_2O outlet (blue).
- On an anaesthetic machine the cylinder yoke, into which the cylinder fits, is protected by the *'pin-index'* system.[3]
- The pin-index system is a series of holes and pins designed to make sure that the wrong cylinder cannot be fitted to the wrong attachment.
- The holes drilled in to the cylinder valve must correspond with the pins that are located on the cylinder yoke of the anaesthetic machine.
- Each medical gas cylinder used on the anaesthetic machine has its own unique pin-index code so only the correct gas can be connected to the correct cylinder yoke.[3]

References

1. Al-Shaikh B and Stacey S (2002). *Essentials of Anaesthetic Equipment*. Churchill Livingstone: London.

2. Association of Anaesthetists of Great Britain and Ireland (2004). *Checking anaesthetic equipment*. AAGBI: London.

3. Ince CS, Skinner AC, and Taft E (2000). Scientific principles in relation to the anaesthetic machine. In Ince CS and Davey A (eds). *Fundamentals of Operating Department Practice*. Greenwich Medical Media: London.

Ventilators

Ventilation of the lungs can be performed without any equipment at all. Today, artificial ventilation is used on a daily basis as part of an anaesthetic technique. To aid this, a range of ventilators have been developed and many are multifunctional.

During general anaesthesia it may be necessary to paralyse and ventilate the patient. Ventilators are used to provide intermittent positive pressure ventilation (IPPV). During spontaneous respiration, gas moves into the lungs by negative intrathoracic pressure but this process is reversed for IPPV. Anaesthetic/medical ventilators should be simple, robust, and economical to purchase and use.[1]

Modern anaesthetic ventilators incorporate the following features (adapted from Al-Shaikh and Stacey[1]):
• Volume cycling—predetermined tidal volume.
• Time cycling—predetermined inspiratory rate.
• Pressure cycling—predetermined pressure is reached.
• Flow cycling—predetermined flow is reached during inspiration when it switches to exhalation.
• Either gas or electrically powered.
• Pressure generator—produces inspiration by generating a predetermined pressure.
• Flow generator—produces inspiration by a predetermined flow of gas.
• Should be easy to clean and sterilise.

Pressure generator ventilators cannot compensate if there is a change in the patient's chest compliance; however, they are able to compensate if a leak is detected. A flow generator can compensate to compliance changes but not leaks within the system.

The modern anaesthetic machine incorporates a 'bag in a bottle ventilator' which is a time cycled ventilator consisting of bellows that collapse delivering the fresh gas flow from within the bellows, and then the driving gas (compressed air) returns the bellows to the ascending position in readiness for the next cycle. The ventilator can generate within the chamber a tidal volume of 0–1500mL. A paediatric version is also available generating tidal volume 0–400mL.

Safety systems

During anaesthesia it is vitally important that both the patient and the equipment used are monitored closely. The complexity of anaesthesia depends on a variety of factors including (adapted from Gwinnutt[2]):
• Type of operation and surgical technique.
• Anaesthetic technique.
• Patient's past medical history and/or pre-existing conditions.
• Anaesthetist's preferences.
• Equipment available and anaesthetist's familiarisation with the equipment.

References and further reading

1. Al-Shaikh B and Stacey S (2002). Essentials of Anaesthetic Equipment. Churchill Livingstone: London.

2. Gwinnutt, C. (2004). *Lecture notes: Clinical Anaesthesia*. Blackwell Publishing: Oxford.

Ince CS, Skinner AC, and Taft E (2000). Scientific principles in relation to the anaesthetic machine. In Ince CS and Davey A (eds). *Fundamentals of Operating Department Practice*. Greenwich Medical Media: Greenwich.

Vaporisers

Inhalational anaesthetic agents (volatiles) are used for the induction and maintenance of anaesthesia and form the basis of modern day anaesthetic practice.[1] Historically, in the early days of anaesthesia, vapours were administered without a vaporiser; ether was administered by the drop method where a cloth was placed over the patient's face and the agent was dripped onto it. The invention of the Schimmelbush mask helped to improve this system which lifted the cloth off the patient's face, enabling air to circulate. This method was extremely dangerous and inaccurate.[1]

Basic principles of vaporisers

- A vaporiser is a device that adds the necessary concentration of volatile anaesthetic vapour to the stream of anaesthetic carrying gas.
- Vaporisers are flow and temperature compensated so they are unaffected by positive pressure ventilation.
- All volatile anaesthetic agents have different physical properties and therefore each vaporiser is agent specific.
- A vaporiser functions by dividing the carrying gas flow into two streams. One stream is directed into the vaporising chamber, the other into the bypass chamber. This is known as the 'splitting ratio'. Gas that leaves the vaporising chamber is fully saturated with the volatile agent of choice. The dial on the vaporiser which can be adjusted by the anaesthetist alters the proportion of gas entering the bypass chamber which in turn can alter the final concentration leaving the outlet.[2]
- All vaporisers used today have a colour-coded 'key filler' system and supply bottle so that each vaporiser can only be replenished with the fluid intended for that particular vaporiser.[3]
- Vaporisers are usually sited on the backbar of the anaesthetic machine. The Selectatec™ system allows the various vaporisers to be removed easily for any reasons, e.g. so they can be refilled or if faulty. It also ensures that only one vaporiser can be used at a time. A combination of vaporiser designs is hazardous and should be strongly discouraged.

There are four types of vaporisers currently in use:[2]
- Plenum.
- Draw-over.
- Gas blenders.
- Computer controlled.

The plenum vaporiser

This is the most frequently used vaporiser in the UK. They are agent specific, efficient, variable, and unidirectional. They are used outside the breathing system. Features of modern plenum vaporisers include (adapted from Eales and Cooper[2]):
- Flow and temperature compensated.
- Consistent output.
- One-hand, easily-operated dial.
- Clear indication of fill level.
- 'Easy-fil™' filler, reduces leaks, agent specific.

The draw-over vaporiser

This is mainly used by the armed forces as part of the tri-service anaesthetic equipment and in remote areas. The draw-over vaporisers are used within the breathing circuit. They have a low resistance to flow and are relatively efficient. Examples include the Oxford Miniature Vaporiser (OMV), simple and robust hence its use as tri-service anaesthetic equipment.

Gas blender

Gas blenders are used to administer desflurane only. They require an external power supply which enables the desflurane to be heated to 39°C and pressurizes it to 1500mmHg (about 2 atmospheres). This means that there is a constant stream of vapour under pressure flowing out of the chamber and blending with the fresh gas flow.

Computer controlled

Computer-controlled vaporisers are found on certain anaesthetic machines and they consist of a central processing unit, assigned by a magnetic code to each volatile agent, which measures and adjusts the gas flow. The volatile agent of choice is adjusted by regulating the flow of gas through the processor.

Safety

According to Ince *et al.*[4] it is important to observe the following important safety precautions:

- Do not carry the vaporiser by the dial.
- Check that the mounting point 'O' rings on the Selectatec™ manifold are intact and undamaged and that the mating surfaces are clean.
- Make sure that the vaporiser control knob is in the 'off' position and the locking lever is in the 'on' position.
- Lower the vaporiser onto the manifold and move the locking lever to the 'lock' position.
- Make sure vaporiser is properly seated.
- Leak test the system with the vaporiser off and then turned on. A leak can be catastrophic for the patient.

References

1. Haslam GM and Forrest FC (2004). Principles of anaesthetic vaporisers. *Anaesthesia and Intensive Care Medicine* **5**(3), 88–91.

2. Eales M and Cooper R (2007). Principles of anaesthetic vaporisers. *Anaesthesia and Intensive Care Medicine* **8**(3) 111–15.

3. Al-Shaikh B and Stacey S (2002). *Essentials of Anaesthetic Equipment*. Churchill Livingstone: London.

4. Ince CS, Skinner AC, and Taft E (2000). Scientific principles in relation to the anaesthetic machine. In Ince CS and Davey A (eds). *Fundamentals of Operating Department Practice*, p.85. Greenwich Medical Media: London.

Breathing systems

To enable an anaesthetic mixture to be delivered to the patient, anaesthetic breathing systems are employed. They are fundamental in coupling the patient's respiratory system to the anaesthetic machine. Different breathing systems exist but the ideal features should include:[1]

- Efficient elimination of expired CO_2.
- Low resistance to gas flow.
- Safety and robustness.
- Low dead space.
- Light and easy to use.

Non-rebreathing systems

Consist of unidirectional valves to direct exhaled gases away from the patient. These systems are seldom used in anaesthesia because of valve problems but are used in the transportation of critically ill patients.

Rebreathing systems

Are widely used in anaesthesia and in 1954, WW Mapleson described the theory of anaesthetic breathing circuits into open, semi-open, and semi closed. The five classifications—A, B, C, D, and E (see Fig. 8.1)—are the mainstay of all modern day anaesthetic breathing systems. B and C are seldom used in anaesthesia and have poor performance.

Mapleson A

Commonly known as 'Magill' or 'Lack' consists of corrugated tubing or coaxial system with an Adjustable pressure limiting (APL) at patient end with a 2L reservoir bag at anaesthetic machine end. A simple system but can prove cumbersome and not suitable for use when ventilation is required. The modern version of this system, the Lack, which is coaxial or parallel and the APL valve is at the anaesthetic machine end. A very good system for spontaneous breathing.

Mapleson D

Commonly known today as a 'Bain' coaxial system, inefficient for spontaneous breathing because the exhaled gas passes into the reservoir bag and there is a chance of rebreathing unless fresh gas flow is high. Good for IPPV and is useful if anaesthesia access to the patient is compromised i.e. head and neck surgery.

Mapleson E and F

Commonly known today as Ayre's T Piece (E) (Phillip Ayre, 1937) and Jackson Rees Modification (F) (Dr Jackson Rees). These systems are used for paediatric patients up to 25–30kg body weight[2] because of their lack of resistance and limited 'dead space', and their valveless state. They are suitable for spontaneous and controlled ventilation.

As there is no APL valve with these systems then scavenging of waste anaesthetic gases can be problematic. Anaesthetists and competent anaesthetic assistants have devised various techniques for this to occur. Certain manufacturers have designed paediatric systems with APL valves so that scavenging can occur. However the use of this particular system is debatable.

Circle systems

The advantages of using the circle system is that they use very low fresh gas consumption and volatile anaesthetic agents (saves money), absorb CO_2 (saves pollution), and they warm and humidify anaesthetic gases (maintain normothermia) (adapted from Fenlon[3]). Appropriate monitoring must be used before this system is utilised.[4]

A diagrammatic version of a circle system is shown in Fig. 8.2.

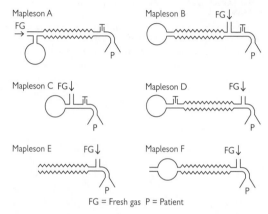

FG = Fresh gas   P = Patient

Fig. 8.1 Breathing circuits. Reproduced with permission from Allman KG and Wilson IH (eds) (2006). *Oxford Handbook of Anaesthesia* (2nd edn). Oxford University Press, Oxford.

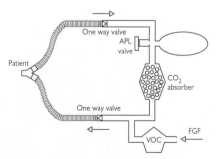

Fig. 8.2 Circle breathing system with CO_2 absorption and VOC.

References and further reading

1. Ince CS, Skinner AC, and Taft E (2000). Scientific principles in relation to the anaesthetic machine. In Ince CS and Davey A (eds). *Fundamentals of Operating Department Practice*. Greenwich Medical Media: London.

2. Al-Shaikh B and Stacey S (2002). *Essentials of Anaesthetic Equipment*. Churchill Livingstone: London.

3. Fenlon S (2005). Equipment for paediatric anaesthesia. In Davey A and Diba A (eds). *Ward's Anaesthetic Equipment*. Elsevier Saunders: London.

4. Association of Anaesthetists of Great Britain and Ireland (2004). *Checking anaesthetic equipment*. AAGBI: London.

Association of Anaesthetists of Great Britain and Ireland (2007). *Recommendations for standards of monitoring during anaesthesia and recovery* (4th edn). AAGBI: London.

Lockwood GG (2007). Circle systems. *Anaesthesia and Intensive Care Medicine* **10**(4) 215–21.

Lovell, T (2007). Breathing systems. *Anaesthesia and Intensive Care Medicine* **8**(3) 102–6.

Humidifiers

Dry anaesthetic gases can affect the cells lining of the respiratory tract. Humidification devices used in anaesthesia and anaesthetic breathing systems are used as a counter to the heat lost to vaporise water in the airway.

The main humidifiers used in anaesthesia are capable of providing microbiological protection for the patient. They are single-patient use and should be positioned as close to the patient's mouth as possible, normally between the catheter mount, which is connected to the ET or other airway adjunct, e.g. LMA, and the anaesthetic breathing system of choice.

The majority of humidifiers used in the clinical area have a provision for connection of a sampling tube for gas and vapour concentration analysers. HME humidifiers are compact, passive, inexpensive, and are the most appropriate for clinical situations.

They function by allowing condensation of water vapour exhalation. They contain a hygroscopic or hydrophobic element as well as a bacterial filter.[1]

Hygroscopic membrane HMEs

Hygroscopic membrane HMEs have the following characteristics (adapted from Poolacherla and Nickells[2]):
- Foam, paper, or wool-like material.
- Coated with moisture-retaining chemicals.
- Impregnated with bactericide.
- Subjected to electrical field to increase its polarity.
- More efficient than hydrophobic HMEs.

Hydrophobic membrane HMEs

Hydrophobic membrane HMEs have the following characteristics (adapted from Poolacherla and Nickells[2]):
- Folded ceramic fibre.
- Surface area must be high.
- Membrane is pleated.
- Low thermal conductivity.
- Allows passage of water vapour.
- Can use nebulisation.
- Performance impaired with high ambient temperatures.

The use of low fresh gas flows in a circle system helps to conserve heat and moisture. The reaction of the soda lime and CO_2 produces heat and moisture.[1]

Heated humidifiers are used in the critical care setting when ventilatory assistance may be required for a number of days rather than hours. They utilise the same principles as vaporisers in the fact that they heat (45–60°C), power, and can maintain a constant and stable humidification of fresh gas flows.

Safety systems

- HMEs must be checked on regular occasions as an accumulation of water in the filter may cause an increase in airway resistance.[2]
- All humidifier systems increase the number of connections within the anaesthetic circuit and potentially increase the risk of disconnection. To minimise this risk a disconnection alarm should be utilised and all connections must be checked on regular occasions and pushed home and twisted.[1]

References and further reading

1. McKindoe A (2003). Humidification devices. *Anaesthesia and Intensive Care Medicine* **4**(11) 353–4.

2. Poolacherla R and Nickells J (2006). Humidification devices. *Anaesthesia and Intensive Care Medicine* **7**(10), 351–3.

3. Al-Shaikh B and Stacey S (2002). *Essentials of Anaesthetic Equipment*. Churchill Livingstone: London.

Association of Anaesthetists of Great Britain and Ireland (2007). *Recommendations for standards of monitoring during anaesthesia and recovery* (4th edn). AAGBI: London.

Association of Anaesthetists of Great Britain and Ireland (2004). *Checking anaesthetic equipment.* AAGBI: London.

Fluid/blood warmers

Fluid/blood warmers are used to infuse warmed fluids to patients. Previously this was done by immersing an infusion coil in a water bath. This is no longer acceptable as they were messy and an excellent medium for bacterial growth.[1] There are two systems that are currently in use: dry heat warmers and the coaxial fluid heating system.

Dry heat warmers

- These consist of two heated plates in which the plastic insert is sandwiched and primed with a crystalloid (normal saline).
- Newer devices utilise a cassette (Fluido®) which is inserted into the machine and can be transferred with the patient to other areas of care.
- Other dry heat warmers include cylindrical devices that utilise giving-sets extension however these are laborious to use.
- These devices increase the resistance to flow and significantly add to the giving-set dead space.[2]

Coaxial fluid heating system (Hotline®)

- These consist of three lumens within the devise with one lumen carrying the infusate to the patient and the other two lumens carrying water heated to 40°C and stored within the heating case.
- The infusate does not come into contact with the circulating water. The coaxial tubing extends to the IV cannula thus ensuring that the tubing is not exposed to room temperature.[2]

A further development involves the use of a pre-shaped heat exchange coil that is situated within the ducting of a forced air convective warmer.[1] There are methods for rapidly infusing warm fluids but this is not discussed in this section; however, further information can be found in the further reading section and on the Medicines and Healthcare products Regulatory Agency (MHRA) website.[3]

References and further reading

1. Diba A (2005). Infusion equipment and intravenous anaesthesia. In Davey A and Diba A (eds). *Ward's Anaesthetic Equipment*. Elsevier Saunders: London.

2. Al-Shaikh B and Stacey S (2002). *Essentials of Anaesthetic Equipment*. Churchill Livingstone: London.

3. Medicines and Healthcare products Regulatory Agency (MHRA). Available at: ▣ www.mhra. gov.uk/index.htm

Association of Anaesthetists of Great Britain and Ireland (2007). *Recommendations for standards of monitoring during anaesthesia and recovery* (4th edn). AAGBI: London.

Association of Anaesthetists of Great Britain and Ireland (2004). *Checking anaesthetic equipment*. AAGBI: London.

Monitoring

The range of monitoring devices is broad and ever increasing. You should ensure that the monitoring devices used in patient care are fit for purpose whatever the circumstances. In addition to this:

- You should have adequate knowledge of the equipment before its use.
- Calibration of all monitoring equipment should be carried out prior to use when necessary and/or be part of a maintenance programme.
- Monitoring devices are there to keep the team aware of the patient's physiological state, record data, and ensure patient safety.
- Monitors are an adjunct to anaesthesia and are no substitute to patient observation.

Remember: monitor the patient and not the monitor.

The AAGBI[1] have set minimal standards that are acceptable for monitoring patients during anaesthesia and recovery periods and advocate the following:

- Monitoring must be attached before the anaesthetic starts and the patient's physiological state should be continued to be monitored until the patient has recovered.
- All patient physiological data collected must be recorded in the patient's notes. If electronic data is being stored then this should comply with local and national policy including the Data Protection Act.
- If a non-medical member of the perioperative team is recording the patient's vital signs then it should be ensured they have the competencies to translate the data and act appropriately should the need arise.
- The anaesthetist is responsible for ensuring that the monitoring has been checked, that it is fit for use, and alarm limits have been set and are audible.
- Monitoring that is deemed essential for the safe conduct of anaesthesia are, pulse oximeter, NIBP monitor, electrocardiography, airway gases; O_2, CO_2, vapour and airway pressure. Also having available a nerve stimulator and some means of measuring the patient's temperature.

Patients should also be monitored when receiving a local/regional anaesthetic or sedative technique when surgical intervention is undertaken. AAGBI[1] state that the minimum monitoring required in this situation is:

- Pulse oximeter.
- NIBP monitor.
- Electrocardiography.

References and further reading

1. Association of Anaesthetists of Great Britain and Ireland (2007). *Recommendations for standards of monitoring during anaesthesia and recovery* (4th edn). AAGBI: London.

Al-Shaikh B and Stacey S (2002). *Essentials of Anaesthetic Equipment*. Churchill Livingstone: London.

Association of Anaesthetists of Great Britain and Ireland (2004). *Checking anaesthetic equipment*. AAGBI: London.

Davey A and Ince CS (2000). *Fundamentals of operating department practice*. Greenwich Medical Media Ltd.,:London.

Non-invasive monitoring

Non-invasive monitoring that is frequently used within the perioperative environment includes:[1]

- ECG.
- NIBP.
- Pulse oximetry.
- Peripheral nerve stimulators.
- Capnography—end-tidal carbon dioxide analyser.
- Respiratory rate.
- Airway gases.
- Vapours.
- Nerve stimulator.
- Temperature measurement.

ECG

An ECG monitors the electrical activity of the heart and will determine rate, arrhythmias, conduction defects, and ischemia.

- ECG monitoring consists of skin electrodes which use silver and silver chloride along with a conducting gel, an amplifier to boost the signal and filter out other frequencies, and an oscilloscope to display the ECG.
- When placing the electrodes on the skin ensure they are attached properly by first cleaning the skin.
- Attaching the electrodes over bony prominences will reduce the occurrence of artefacts produced by muscular activity such as shivering.
- A 3-lead ECG is normally used during the perioperative phase:
  - Although there are many configurations, the 3-lead used most widely is left arm, right arm, and left leg and the latter is often placed over the apex; this allows lead I, II, and III to be monitored and the anaesthetist can choose which provides the best amplitude.
- CM5 configuration can be used if cardiac ischaemia is a concern.
- The CM5 configuration consists of one lead over manubrium sterni, the second lead normally placed over the left clavicle on a bony prominence, and the third lead in the V5 position over the left ventricle.
- CM5 configuration will detect left ventricular ischemia.
- Electrical interference can be caused by other equipment such as diathermy and mobile phones. Most modern monitors are produced with shielding to limit this interference. The MHRA highlight that mobile phones can adversely affect some medical equipment and therefore the Association for Perioperative Practice[2] recommend that all mobile phones should be switched off in the perioperative environment.
- Diathermy burns can occur at the ECG electrode site in the absence of, or misplacement of, a diathermy plate as the passage of the electrical current from the diathermy can pass through the ECG electrodes.

NIBP

- NIBPs are normally performed with the use of an automatic NIBP measurement device.
- This device gives trend information on systolic, diastolic, mean arterial pressures, and pulse rate.
- It consists of a cuff and tube which connects to an inflation and deflation device.
- A pressure transducer and microprocessor converts the fluctuations in the cuff pressures into a readable BP measurement on the monitor.
- It is essential that the correct size cuff is used, the middle of the cuff bladder should be positioned over the brachial artery, and the cuff should cover at least 2/3 of the patient's upper arm and should be free of kinks and folds. This will ensure the optimum conditions for a correct reading and prevent soft tissue injury to the patient.
- If the cuff is too small it will over-read the BP; equally if the cuff is large it will under-read the BP, though the error is greater when the cuff is too small.
- Atrial fibrillation and other arrhythmias will affect NIBP readings.
- On the initial BP the cuff will inflate to above the previous systolic pressure.
- As the cuff is inflated and deflated the transducer senses the oscillations in the cuff from the returning blood flow
- Mean arterial pressure corresponds to the maximum oscillations at the lowest cuff pressure; systolic pressure corresponds to the rapidly increasing oscillations; and diastolic pressure corresponds to the rapidly decreasing oscillations.

References and further reading

1. Association of Anaesthetists of Great Britain and Ireland (2007). *Recommendations for standards of monitoring during anaesthesia and recovery* (4th edn). AAGBI: London.

2. Association for Perioperative practice (AfPP) (2007). *Standards and recommendations for safe perioperative practice.* AfPP: Harrogate.

Al-Shaikh B and Stacey S (2002). *Essentials of Anaesthetic Equipment.* Churchill Livingstone: London.

Davey A and Ince CS (2000). *Fundamentals of operating department practice.* Greenwich Medical Media Ltd.: London.

Huddesmith J, Wheeler D, and Gupta A (2004). *Core topics in perioperative medicine.* Greenwich Medical Media Ltd.: London.

Pulse oximetry

- This measures the arterial blood O_2 at the arterioles.
- Pulse oximetry is made up of a probe which consists of two light emitting diodes on one side a photodetector on the other, and a microprocessor which displays the O_2 saturation, pulse rate, and a waveform.
- Alarm limits can be set for low and high saturation readings and low and high pulse rates.
- Red and infrared light is emitted from the diodes at 660nm and 940nm, emitting the light at a high frequency of about 30 times per second.
- The red and infrared light from the diodes passes through the skin, tissue, and bone, and a percentage of this light is absorbed.
- The photodetector detects the returning light transmitted through the tissue which the microprocessor is programmed to mathematically analyse into a readable O_2 saturation level.
- Inaccurate readings can be given when the patient is suffering from carbon monoxide poisoning, including smoking, coloured nail varnish, IV injection of certain dyes such as methylene blue, hypoperfusion, and severe vasoconstriction.
- If the oximetry probe becomes disconnected, it can take some time for the peripheral saturation to change; if this occurs, closely observe the patient's colour.
- Inaccurate measurements can be caused by excessive movement, malpositioning of the probe, and external florescent light. Probes have also been known to read a percentage when attached to nothing except a blanket.
- Be aware that probes can also cause pressure damage if left on one site for too long; some manufacturers suggest that the position of the probe should be changed every 2 hours.

Peripheral nerve stimulators

- Peripheral nerve stimulation is used during the anaesthetic phase to monitor the degree of neuromuscular blockade.
- They can also be used to confirm adequate reversal of neuromuscular blockade.
- Two surface electrodes, normally ECG electrodes, are positioned over the nerve and connected via leads to the stimulator which is battery operated. There are also stimulators available with detachable ball electrodes to enable skin contact.
- Supramaximal stimulation is used to stimulate the muscle.
- When supramaximal stimulation is used, contraction of the muscle is observed visually, palpated, or measured by a pressure transducer.
- The most common nerves used are ulna, posterior tibial, facial, and common peroneal.
- There are various methods of monitoring neuromuscular transmission:
  - Twitch—short duration stimulus every 10 seconds.
  - Tetanic stimulation.
  - Train-of-four (ToF)—this is four supra-maximal stimuli of 0.1–0.2ms duration delivered at 2Hz, i.e. 0.5 seconds between.

- Post tetanic count—is used to assess more profound degrees of block.
- Double burst.
- It is essential to remember the smaller the muscle group being stimulated, the more sensitive it is to the muscle relaxant, therefore this might not reflect the true picture of the depth of diaphragmatic block.
- Nerve stimulators can also be used to assist in locating the nerve tract when attempting regional anaesthesia.

Respiratory rate

- Respiratory rate is normally monitored by observation of the patient—calculate the rise and fall of the patient's chest on inhalation and exhalation over a period of 1 minute.
- The adequacy of ventilation is judged clinically by the colouring of the patient and the absence of distress associated with breathing difficulties.
- Patients who are recovering from anaesthesia can be particularly prone to airway obstruction due to secretion or blood in the upper airway.
- The following patients are also at risk of reduced respiratory function:
  - Patients following cardiothoracic surgery.
  - Morbidly obese.
  - Heavy smokers.
  - Neuromuscular blockade administration.
  - Patients with pre-existing pulmonary disorders.
- Anaesthetised patients' respiratory rate and volume are normally monitored by:
  - Pneumotachography—measures gas flow.
  - Pressure monitoring during controlled ventilation.
  - Volume monitoring either using pneumotachography or respirometer (measures tidal and minute volume).

Capnography (end-tidal carbon dioxide analyser)

- Capnography is used to monitor levels of ventilation, confirm tracheal intubation, as a disconnection alarm, and to diagnose lung embolisation and malignant hyperpyrexia.
- It can be performed by either mainstream (within the patient's gas stream) or sidestream analysers (at the distal end of the breathing system via a sampling tube).
- Using the principles of infrared absorption for CO_2, the rise and fall of CO_2 is measure through the respiratory cycle.

References and further reading

Al-Shaikh B and Stacey S (2002). *Essentials of Anaesthetic Equipment*. Churchill Livingstone: London.

Association of Anaesthetists of Great Britain and Ireland (2007). *Recommendations for standards of monitoring during anaesthesia and recovery* (4th edn). AAGBI: London.

Davey A and Ince CS (2000). *Fundamentals of operating department practice*. Greenwich Medical Media Ltd.: London.

Huddesmith J, Wheeler D, and Gupta A (2004). *Core topics in perioperative medicine*. Greenwich Medical Media Ltd.: London.

Invasive monitoring

Invasive arterial pressure

- Invasive arterial pressure monitoring allows for beat-by-beat measurement of the BP with continual accuracy.
- Indications for use would be a patient's condition predisposing towards severe changes in BP during the perioperative period and therefore constant measurement of BP is required, e.g. trauma, pre-existing cardiovascular disease.
- Indications for invasive arterial pressure monitoring may include rapid major haemodynamic instability such as blood loss and large fluid shifts. Also patients undergoing cardiopulmonary bypass as this is the only way to assess if bypass is providing adequate perfusion pressures.
- Arterial blood can also be taken as a sample for arterial blood gas analysis.

Cannula site

- An indwelling arterial cannula is inserted into:
  - Radial artery: first preference if palpable. If radial artery is cannulated then an Allen test should be performed to ensure that there is collateral flow through the ulna artery. In case there is no collateral flow through the ulna artery, radial artery puncture is contraindicated since it can result in a gangrenous finger or loss of the hand from spasm or clotting of the radial artery.
  - Brachial artery: if radial not palpable.
  - Femoral artery: only if access is limited as this site is a potentially dirty area and a risk of infection.
  - Axillary artery: if others unavailable.
  - Dorsalis pedis: if access is limited (e.g. neurosurgery).
- The cannula is then attached to a transducer which has previously been zeroed to atmospheric pressure and set at the sternal angle/mid-axillary line of the patient.
- The current generated in the transducer is then measured and converted electronically and displayed on the monitor as systolic, diastolic, and mean arterial pressures.

Complications

- Infection: as with all invasive procedures strict aseptic technique should be adhered to.
- Arterial injection: arterial lines should be dressed appropriately stating clearly that the line is arterial. Arterial cannulas are specifically designed to eliminate this potential risk as they do not have an injection port.
- Bleeding: it is essential that the cannula is dressed properly and that all connections are tightened to ensure they do not disconnect. Patients can exsanguinate if this goes unnoticed.
- Clotting: though this is reduced with the constant flush device inbuilt to the transducer sets.
- Ischemia distal to the cannula.
- Haematoma: this is normally related to multiple attempts of insertion.

References and further reading

Association of Anaesthetists of Great Britain and Ireland (2007). *Recommendations for standards of monitoring during anaesthesia and recovery* (4th edn). AAGBI: London.

Al-Shaikh B and Stacey S (2002). *Essentials of Anaesthetic Equipment.* Churchill Livingstone: London.

Huddesmith J, Wheeler D, and Gupta A (2004). *Core topics in perioperative medicine.* Greenwich Medical Media Ltd.: London.

Central venous pressure

- CVP measurement is used to closely monitor fluid balance when either significant shifts/losses are anticipated in connection with the planned surgery or if required by the patient's clinical condition.
- It directly measures the filling pressure of the right atrium.
- It can also be used for sampling blood, administering drugs, parental nutrition, and haemofiltration for haemodialysis.
- The Seldinger technique was originally devised for the insertion of venous or arterial catheters for radiological investigations[1] and is now commonly used to insert central venous catheters:
  - A guide wire is inserted into the needle used for venous puncture.
  - The guide wire then allows the needle to be withdrawn and, in succession, dilators and eventually the catheter to be railroaded over the guide wire in to position. The guide wire is then removed.
- Catheters can present as either single lines or up to four ports (quad lines) and can be inserted when the patient is awake under local anaesthetic; this can be unpleasant and patient support is essential.
- Before the central line is used confirmation of the placement of the catheter via x-ray should be confirmed.

Cannula site

- Veins of the arm: these are sometimes described as long lines and are free from complication of direct approaches such as pneumothorax:
  - Median basilica vein.
  - Cephalic vein.
- External jugular vein: can be difficult to place.
- Subclavian vein: high incidence of pneumothorax.
- Internal jugular vein: can produce haematoma if the carotid artery is pierced.
- Femoral vein: high incidence of thrombophlebitis and leg oedema.

Complications

- Guide wire: when the guide wire is being inserted the anesthetic assistant should monitor the patient's ECG. If the guide wire is inserted too far it enters the right atrium of the heart which will cause an increase in cardiac rhythm or ectopic beats; if this occurs the anesthetist should be informed immediately.
- Patient positioning: it is essential that the patient is positioned in a head-down tilt as air can be entrained through the cannula causing an air embolus; the head-down position also enlarges the neck veins.
- Pneumothorax with central vein techniques.
- Haematoma.
- Infection: as with all invasive procedures strict aseptic technique should be adhered to.

Setting up transducers

- A cannula is attached to a column of bubble-free saline (CVP) or heparinised saline (for arterial line) (manometer line) which flows through a transducer to a bag of saline/heparinised saline that is under approximately 300mmHg of pressure via a pressure bag.

- The monometer line and the transducer kit are made from a material that reduces compliance. This is important when considering the recordable trace from the transducer as compliant tubing would cause dampening and therefore reduce the trace. Equally if the materials are too stiff then this would cause resonance.
- Due to the pressure and a constant flushing device, which is built into the transducer set, a constant flush of 3–4mL/hour of saline/hepranised saline is delivered through the cannula. Therefore clotting and backflow through the cannula is prevented. There is also the ability to manually flush the cannula.
- Within the transducer is a diaphragm which is an extremely thin membrane that acts as an interface between the transducer and the column of water.
- As the column of fluid moves with the arterial pulsation over the diaphragm it causes changes in resistance which allows current to flow through the wires of the transducer.
- The transducer is attached via cables to an amplifier, oscilloscope.
- Complications with invasive monitoring equipment include:
  - Dampening of the trace which can be related to changes in the patient's position. Raising the transducer above or below the sterna angle/mid-axillary line of the patient will result in error readings.
  - Air in the transducer set—this is the most common complication.

Oesophageal Doppler

- This technique interprets images gained by Doppler in the oesophagus.
- Oesophageal Doppler allows for continuous monitoring of the left and right ventricle as well as the detection of early myocardial ischemia.
- The probe with manipulation can also view cardiac valves, coronary vessels, and coronary grafts.
- Visualisation of the cardiac chambers, the aorta, vena cava, and pulmonary arteries can also be achieved.
- Patients need to be adequately sedated or intubated though a suprasternal probe is available and can be used on awake patients.

Complications

- The probe can cause damage to the oesophagus and burns.
- The readings and their interpretation are dependent on operator expertise.
- Insertion of the probe is not recommended in patients with pharygo-oesophageal pathology.

References and further reading

1. Simpson PJ and Popart MT (2002). Understanding anaesthesia (4th edn). Butterworth-Heinemann: Oxford.

Al-Shaikh B and Stacey S (2002). Essentials of anaesthetic equipment (2nd Ed). Churchill Livingstone: London.

Davey A and Ince CS (2000). Fundamentals of operating department practice. Greenwich Medical Media Ltd.: London.

Huddesmith J, Wheeler D, and Gupta A (2004). Core topics in perioperative medicine. Greenwich Medical Media Ltd.: London.

Monitoring obese patients

The AAGBI recommend that monitoring the following is essential at the induction of anaesthesia for *all patients*:
- ECG.
- NIBP.
- SpO_2.
- Airway gas.

ECG

A 3-lead ECG, referred to as standard limb leads, is generally used during anaesthesia.
- The electrodes are commonly placed on the right arm (red) and left arm (yellow) with a third, left leg (black/dark green), placed more commonly on the left side of the thorax.
- With obese patients it may be necessary to relocate the electrodes in order to obtain a better trace.
- One alternative to the above is to place the electrodes on the arms of the patient e.g. red to right forearm, with yellow and black either aspect of the left forearm
- This configuration may also be useful when dealing with agitated patients or children as it is less intrusive than rearranging clothing to apply the electrodes in a more conventional layout.

NIBP

There are many sizes of cuffs available for today's monitors. They range in length and width to fit babies through to large adults, therefore a cuff should be chosen that fits the patient comfortably i.e. is long enough to encompass the limb and that the width does not impede joint movement.
- Practitioners should ensure that whatever the cuff size, that it is placed correctly over the artery, failure to do so might cause an incorrect reading, or appear as a fault on the monitor screen.
- Where there is a deep layer of body fat the NIBP will often be difficult or sometimes impossible to record; in this situation the practitioner should consider a different size cuff, and/or an alternative placement sites e.g. the patient's forearm in favour of the upper arm, or the calf area where sometimes leaner tissue can be located.
- Failure to obtain readings using this method may result in having to apply invasive monitoring techniques.

When dealing with patients who are agitated, or children, it might be wise not to attach the monitoring (unless medically contraindicated) until immediately after the induction of anaesthesia so as not to further upset the patient.

SpO$_2$

Obese patients will often have large fingers, which will often lead to inaccurate SpO$_2$ readings of both the pulse and saturation.

• In these situations alternative probe placement sites should be considered e.g. the toes.
• The use of a smaller multi-use pulse oximeter probe should also be considered for other areas that may be suitable e.g. the ear lobe

Airway gas

Monitoring the airway gas gives a clear indication that the patient's airway is patent.

• The digitalised wave form of the capnograph signifies that the patent's lung function is good, and that gaseous exchange is taking place.
• The measurement is obtained via the capnograph sensor placed within the patient's anaesthetic circuit and attached to the anaesthetic machine.
• When an obese patient lies in the supine position, their abdominal contents push up their diaphragm, restricting its movement—if this is the case, the patient should be positioned 'sitting up' or tilt the head.

References

Association of Anaesthetists of Great Britain and Ireland (2007). *Perioperative management of the morbidly obese patient.* AAGBI: London.

Association of Anaesthetists of Great Britain and Ireland (2007). *Recommendations for standards of monitoring during anaesthesia and recovery* (4th edn). AAGBI: London.

Association of Anaesthetists of Great Britain and Ireland (2004). *Checking anaesthetic equipment.* AAGBI: London.

Association of Anaesthetists of Great Britain and Ireland (2001). *Preoperative assessment: the role of the anaesthetist.* AAGBI: London.

National Obesity Forum. Available from: www.nationalobesityforum.org.uk

National Obesity Care Pathway (2005). Available from: http://nationalobesityforum.org.uk/images/stories/Obesity_Care_Path.pdf

Royal College of Anaesthetists (2004). *Guidelines for the Provision of Anaesthetic Services.* RCoA: London.

Arterial blood gases

Definition

An arterial blood gas is a set of tests performed on a sample of arterial blood. Results from this test provide the practitioner with information about:

- Adequacy and extent of gas exchange in the lungs.[1]
- Acid–base balance

Additionally, the test may provide fractional O_2 saturation SaO_2, and may also provide serum concentrations of the electrolytes Na^+, K^+, blood glucose, and serum lactate.

The sample

A sample of 3–4mL of arterial blood is drawn into a heparinised syringe (commercially available syringes with freeze-dried heparin are commonly used). The blood sample is obtained in two ways:

- An arterial 'stab'—usually the radial artery.
- From an indwelling arterial catheter.

Precautions

- The blood sample should be labelled appropriately (if going to a lab for analysis):
- Include FiO_2 on the request.
- Include patient temperature on the request.
- The sample should be fresh—continued cellular metabolism can affect the result.
- No air bubbles should be present—air bubbles can dissolve in the plasma which will affect the result.

Result interpretation

This may appear a little daunting, but with the adoption of a systematic approach can be readily achieved.

Normal ranges[2]

- PaO_2:   12–15KPa (90–110 mmHg).
- $PaCO_2$:   4.5–6KPa (34–46 mmHg).
- HCO_3:   21–27.5mmol/L.
- H^+ ions   36–44nmol/L (pH 7.35–7.45).

Remember to use your laboratory's reference values.

A five-step approach to result interpretation[3]

Firstly, ensure that the result is for your patient!

- Step 1: what is the PaO_2? Is the patient hypoxic?
- Step 2: look at the pH, is the patient acidaemic (pH <7.35) or alkalaemic (pH >7.45)?
- Step 3: look at $PaCO_2$, <4KPa= respiratory alkalosis, >6KPa= respiratory acidosis.
- Step 4: look at HCO_3, <21= metabolic acidosis, >27.5 = metabolic alkalosis.
- Step 5: determine compensation.

The body attempts to maintain pH within the normal range by compensation. The body compensates for acid–base disturbances as follows:
- If the primary cause is metabolic, the respiratory system will compensate by increasing or decreasing excretion of CO_2.
- If the primary cause is respiratory the renal system compensates by excretion or reabsorption of bicarbonate and acidification of urine.

References

1. Rempher K and Morton GM (2005). Patient assessment: Respiratory system. In Morton PG, Fontaine DK, Hudak GM, *et al.* (eds). *Critical Care Nursing A Holistic Approach* (8th edn), p.492–516. Lippencott Williams and Wilkins: Philadelphia.

2. Waugh A and Grant A (2006). *Ross and Wilson Anatomy and Physiology in Health and Illness* (10th edn). Churchill Livingstone: Edinburgh.

3. Resuscitation Council UK (2006). *Advanced Life Support* (5th edn). Resuscitation Council UK: London.

Acid–base balance

Definition

Normal cellular activity within the body requires that the balance between acids and bases in body fluids is tightly controlled.[1] Usefully, the balance between acids and bases is reflected in the pH of the extracellular fluid.[2]

Measuring pH

- The normal range for the pH of blood is between 7.35 and 7.45.[2]
- Deviation from this range can have major effects on body systems, especially the CNS and the cardiovascular system.[1]

Common terms

- An acid is a substance that can donate a hydrogen ion when in solution e.g. hydrochloric acid (a strong acid) or carbonic acid (a weak acid).
- A base is a substance that can accept a hydrogen ion from a solution e.g. bicarbonate.
- Acidaemia is said to exist when the pH of the blood is <7.35.
- Alkalaemia is said to exist when the pH of the blood is >7.45.
- The term acidosis refers to the process that is causing the acidaemia.
- The term alkalosis refers to the process that is causing the alkalaemia.[3]
- The relatively constant balance between acids and bases is maintained by three systems:
  - Buffers.
  - The respiratory system.
  - The renal system.

Determining acid–base balance

Acid–base balance is determined by completing steps 3–5 of the arterial blood gas analysis (📖 see A five-step approach to result interpretation, p.160).

Common causes of acid–base disturbances

- Acidosis is more common than alkalosis.
- Respiratory acidosis is caused by an increase in CO_2—e.g. reduced conscious level, head injury, chest trauma, chest infection, inadequate ventilation, atelectasis.
- Respiratory alkalosis is caused by a decrease in CO_2— e.g. hyperventilation, fear, pain.
- Metabolic acidosis—e.g. renal failure, ketoacidosis, severe diarrhoea.
- Metabolic alkalosis—e.g. overuse of antacids, GI fistula losses, prolonged NG free drainage.

Treatment of acid–base disturbances

The usual treatment is to try and correct the underlying cause, e.g. hypoventilation following early extubation with a decreased respiratory rate could cause a respiratory acidosis; the treatment would be to ensure adequate ventilation.

A patient who is hypovolaemic may develop a metabolic acidosis because of poor peripheral circulation, resulting in a build up of metabolic acids e.g. lactic acid. Treatment here would be to ensure adequate circulation through the administration of fluids.

References

1. Waugh A and Grant A (2006). *Ross and Wilson Anatomy and Physiology in Health and Illness* (10th edn). Churchill Livingstone: Edinburgh.

2. Porth C (2008). *Essentials of Pathophysiology* (2nd edn). Lippincott, Williams and Wilkins: Philadelphia.

3. Rempher K and Morton GM (2005). Patient assessment: Respiratory system In Morton PG, Fontaine DK, Hudak GM, et al. (eds). *Critical Care Nursing: A Holistic Approach* (8th edn). Lippencott Williams and Wilkins: Philadelphia.

Medical gas cylinders

Identification of colour-coded cylinders

- All medical gas cylinders make use of a system of a unique colouring which assists in the identification of their contents.
- From July 2006 all new medical gas cylinders in the UK have been coloured according to the new standard BS EN1089:3.
- *Caution:* full transition to the new system is expected to take until 2010.
- Colour alone must **never** be used to identify contents of a cylinder
- Labels on the cylinder/cylinder collar **must** be the primary method of identifying contents.
- **Never** use a cylinder unless the contents can be clearly identified.
- An empty cylinder weight is referred to as 'Tare Weight'.

Checking of cylinders and its contents

Every cylinder has a number of other identifying markings on the cylinder shoulder/valve block. These markings contain the following information:
- Name and chemical symbol of the gas/mixture contained.
- Cylinder size/capacity.
- Empty cylinder weight.
- Maximum working pressure and test pressure.

Cylinders also have plastic collars attached that contain:
- Directions for use.
- Storage and handling instructions.
- Appropriate hazard warning notice.
- Shelf life and expiry date.
- Batch number.
- Product licence number.

In addition, cylinders are supplied with a red or white plastic safety seal that covers the gas outlet, held in place by clear plastic shrink wrap. This prevents dust or other foreign bodies from entering the gas outlet, and also acts as a visual safety indicator.

References

Allman KG and Wilson IH (eds) (2006). *Oxford Handbook of Anaesthesia* (2nd edn). Oxford University Press: Oxford.

Al-Shaikh B and Stacey S (2002). *Essentials of Anaesthetic Equipment*. Churchill Livingstone: London.

Association of Anaesthetists of Great Britain and Ireland (2004). *Checking anaesthetic equipment.* AAGBI: London.

Royal College of Anaesthetists (2004). *Guidelines for the Provision of Anaesthetic Services*. RCoA: London.

Attaching cylinders to pin index system on an anaesthetic machine

- The pin index safety system (BS EN 850) is an *almost* foolproof safety system which prevents the connection of cylinders at the wrong location.
- System comprises of a pair of locating holes beneath the gas outlet of the cylinder valve block which correspond to a pair of pins located at the inlet connection of the relevant machine.
- Pin/hole positions are unique for each gas and therefore prevent incorrect connection of cylinders.

To attach a gas cylinder to any piece of equipment—anaesthetic machine, insufflator or regulator:
- The shrink wrap covered seal is removed.
- The valve opened momentarily to blow away any foreign bodies or debris.
- The cylinder is then securely attached to the relevant piece of equipment by offering up the pin index holes on cylinder block to the corresponding pins located on the machine yolk taking care not to force the fit.
- The cylinder is then secured to the machine yolk by the appropriate means.
- The valve is slowly opened by two anti-clockwise turns of the spindle.

In the event of a leak—usually an audible hiss or an unexplained loss of gas/drop in pressure—then:
- Check that the locking screw is sufficiently tight.

If the leak remains after tightening:
- The cylinder should be turned off and removed from the piece of equipment.
- The sealing washer between the cylinder and the equipment i.e. the bodock washer or the rubber 'O' ring should be checked for damage and replaced as necessary.

If the problem remains consider replacing the cylinder and/or the particular piece of equipment.

Never force an ill-fitting cylinder:
- It may be the incorrect type/size cylinder.
- Attempts to force it may cause the index pins to be bent out of shape or dislodged, preventing the attachment of another cylinder or allowing the connection of an incorrect cylinder with potentially disastrous results.

Safe storage of cylinders
- Under cover, preferably inside, dry, clean environment avoiding extremes of temperature.
- Not near combustible material or sources of heat.
- Medical gases should be stored separately from other gases.
- Where more than one type of gas is stored in a location, gases should be segregated.

- Under no circumstance should cylinders be repainted, markings on the cylinder/valve block obscured, or labels be removed.
- F-size cylinders should be stored vertically, E-size and smaller stored horizontally.

Pipeline gases

- Whilst cylinders provide a more mobile form of gas supply, the majority of gas supplied within the perioperative setting is by means of pipelines fed by either bulk tanks or large cylinder manifolds.
- The colour coding used on cylinders also extends to pipeline supplies, with pipes and connection points taking on the same colour as the relevant cylinder shoulder.
- Pipeline connections also make use of a unique interface to prevent the incorrect connections.
- Only wall mounted connection points and associated pipelines that are compliant with HTM 02-01 should be used for delivery of medical gases to patients.

References

Allman KG and Wilson IH (eds) (2006). *Oxford Handbook of Anaesthesia* (2nd edn). Oxford University Press: Oxford.

Al-Shaikh B and Stacey S (2002). *Essentials of Anaesthetic Equipment.* Churchill Livingstone: London.

Association of Anaesthetists of Great Britain and Ireland (2004). *Checking anaesthetic equipment.* AAGBI: London.

Royal College of Anaesthetists (2004). *Guidelines for the Provision of Anaesthetic Services.* RCoA: London.

Simpson J and Popat M (2002). *Understanding anaesthesia.* Butterworth-Heinemann: Edinburgh.

Scientific principles

Heat and humans

The difference between heat and temperature

Although, in everyday language, heat and temperature are considered to be the same, strictly speaking they are not:

- **Heat** is a measurement of the *total energy* (kinetic and potential) of the molecules or atoms making up a substance. This energy can be transferred from a hotter substance to a colder substance. The heat of a body depends both upon its temperature and mass
- **Temperature** is a measurement of the *average kinetic energy* of individual molecules or atoms of a substance; temperature can be regarded as the relative degree of 'hotness' or 'coldness' of a body.

Body temperature

Although normal body temperature is usually regarded as an oral temperature of approx 37°C, a range of values of temperature can be observed both in, and between, 'normal' individuals (±0.6°C). 'Normal' body temperature also varies with:

- Time of day—up to approx 1°C between early morning and late afternoon/early evening.
- Menstrual cycle—temperature drops immediately prior to ovulation.
- Age—temperature declines with age.
- External temperature.
- Exercise.

Temperature also varies between different regions of the human body, e.g.:

- Oral body temperature averages between 36.4°C and 37.6°C.
- Tympanic temperature is usually between 0.3°C and 0.6°C higher than oral temperature.
- Axillary temperature is usually between 0.3°C and 0.6°C lower than oral temperature.
- Rectal temperature is usually between 0.3°C and 0.6°C higher than oral temperature.

The regulation of body temperature

- All heat in the body is produced by processes that occur in the cells— i.e. cellular metabolism—in a process known as thermogenesis.
- In thermogenesis the chemical energy contained in digested food is converted into other forms of energy, substantially heat.
- The amount of heat production in a person at any time is determined by the speed with which energy is released from foods ——the metabolic rate—and is measured in watts.
- All tissues produce heat, but those in which rapid chemical reactions occur—e.g. brain, liver—produce large amounts of heat with the consequence that the temperature of these organs is usually approximately 1°C higher than the rest of the body.
- As the generation of heat within the body is continuous (but not constant) the body must lose heat energy at a rate that ensures no build up of heat and a corresponding increase in body temperature.

- In normal circumstances the heat lost from the body equals the heat gained from cellular metabolism and other sources—temperature homeostasis.
- Normal regulation of the body's temperature is effected by the thermoregulatory centres in the hypothalamus.
- The temperature of blood pumping through the brain is constantly monitored together with information from temperature receptors in the skin. The body then adjusts its temperature in response to this information and does so in a variety of ways:

Ways in which body temperature can be increased
- Vasoconstriction: constriction of fine blood vessels of the skin; this reduces blood flow to the skin and, therefore, reduces the amount of heat lost.
- Shivering: contractions of the skeletal muscles producing heat energy.
- Piloerection: erector pili muscles contract causing body hairs to stand on end, trapping an insulating layer of warm air next to the skin.
- Sympathetic metabolic stimulation: body cells increase the rate of heat production as a result of signals from the nervous system.

Ways in which body temperature can be decreased
- Vasodilation: blood vessels in the skin dilate, increasing blood flow to the skin and facilitating heat loss.
- Restriction of heat production mechanisms: e.g. shivering, chemical reactions.
- Erector pili muscles relax: lowers skin hairs and allows air to circulate over skin.
- Perspiration: glands in the skin secrete sweat onto the surface of the skin which then evaporates through the action of body heat.

Thermoregulation abnormalities
Despite the fact that, in normal circumstances, body temperature is regulated to a very high degree, situations can arise where these control mechanisms fail or are inadequate, e.g. at extremes of age or as a result of prolonged anaesthesia. These circumstances include:
- Malfunction of the hypothalamus as a result of cerebral trauma, e.g. oedema resulting from head injury, cerebrovascular accidents, brain surgery.
- Effects of toxic substances, e.g. bacterial or viral infections, drugs (including anaesthetic agents).
- Dehydration: with consequent loss of sweating ability.
- Prolonged exposure to high/low temperatures.

Such circumstances can give rise to hyperthermia or hypothermia:
- *Hyperthermia:* core body temperature consistently above the normal range.
  - Hyperthermia is usually caused by overexposure to a hot environment or as a result of pathogenic infection.
  - It can also arise, in susceptible patients, as a result of exposure to some anaesthetic agents such as halothane and muscle relaxants (e.g. suxamethonium) and occasionally progresses to the potentially fatal condition of malignant hyperthermia.

- *Hypothermia*: core body temperature consistently below the normal range such that normal metabolism is not possible.
  - Hypothermia is a common (particularly at the extremes of age) and potentially serious complication during anaesthesia and surgery.
  - It is associated with numerous perioperative complications including myocardial ischaemia, the impairment of normal coagulation, and a substantially increased risk of wound infection.
  - It arises for a number of reasons, including, as a result of general anaesthesia:
    —depression of the thermoregulatory centre.
    —decrease in metabolic rate.
    —increase in vasodilation.
  - Spinal and epidural anaesthesia can cause hypothermia through vasodilation and loss of muscle tone.
  - Hypothermia also arises as a result of exposure of body surfaces and cavities to the operating theatre environment, which tends to be cool and low in humidity.
  - Hypothermia can also be deliberately induced for some surgery— temperatures 1–3°C below normal provide substantial protection against cerebral ischaemia and hypoxaemia.

The transmission of heat

There are, essentially, four physical processes by which heat can be transferred (lost or gained):

- *Conduction:* the process by which heat is transmitted through a substance (solid, liquid, gas) or from one substance to another. Conduction is due to molecules colliding with other and transferring their heat energy through the substance or between substances. Conduction varies with the conducting substance; it is greatest in solids and least in gases. For conduction to occur between substances there must be direct contact; in normal circumstances conduction accounts for approximately 2–3% of the body's heat loss, but it is also possible to gain heat by conduction (e.g. warm bath).
- *Convection:* the process by which heat is transferred in a fluid (liquid or gas) by the movement of molecules from cooler, relatively high density, regions of the fluid to warmer, relatively low density regions. Convection does not occur in solids. Normally, convection accounts for approximately 10–15% of the body's heat loss.
- *Radiation:* the process by which heat is lost by the emission of electromagnetic (infrared) radiation from a body. The greater the difference in temperature between the body and the surrounding environment, the greater is the loss of heat from the body by radiation. Radiation does not depend on any substance, i.e. it does not depend on the movement of molecules. In normal circumstances approximately 60% of the body's heat loss is through radiation, but the body may also gain heat by radiation (e.g. sunbathing, proximity to fire).
- *Evaporation:* the process by which heat is transferred by the transformation of a liquid into a vapour and is one of the processes by which the human body loses heat during sweating. Typically, one might

expect 20% of the body's total heat loss to be through evaporation although the rate at which evaporation occurs depends upon:

• Surface area.
• Convection currents.
• Atmospheric humidity.
• The type of liquid.
• Temperature of liquid.

Although heat loss through convection and radiation mainly occur via the skin, these processes also occur in the lungs. Inhaled air is usually cooler and dryer than the internal surface of the lung; in warming and moisturising the inhaled air, the body loses heat energy when the air is exhaled.

Electricity

Static and dynamic electricity

Electricity of all kinds involves electrons—the negatively charged particles found in all atoms—but it is important to distinguish between static electricity and dynamic electricity.

- *Static electricity,* so called because it builds in one place, is caused primarily by friction.
  - As materials are rubbed together, electrons are removed from one material (so that it becomes positively charged) and deposited on the other (which becomes negatively charged).
  - Static electricity builds up on door handles and other metal objects in rooms which have synthetic carpets, on synthetic clothing, and on the bodies of motor vehicles as a result of the friction caused by moving air.
  - The static normally discharges upon touch, causing a spark which can ignite flammable gases, causing explosions and/or fires.
  - To reduce this risk in theatres, cotton clothes are used, and anti-static materials are incorporated into equipment to reduce the build-up of static electricity.
  - Maintaining a high relative humidity also reduces the risks of static electricity accumulating.
  - Static electricity has practical uses, e.g. in photocopiers, inkjet printers, in reducing pollution by removing particles of smoke, dirt, and dust from the air, and in paint spraying cars.
- *Dynamic electricity* is caused by the flow of electrons, through a conductor, from point of higher concentration (higher potential) to a point of lower concentration (lower potential), i.e. an electric current—which can be direct current (DC) or alternating current (AC).

Direct and alternating current

- *DC* is current that travels in a circuit in one direction only.
  - It is produced by sources such as batteries, dynamos, and solar cells and is commonly used to power small electrical devices, e.g. radios, torches, pacemakers.
  - DC can also be produced from an AC supply by using a rectifier.
- *AC* is current that cyclically changes in size and direction, typically at 50 or 60 Hz (cycles per second).
  - It is the form of electricity that is routinely supplied to industry and domestic buildings.
  - AC possesses one main advantages compared with DC; AC allows transformers to be used to increase or decrease voltages depending upon purposes.
  - AC can be converted into DC by using an electrical inverter.

Some electrical terms

- *Current:* the rate of flow of electrons (electrical charge) between two points in one second (measured in amperes).
- *Current density:* current flowing/unit area.
- *Voltage:* also known as potential difference—the difference in electrical charge between two points (measured in volts).

- *Resistance:* the opposition to the flow of electrons (measured in ohms). Resistance of a wire depends upon its diameter, length, and material.
- *Circuit:* the continuous pathway followed by electricity from the source of generation to its destination and back.
- *Electrical power:* the rate of flow of energy, or the work done per second in causing electrical charge to flow (measured in watts).
- *Insulator:* a material that resists the flow of electric current; an object intended to support or separate electrical conductors without current passing through itself.
- *Conductor:* a material that allows the flow of electric charge (current) through it.
- *Semi-conductor:* a substance, usually a solid chemical element or compound, which can conduct electricity under certain conditions only; this property makes it a good medium for the control of electrical current.

Physiological effects of electricity

- The physiological effects of electricity on the human body depend upon the amount of current flowing and upon the path the current takes through the body (Table 9.1).
- Although the current flowing depends upon the voltage applied and the resistance of the path taken, it is the size of current that is the main factor in classifying the potential hazards.
- The frequency of the current also impacts upon the physiological effects, with very high frequencies producing heat rather than muscular contractions, a fact that allows their use in electrosurgery.
- Note that the heart is extremely sensitive to frequencies of 50–60Hz—frequencies at which industrial and domestic supplies are normally delivered.
- The most common type of electric shock received by humans is *macro-shock*, where the electric current travels through body tissues to the heart only after overcoming the relatively high resistance offered by dry, intact skin. In such circumstances, Table 9.1 identifies that currents above 10mA may produce sustained muscular contraction, whereas currents greater than approximately 100mA have the potential for causing death as a result of inducing ventricular fibrillation.
- *Micro-shock*, on the other hand, occurs when current flows directly to the heart muscle, e.g. via pacemaker wires, catheters. The size of the current necessary to cause ventricular fibrillation in such a situation is many times smaller than in normal circumstances and may be as little as 20μA.

Table 9.1 Physiological effects of electricity*

Current (at 60Hz)	Physiological effect
1mA	Threshold of perception
5mA	Considered the maximum harmless current
10–20mA	Beginning of sustained muscular contraction (cannot let go of electrical contacts)
50mA	Pain, possible fainting and exhaustion. Cardiac and respiratory functions continue
100–300mA	Ventricular fibrillation—fatal if sustained. Respiratory function continues
6A	Sustained ventricular contraction followed by normal heart rhythm if current stops (defibrillator). Temporary respiratory paralysis. Potential burns

*Adapted from Nave CR and Nave BC (1985). *Physics for Health Sciences*. WB Saunders: Philadelphia.

Gases and the gas laws

Atmospheric pressure

Air is made up of a mixture of gases (see Table 9.2).

Table 9.2 Composition of air

Component	Percentage by volume	Partial pressure (kPa)
Nitrogen (N_2)	78.08	79.10
Oxygen (O_2)	20.95	21.21
Argon (A)	0.93	0.95
Carbon dioxide (CO_2)	0.03	0.04
Total	99.99	101.30

There are other gases present in the atmosphere in very small amounts, e.g. neon, helium, krypton, xenon. Also present is water vapour, which varies in concentration from almost 0% in the cold, dry regions of the Antarctic, for example, to 4% in humid tropical areas.

The term 'partial pressure' refers to the contribution that each gas makes to the total pressure exerted by the atmosphere.

The gas laws

Boyle's law can be expressed:
The volume of a given mass of gas is inversely proportional to the pressure to which it is subjected provided that the temperature remains constant.

Volume (V) $\propto$ 1/pressure (P) (for constant temperature)

or $\qquad\qquad$ P x V = constant

Boyle's law is commonly used to predict the result of introducing a change in the volume or pressure of a fixed mass of gas. The original and final volumes (V_1 and V_2) and pressures (P_1 and P_2) of the fixed mass of gas are related by the equation:

P1 x V1 = P2 x V2 = constant

Charles' law can be expressed:
The volume of a given mass of gas is directly proportional to its absolute temperature (in Kelvin), provided that the pressure remains constant.

Volume (V) $\propto$ temperature (T) (at constant pressure)
or $\qquad$ V/T = constant

If a change is introduced to the volume or absolute temperature of a fixed amount of gas, then the original and final volumes (V_1 and V_2) and absolute temperatures (T_1 and T_2) are related by the equation:

$V_1/T_1 = V_2/T_2$ = constant

Gay-Lussac's law can be expressed:
The pressure of a given mass of gas is directly proportional to its absolute temperature (in Kelvin), provided that the volume is constant.

Pressure (P) $\propto$ temperature (T) (at constant volume)

or $\qquad$ P/T = constant

If a change is introduced to the pressure or absolute temperature of a fixed amount of gas, then the original and final pressures (P_1 and P_2) and absolute temperatures (T_1 and T_2) are related by the equation:

$P_1/T_1 = P_2/T_2$ = constant

The general gas law can be expressed:
The product of the pressure and volume of a given mass of gas is directly proportional to its absolute temperature (in Kelvin)

Pressure (P) x volume (V) $\propto$ temperature (T)

or $\qquad$ P x V/T = constant

If a change is introduced to the pressure, volume or absolute temperature (in Kelvin) of a fixed amount of gas, then the original and final pressures (P_1 and P_2), volumes (V_1 and V_2) and absolute temperatures (T_1 and T_2) are related by the equation:

P_1 x $V_1/T_1 = P_2$ x V_2/T_2 = constant

Dalton's law can be expressed:
The partial pressure of a gas in a gas mixture is the pressure that this gas would exert alone if it occupied the total volume of the mixture in the absence of other components.

$P_{total} = p_a + p_b + p_c + \ ....$

where p_a, p_b, p_c...... are the partial pressures of gases in a gas mixture.

Henry's law can be expressed:
The amount of a gas that will dissolve in a given type and volume of a liquid at a given temperature is directly proportional to the partial pressure of the gas in equilibrium with that liquid.

Concentration $\propto$ partial pressure (at constant temperature)

or $\qquad$ C/p = constant

The breathing process

During *inspiration*, the sternum moves outwards and upwards, the ribs lift and rotate outwards and the diaphragm contracts, flattens, and descends towards the abdomen.

- The net result of these movements is an increase in the volume of the thoracic cavity, which consequently causes the pressure in the thoracic cavity to decrease (Boyle's law) to below atmospheric pressure.
- The resulting pressure gradient causes air to travel down the trachea and into the lungs until the air within the lungs reaches atmospheric pressure.

During *expiration* the opposite movements occur:

- This serves to decrease the volume of the thoracic cavity, so that the pressure is increased above atmospheric pressure.
- This increase in pressure creates a pressure gradient and forces the gases in the lungs back into the atmosphere.

Inhalation is an active process—involving muscle contraction—and as such involves work being done (the work of breathing). This work can be regarded as consisting of three components: the work necessary to expand the lungs against their elastic forces; the work that is required to overcome the viscosity of the lungs and chest wall; and the work required in moving air into the lungs against the resistance of the airway. Exhalation, however, (in normal breathing) is passive—involving muscle relaxation, the recoil of the lungs, ribs, and sternum—and as such does not require work to be done. During exercise, however, exhalation can be an active process.

Positive and negative pressures

When considering pressures in the lungs and thorax, the terms 'negative pressure' and 'positive pressure' are often used. This is done for convenience and means that all pressures involved are compared with, and expressed relative to, normal atmospheric pressure (101.3kPa). So:

- Any pressure *above* normal atmospheric pressure is regarded as positive pressure, e.g. a pressure of +0.3kPa is the same as 101.6kPa
- Any pressure *below* normal atmospheric pressure is regarded as negative pressure, e.g. a pressure of –0.3kPa is the same as 101kPa)

Although relatively small, these pressure differences are more than enough to form a 'pressure gradient,' and enable the gases involved in inhalation and exhalation to move in the required direction.

The pressures involved in breathing

Intra-alveolar pressure is the same as the pressure everywhere in the lungs, and varies between –0.4kPa during inspiration to +0.4kPa during expiration.

Intrapleural pressure is the pressure between the lungs and the pleural sac which surrounds them.

- Because of the elastic nature of lung tissue, lungs constantly tend to move towards a state of collapse, and it is the negative pressure in the intrapleural spaces that stops them collapsing.

- Intrapleural pressure normally varies between −1.1kPa during inspiration and −0.3kPa during expiration.
- This negative pressure must be maintained at all times (even after expiration, when the lungs are at their smallest, and the alveoli are at atmospheric pressure) to ensure that atmospheric pressure continues to push the lungs outwards against the pleural sac and chest wall to prevent the lungs from collapsing.

Gas exchange (Table 9.3)

- Differences in the partial pressures of inspired, alveolar, and expired air promote free interchange of gases within the lungs—most importantly O_2 and CO_2.
- The partial pressure of O_2 in the atmosphere (i.e. inspired air) is approximately 21.3kPa, whereas the partial pressure of O_2 in the air in the alveoli is approximately 14kPa. This pressure gradient means that O_2 passes from the inspired air to the alveoli.
- The reverse is true for CO_2—the partial pressure of CO_2 in alveolar air (approximately 5.3kPa) is much higher than the partial pressure of CO_2 in the atmosphere (approximately 0.03kPa); CO_2, therefore, passes from the alveolar air to expired air.
- O_2 passes from the alveolar air of the lungs (partial pressure approximately 14kPa) into the blood in the pulmonary capillaries (partial pressure approximately 5.3kPa) because of the pressure gradient between alveolar air and that in the capillaries.
- Similarly, there is a pressure gradient between CO_2 in the capillaries (partial pressure approximately 6kPa) and in alveolar air (partial pressure approximately 5.3kPa) and so CO_2 is transferred from blood into air in the alveoli.
- At the tissue capillaries, pressure gradients force O_2 from blood (partial pressure approximately 14kPa) into tissue (partial pressure approximately 5.3kPa) and CO_2 from tissue (partial pressure approximately 6kPa) back into blood (partial pressure approximately 5.3kPa).

Table 9.3 Gas exchange

Location	Partial pressure O_2 (pO_2) (kPa)	Partial pressure CO_2 (pCO_2) (kPa)
Atmosphere	21.3	0.03
Alveoli	14.0	5.3
Pulmonary artery	5.3	6.0
Pulmonary vein	14.0	5.3
Systemic artery	14.0	5.3
Systemic vein	5.3	6.0

SI units

All systems of weights and measures are linked through a number of international agreements that support the International System of Units. This system is the SI, derived from the French 'Système International d'Unités'.

Base SI units

Central to the SI are seven base units—for seven base quantities that are assumed to be mutually independent. The base units are able to be defined without reference to any other units (Table 9.4)

Table 9.4 Base SI units

Unit	Measure of	Symbol
Metre	Length	m
Kilogram	Mass	kg
Second	Time	s
Ampere	Electric current	A or amp
Kelvin	Temperature	K
Mole	Amount of substance	mol
Candela	Luminous intensity	cd

SI derived units

Other SI units—SI derived units—are able to be defined in terms of the seven base units (Table 9.5).

Table 9.5 SI derived units

Unit	Measure of	Symbol
Square metre	Area	m^2
Cubic metre	Volume	m^3
Kilogram per cubic metre	Mass density	kg/m^3
Cubic metre per kilogram	Specific volume	m^3/kg
Mole per cubic metre	Amount of substance concentration	mol/m^3
Metre per second	Velocity	m/s
Metre per second squared	Acceleration	m/s^2
Ampere per square metre	Current density	A/m^2
Candela per square metre	Luminance	cd/m^2

Special names and symbols

For convenience and to enhance understanding, a number of SI derived units have been given special names and symbols, see Table 9.6.

Table 9.6 Special names and symbols

Unit	Measure of	Symbol	Expressed in terms of other SI units
Newton	Force	N	–
Pascal	Pressure	Pa	N/m^2
Hertz	Frequency	Hz	$1/s$
Joule	Energy	J	Nm
Watt	Power	W	J/s
Degree Celsius	Temperature	°C	–
Coulomb	Charge	C	–
Volt	Potential	V	W/A
Farad	Capacitance	F	C/V
Ohm	Resistance		V/A
Siemens	Conductance	S	A/V
Becquerel	Activity (of a radionuclide)	Bq	$1/s$
Sievert	Dose equivalent	Sv	J/kg

Multiplying prefixes

Some of the units used within the SI are either too large or too small to be useful in everyday life (e.g. the metre is too small when measuring very large distances (e.g. distance from the Earth to the moon), but too large when measuring very small distances (e.g. the diameter of a human hair) so the system employs a standard set of multiplying prefixes to convert units to a more convenient size (see Table 9.7).

Note: the kilogram is the only SI unit that has a prefix as part of its name and symbol. Because multiple prefixes are not allowed, in the case of the kilogram, prefixes are used with the unit name 'gram' (symbol 'g') so, 10^{-6} kg is not written as 1μkg (1 microkilogram), but as 1mg (1 milligram). Otherwise, any SI prefix may be used with any SI unit.

Table 9.7 Multiplying prefixes

Prefix	Symbol	Multiplying factor
Tera	T	1,000,000,000,000 (10^{12})
Giga	G	1,000,000,000 (10^{9})
Mega	M	1,000,000 (10^{6})
Kilo-	k	1,000 (10^{3})
Hecto-	h	100 (10^{2})
Deka-	da	10 (10^{1})
Deci-	d	0.1 (10^{-1})
Centi-	c	0.01 (10^{-2})
Milli-	m	0.001 (10^{-3})
Micro-	μ	0.000001 (10^{-6})
Nano-	n	0.000000001 (10^{-9})
Pico-	p	0.000000000001 (10^{-12})

Airway management

The importance of airway management

- Maintaining adequate oxygenation is the number one priority for all members of the anaesthetic team.
- Airway management requires that:
  - There is a clear pathway between the O_2 supply and the patient's lungs.
  - The patient's lungs are protected from the risk of aspiration.
- If there is no respiration or ventilation then subsequently there will be no oxygenation and the patient's circulation and all other vital processes will cease.
- Failure to adequately maintain the airway is responsible for approximately 30% of deaths associated with anaesthesia.
- Remember, it is oxygenation, and not intubation, which keeps patients alive and this can be achieved through simple bag and mask hand ventilation.

References and further reading

Allman KG and Wilson IH (eds) (2006). *Oxford Handbook of Anaesthesia* (2nd edn). Oxford University Press: Oxford.

Association of Anaesthetists of Great Britain and Ireland (2004). *Checking anaesthetic equipment*. AAGBI: London.

Royal College of Anaesthetists (2004). *Guidelines for the Provision of Anaesthetic Services*. RCoA: London.

The role of the anaesthetic practitioner in airway management

It is essential that all equipment is prepared and checked prior to the commencement of all operating lists, even when patients may only require regional or local anaesthetic techniques.

Routine checking must include:

- O_2 supply, tug test of pipelines, and cylinder availability with sufficient contents in case of pipeline failure.
- Anaesthetic machine and ventilator checks as per the current AAGBI recommendations.[1]
- The availability and integrity of breathing circuits and HME filters, including a self-inflating resuscitation bag. Self-inflating resuscitation bags can be used to effectively ventilate patients even if the O_2 supply fails as most patients can survive if ventilated with air.
- Suction apparatus connected and able to generate a vacuum with all tubing attached and both pharyngeal and bronchial suction catheters available.
- A range of appropriately sized facemasks available. Clear masks are considered advantageous as vomit or secretions can be more quickly detected and managed.
- Airways in a range of types and sizes. Both oral and nasal airway may be used routinely and should remain in their packaging prior to use in order to reduce the risk of cross infection.
- Laryngeal mask airways (LMAs) are essential and all sizes must be available. Disposable LMAs are recommended unless adequate facilities are available for decontamination and sterilisation; this is particularly important with the concern of prion disease.
- A prion is an abnormal, transmissible agent that is able to induce abnormal folding of normal cellular prion proteins in the brain, leading to brain damage and the characteristic signs and symptoms of the disease. Prion diseases usually progress rapidly and are always fatal.
  - Prion diseases, also known as transmissible spongiform encephalopathies (TSEs) are a group of progressive neurodegenerative conditions that exist in both humans and animals.
  - Human prion disease can include Creutzfeldt–Jakob disease (CJD) or variant Creutzfeldt–Jakob disease (vCJD).
  - Animal prion disease can include scrapie, bovine spongiform encephalopathy (BSE) and chronic wasting disease (CWD).
  - Whilst prion disease is not contagious, CNS tissues that include brain, spinal cord, and eye tissue are considered to be extremely infectious and are a cause for concern for those directly handling infected tissue. Although there is no evidence that blood is infectious, special infection precautions should be taken by those handling blood or blood products.
  - A tonsil biopsy is used to diagnose vCJD.
- The move towards single-use devices accelerated following the recognition that prion diseases (causing vCJD) were potentially transmissible despite current disinfection and sterilising techniques. The extent of this risk is at present unproven and considered exceptionally low.[2]

- A laryngoscope, Macintosh long (4) and short (3) blades need to be available, their bulbs tested and checked for brightness. The location of a McCoy laryngoscope blade and short laryngoscope handle should be noted.
- Sterile unopened ET tubes, of the anticipated size plus one size smaller/larger close to hand. A syringe for cuff inflation is needed and the use of a cuff pressure gauge is recommended to avoid inflation pressures >30cm H_2O causing ischaemia of the tracheal lining with the potential to cause permanent damage.
- A disposable bougie needs to be readily accessible to assist with intubation should the view of the larynx be incomplete or the passage of the ET tube be obscured in any way.
- Lubricants should be water based and sterile for the lubrication of airways, LMAs, and ET tubes.
- A selection of tapes and ties to secure the position of airway management devices used, noting any patient allergies prior to use.
- Patient monitoring should be switched on and all patient connection devices checked for availability, integrity, and cleanliness. These must include SaO_2, NIBP, ECG, and invasive monitoring sets and connectors.
- Gas analysis monitoring devices must be switched on and patient sampling lines connected into the patient breathing circuits, usually via the single-use HME filter.
- Patient beds, trolleys, and operating tables need to be charged if electrically operated; the brakes, rise, and fall mechanism and the head end tip all in working order.
- Patients must be positioned within easy reach of the anaesthetist at the head end of the bed, trolley, or operating table with the height adjusted to a comfortable working height for the anaesthetist managing the airway.
- All patients will need a pillow positioned just under the head and neck to allow head extension and neck flexion.

Good preoperative preparation, assessment of the operating list, checking of equipment and planning are all essential for successful outcomes in airway management.

References

1. Association of Anaesthetists of Great Britain and Ireland (2004). *Checking anaesthetic equipment.* AAGBI: London.

2. Cook T and Walton B (2005). *The laryngeal mask airway.* Anaesthesia **20**, 32–42.

Further reading

Allman KG and Wilson IH (eds) (2006). *Oxford Handbook of Anaesthesia* (2nd edn). Oxford University Press: Oxford.

National Prion Clinic. Available from: ⌨ www.uclh.nhs.uk/

Royal College of Anaesthetists (2004). *Guidelines for the Provision of Anaesthetic Services.* RCoA: London.

Maintaining the airway

One of the top priorities during anaesthetics must be to maintain a patent airway, free from secretions. To this end the anaesthetic practitioner must be familiar with the following equipment and techniques:

Patient positioning

- A pillow must be positioned under the patient's head and neck but not too far under the shoulders.
- This position, with the neck flexed and the head extended, commonly referred to as the 'sniffing the morning air' position, will permit a straight line of vision from the patient's mouth to their vocal cords with the aid of a laryngoscope.
- Caution should be applied if potential cervical spine injury exists.

Head tilt and chin lift

- In the unconscious patient the tongue can obstruct the airway.
- This can usually be avoided by placing one hand on the patient's forehead then tilting the head backwards while lifting the patient's chin firmly with the finger tips of the other hand.

Jaw thrust

- When obstruction is not alleviated by the simple head tilt and chin lift then the jaw thrust may be needed.
- The practitioner displaces the posterior aspect of the mandible (angle of the jaw) upwards and forwards aiming to get the lower teeth in front of the upper teeth.
- This manoeuvre pulls forward the tongue and lifts it off the back of the pharynx, securing the patient's airway for either spontaneous respiration or bag and mask hand ventilation.

Removal of secretions or vomit

- Suction must be immediately available for use, usually with a Yankauer pharyngeal sucker attached.
- Trauma and bleeding can be avoided by only applying suction to the airway under direct vision.

Facemasks

- Facemasks are available in a range of paediatric and adult sizes and must be selected to fit over the bridge of the nose onto the cleft of the chin.
- Holding a facemask is a skill, which the anaesthetic practitioner must practice and master.
- The thumb and index finger are used to press the mask against the patient's face and a tight seal is then achieved by the remaining three fingers, placed on the mandible, lifting the patient's face into the mask whilst maintaining a head tilt and jaw thrust at the same time.
- Holding a facemask may require two hands with a second person, if required to squeeze the bag to provide ventilation.

Oropharyngeal airway

- The Guedel airway is the most commonly used airway.
- They are colour coded and available in adult and paediatric sizes.
- The appropriate sized airway for an adult patient may be chosen to correspond to the distance from the patient's incisor teeth down to the angle of their jaw.
- Airways should be lubricated prior to use and then, in adults, be inserted into the patient's mouth upside down and then rotated through 180° into the oropharynx.

Nasopharyngeal airway

- These airways are softer than oropharyngeal airways and typically are better tolerated by the semiconscious patient.
- They are available in a wide range of sizes denoted by their diameter.
- The most appropriate size will usually correspond with the diameter of the patient's little finger.
- The nasopharyngeal airway needs to be well lubricated prior to the insertion of the bevelled end into the nostril.
- Advancing it requires a gentle twisting action, pushing gently in a posterior direction.
- A safety pin inserted through the flanged end of the nasopharyngeal airway prior to insertion, can prevent it from slipping too far into the patient's nose.

References and further reading

Allman KG and Wilson IH (eds) (2006). *Oxford Handbook of Anaesthesia* (2nd edn). Oxford University Press: Oxford.

Difficult Airway Society Guidelines (2004). Available at: ⊠ www.das.uk.com/guidelines/guideline-shome.html

Latto IP, and Vaughan RS (eds) (1997). *Difficulties in Tracheal Intubation* (2nd edn). Saunders: London.

Royal College of Anaesthetists (2004). *Guidelines for the Provision of Anaesthetic Services*. RCoA: London.

Endotracheal tubes: overview

The cuffed ET tube is regarded as the most reliable way of maintaining a patient's airway by protecting the trachea from contamination and facilitating IPPV. Cuffed ET tubes are all single use and available in sizes 2–10mm internal diameter and have the following safety feature incorporated into their design:

- ET tubes have a radiopaque line for x-ray detection.
- At the distal end of the ET tube there is an additional hole called Murphy's eye. This will allow ventilation to continue if the end of the tube becomes obstructed. The most common reason for the obstruction is that the tube is inserted too far and impinges on the carina or bronchus wall.
- ET tubes now have high volume, low pressure cuffs with a pilot balloon, which when inflated seals off the trachea, reducing the risk of tracheal contamination. The low-pressure cuff is designed to reduce the risk of prolonged pressure from the cuff on the tracheal lining, which may cause ischaemia of the tracheal mucosa.

The role of the anaesthetic practitioner

- An appropriate selection of different sized ET tubes must be available for immediate use. One size smaller than anticipated should always be within reach.
- ET tubes should be kept sterile within their wrappers until required to minimise the risks of cross infection.
- The lumen of the ET tube and the cuff must be checked prior to use.
- The ET tube is lubricated with a sterile, water-soluble lubricant immediately prior to insertion.
- When the ET tube is situated in the trachea the cuff is inflated with the minimum amount of air to achieve a seal within the trachea with no air leak. The cuff pressure must not exceed 30cm H_2O and can be checked with a pressure gauge designed for the purpose, if available.
- The position of the ET tube needs to be secured either with ties or tape according to the anaesthetist's preference.
- Patient documentation must be completed recording the type and size of ET tube used, noting the method of insertion, and the type of tape or ties used to secure.

References and further reading

Allman KG and Wilson IH (eds) (2006). *Oxford Handbook of Anaesthesia* (2nd edn). Oxford University Press: Oxford.

Al-Shaikh B and Stacey S (2002). *Essentials of Anaesthetic Equipment.* Churchill Livingstone: London.

Berg S (2006). Paediatric and neonatal anaesthesia. In Allman KG and Wilson IH (eds) (2006). *Oxford Handbook of Anaesthesia* (2nd edn). Oxford University Press: Oxford.

Latto IP and Vaughan RS (eds) (1997). *Difficulties in tracheal intubation* (2nd edn). Saunders: London.

Types of endotracheal tubes

This is only a small selection of the large variety of ET tubes available.

Cuffed ET tubes

- Cuffed tubes, when inflated, provide an airtight seal between the seal and the tracheal wall.
- The airtight seal protects the patient's airway from aspiration and allows ventilation during IPPV.
- Following intubation, the cuff is inflated until no gas leak is audible.
- The narrowest point in an adult airway is the glottis so cuffed tubes are used to achieve an airtight seal.[1]

Uncuffed ET tubes

- The paediatric trachea is conical where the narrowest part is at the level of the cricoid ring, and the only part of the airway completely surrounded by cartilage.
- If the tracheal tube is too large, it will compress the tracheal epithelium at this level, leading to ischaemia with consequent scarring and the possibility of sub-glottic stenosis.[2]
- A correctly sized tube is one where ventilation is adequate but a small audible leak of air is present when positive pressure is applied
- Avoid the use of catheter mounts for paediatric patients due to the large dead space involved.[2]

Reinforced ET tubes

- These have a nylon or metal spiral embedded within the wall of the ET tube.
- These are used to reduce the risk of an obstructed airway caused by the kinking of the ET tube e.g. when turning a patient prone, or during maxilla-facial/neurosurgery.
- They are less rigid than the standard ET tubes and may need a stylet to aid insertion.
- Meticulous positioning and fixing of these tubes is essential to ensure the airway is maintained.

Preformed ET tubes

- These can be north or south facing and are used to direct the breathing circuits, when connected to the ET tube, away from the surgical site e.g. ENT or plastic surgery.
- Both are available as cuffed or uncuffed tubes.
- Some paediatric anaesthetists, because of the ease with which they can be made secure, favour the use of uncuffed north-facing ET tubes.

Double lumen ET tubes

- These are exactly what they say they are and are two tubes in one.
- They are available in a large variety of types and sizes, all available as either left or right-sided tubes.
- They are intended to intubate one or other of the main bronchi as well as the trachea.
- They are designed to facilitate single lung ventilation allowing the collapse of one lung during thoracic surgery.

- When inserted their exact position is usually confirmed with the aid of a fibreoptic bronchoscope prior to surgery to ensure that one lung ventilation is possible when required.

Laser resistant ET tubes

- These are designed for airway management during laser surgery to the larynx.
- These tubes have a metal foil, which is non-flammable and therefore able to reduce the combustion risk during surgery.
- Sterile saline also needs to be used to inflate the ET tube cuff throughout the procedure.

References and further reading

1. Al-Shaikh B and Stacey S (2002). *Essentials of Anaesthetic Equipment.* Churchill Livingstone: London.

2. Berg S (2006). Paediatric and neonatal anaesthesia. In Allman KG and Wilson IH (eds) (2006). *Oxford Handbook of Anaesthesia* (2nd edn). Oxford University Press: Oxford.

Allman KG and Wilson IH (eds) (2006). *Oxford Handbook of Anaesthesia* (2nd edn). Oxford University Press: Oxford.

Anaesthesia UK. Available at: ☒ www.frca.co.uk/default.aspx

Latto IP and Vaughan RS (eds) (1997). *Difficulties in Tracheal Intubation* (2nd edn). Saunders: London.

Laryngeal mask airway

The first LMA was described by Dr Archie Brain, a London anaesthetist, in 1983. The LMA provides a less traumatic alternative to ET intubation but also, when used in place of a facemask, gives better airway control.

It can be used for both spontaneous respiration and positive pressure ventilation, *but it must be remembered that the LMA does not protect the lungs from aspiration.*

- The LMA is available in sizes 1–6 and size selection is based upon the weight of the patient.
- The amount of air needed for cuff inflation increases with tube size. The LMA cuff must be deflated, wrinkle free, and well lubricated on the posterior surface prior to insertion.
- The assistant may be required to open the patient's mouth as widely as possible using a jaw thrust.
- Once in place, the LMA cuff will need inflating gently at which point the LMA will usually lift slightly within the pharynx.
- After this readjustment the LMA can be connected to the breathing filter and circuit.
- Once in position the efficacy of ventilation must be assessed by clinical observation, appropriate tidal volumes, and end-tidal CO_2 (Table 10.1).

Table 10.1 LMA selection and cuff volume guide

LMA size	Patient weight (kg)	Cuff volume (mL)
1	0–5	2–4
1.5	5–10	5–7
2	10–20	7–10
2.5	20–30	12–14
3	30–50	15–20
4	50–70	20–30
5	70–100	30–40
6	>100	< 50

Reinforced laryngeal mask airway (RLMA)
- The RLMA was developed with a coil inside the wall of the LMA to prevent inadvertent kinking of the device when in use.
- It is used when surgery is in close proximity to the airway or when the airway may need to be covered by the surgical drapes.
- The technique for insertion is the same as the standard LMA but meticulous attention must be paid to securing the device once in position.

Intubating laryngeal mask airway (ILMA)
The ILMA was developed to make a device through which intubation was possible as it was previously impossible through an LMA.

- It is useful in the management of both anticipated and unexpectedly difficult cases of intubation and such use is now recommended in various difficult airway management algorithms.
- The ILMA is currently a reusable device and is available in adult sizes 3–5.
- The aperture of the ILMA is designed for the insertion of a well-lubricated size 8mm ET tube through it.
- It is also possible to ventilate via the ILMA during the intubation process, if the patient should require it.

Proseal laryngeal mask airway (PLMA)

- The PLMA is the most recent development of the LMA and has been developed to offer improved performance with IPPV.
- It has a double cuff to allow increased cuff pressures with an improved laryngeal seal.
- The PLMA has an additional drain tube, which is intended to allow the separation of the respiratory and the alimentary tracts, providing a way of escape for any unexpected gastric contents.
- The PLMA is available as a reusable and single-use device in adult sizes 3–5.
- Unlike the other LMAs the PLMA has an introducer, which when attached gives additional rigidity to aid insertion.
- When the PLMA is correctly inserted, the drain tube should be directly above and in line with the oesophagus allowing a lubricated NG tube to be passed through the drain tube into the stomach through which gastric contents may be aspirated.
- *However it must be noted that there still remains the risk of gastric aspiration while the PLMA is in situ.*

References and further reading

Allman KG and Wilson IH (eds) (2006). *Oxford Handbook of Anaesthesia* (2nd edn). Oxford University Press: Oxford.

Brain AIJ (1993). *The Intravent laryngeal mask: Instruction manual* (2nd edn). Intravent: Henley-on-Thames.

Calder I and Pearce A (eds)(2004). *Core Topics in Airway Management.* Cambridge University Press: Cambridge.

Intavent Orthofix. Available at: http://www.intaventorthofix.com/index.html

Latto IP and Vaughan RS (eds) (1997). *Difficulties in Tracheal Intubation* (2nd edn). Saunders: London.

Royal College of Anaesthetists (2004). *Guidelines for the Provision of Anaesthetic Services.* RCoA: London.

Wharton NM, Gibbison B, Gabbott DA, *et al.* (2008). I-gel insertion by novices in manikins and patients. *Anaesthesia* **63**(9) 991–5.

Additional supraglottic devices

Combitube: has a dual tube with dual cuffs, designed to straddle the larynx and can allow ventilation from holes between the two cuffs, or act simply as a tracheal tube.[1]

Laryngeal tube (LT): is based on the combitube and has a single blind-ending tube, with distal and proximal cuffs; ventilation occurs via holes between the cuffs. It is easy to insert and atraumatic.[1]

I-gel: this is a new cuffless polymer airway of similar in design to the PLMA. It is a single use, supraglottic airway management device designed to create a non-inflatable, anatomical seal of the pharyngeal, laryngeal, and perilaryngeal structures whilst avoiding compression trauma. There is potential for the i-gel to have a role for use during cardiopulmonary resuscitation and perhaps when tracheal intubation fails.[2]

Streamlined liner of the pharynx airway (SLIPA): is a cuffless airway with the body of the SLIPA acting as a reservoir if regurgitation occurs. This airway is sized by matching the external diameter of the patient's larynx to the 'size' of the device.[1]

Cobra perilaryngeal airway (CobraPLA): is similar to the LT. It has a bullet tip as opposed to a distal balloon and is designed to sit higher in the airway than the LT.[1]

References and further reading

1. Jackson K and Cook T (2006). Equipment for airway management. *Anaesthesia and Intensive Care Medicine* **7**(10) 356–9.

2. Wharton NM, Gibbison B, Gabbott DA, et al. (2008). I-gel insertion by novices in manikins and patients. *Anaesthesia* **63**(9) 991–5.

Allman KG and Wilson IH (eds) (2006). *Oxford Handbook of Anaesthesia* (2nd edn). Oxford University Press: Oxford.

Calder I and Pearce A (eds) (2004). *Core Topics in Airway Management*. Cambridge University Press: Cambridge.

Difficult Airway Society Guidelines (2004). Available at: ▣ www.das.uk.com/guidelines/guideline-shome.html

Intavent Orthofix. Available at: ▣ http://www.intaventorthofix.com/index.html

Latto IP and Vaughan RS (eds) (1997). *Difficulties in Tracheal Intubation* (2nd edn). Saunders: London.

Royal College of Anaesthetists (2004). *Guidelines for the Provision of Anaesthetic Services*. RCoA: London.

Wharton NM, Gibbison B, Gabbott DA, et al. (2008). I-gel insertion by novices in manikins and patients. *Anaesthesia* **63**(9) 991–5.

Difficult airway assessment

An airway, which is difficult to manage, is created by both anatomical and clinical factors that complicate, for the skilled practitioner, either ventilation administered via a facemask and/or ET intubation. Predicting which patients will prove difficult to ventilate, intubate, or both, is complex and the subject of much debate. However airway evaluation is a skill that needs to be learnt for the benefit of patient safety. There are many methods and predictive scoring systems described in the literature. Only one method each for ventilation and intubation will be explored here.

> It is advisable to know one system well, to remember it and to use it.

Airway difficulties can be separated into categories:
• Difficult to ventilate.
• Difficult to intubate.
• Both of these.

Difficult mask ventilation (DMV)

DMV occurs when the unassisted anaesthetist fails to maintain the oxygen saturation of a patient with bag and mask hand ventilation. The incidence of DMV is not uncommon and may occur in approx. 5% of patients. There are five predictors of DMV and the acronym *OBESE* can be used to remember these:
  • Obesity.
  • Bearded.
  • Elderly (>55 years old).
  • Snorers.
  • Edentulous.

When a patient presents with two or more of the above features, then there is a likelihood of DMV.

Difficult intubation

The incidence of difficult intubation is estimated at 1–3% of patients who require ET intubation. It is important to assess all patients' airways preoperatively to predict possible intubation difficulties prior to anaesthesia. This will ensure that the appropriate skill mix of staff and all necessary equipment will be readily available to implement the planned intubation technique e.g. awake fibreoptic intubation. One commonly used acronym, *LEMON*, can be a helpful way to remember the predictors for intubation difficulties. The greater the number of unusual anatomical features a patient has the greater the likelihood of intubation difficulties.
• **Look** externally for any abnormalities to the facial shape. These may include a receding jaw, short or thick neck, protruding teeth, narrow mouth opening, obesity, or other face/neck pathology.
• **Evaluate** the jaw.
  • Patients should be able to open their mouths sufficiently to place 3 of their fingers between their upper and lower teeth.
  • Thyromental distance, the distance from the thyroid notch to the tip of the jaw when the patient's head is extended is usually >6.5 cm.

- Patients are usually able to place their bottom teeth in front of their top teeth (jaw protrusion).
- *Mallampati* is a scoring system, first described in 1985, based upon the available view of the patient's oropharynx. The patient is sat down with their head held in a neutral position and asked to open their mouth wide and to protrude their tongue maximally. What is then visible is categorised and this is illustrated in Fig. 10.1. The less the anaesthetist is able to view, the greater the likelihood of intubation difficulties.
- *Obstruction* to the airway can be caused by foreign body, tumour abscess, swelling, or haematoma.
- *Neck mobility*, patients should be able to tilt their heads backwards through the movement of the atlanto occipital (AO) joint. On examination of the patient lying down, one finger of one hand is placed onto the occiput and one finger of the other hand is placed onto the chin; the patient is then asked to tip their head backwards resulting in the finger on the chin usually being lifted higher than the finger placed onto the occiput. Restricted neck movement may be caused by cervical spondylosis, rheumatoid arthritis, or cervical nerve compression.

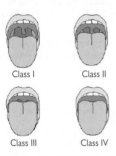

Class I

Class II

Class III

Class IV

Class I: visualisation of the soft palate, uvula, fauces, anterior and posterior tonsillar pillars

Class II: visualisation of the soft palate, fauces and uvula

Class III: visualisation of the soft palate and the base of the uvula

Class IV: soft palate is not visible at all

Fig. 10.1 Mallampati classification. Reproduced with permission from Allman KG and Wilson IH (eds) (2006). *Oxford Handbook of Anaesthesia* (2nd edn). Oxford University Press: Oxford.

References and further reading

Allman KG and Wilson IH (eds) (2006). *Oxford Handbook of Anaesthesia* (2nd edn). Oxford University Press: Oxford.

Langeron O, Masso E, Huraux C, *et al.* (2000). Prediction of difficult mask ventilation. *Anaesthesiology* **92**,1229–36.

Mallampati SR, Gugino LD, Desai S, *et al.* (1983). Clinical signs to predict difficult tracheal intubation. *Canadian Anaesthetists Society Journal* **30**, 316–17.

Rapid sequence induction (RSI)

- The aim of RSI is to secure a patient's airway as quickly as possible, avoiding any soiling of the lungs from gastric contents through the application of cricoid pressure or Sellick's manoeuvre as it is sometimes called.
- Pulmonary aspiration of gastric contents, even in quantities as low as 30mL, is associated with significant morbidity and mortality.
- Cricoid pressure is widely accepted as standard practice in the UK and USA but it is controversial and not as widely practised in continental Europe. It is possible that poorly applied cricoid pressure can obscure the anaesthetist's view of the larynx and make intubation in urgent circumstances more difficult.

Indications

- Inadequate preoperative fasting, <6 hours solid food, <4 hours breast milk, and <2 hours clear fluids.
- Delayed gastric empting e.g. due to trauma, an acute abdomen, opioids or poorly controlled diabetes.
- Oesophageal sphincter incompetence e.g. caused by gastric reflux or pregnancy.

Preparation

Patient monitoring needs to be attached (ECG, NIBP, SAO$_2$) with base line recording noted. An IVI must be sited and connected to a free-flowing infusion.

Equipment

- Patient needs to be positioned on a tipping trolley or operating table.
- Suction connected, switched on, and easily accessible, e.g. under the pillow by the right hand of the anaesthetist.
- Selection of ET tubes, cut if necessary, the cuff of the chosen ET tube checked with an air filled 10mL syringe attached to the pilot balloon.
- Laryngoscopes ($\times$ 2) checked with both long and short blades available. The laryngoscope of choice must be placed within easy reach of the left hand of the anaesthetist.
- Bougie must be instantly available to railroad the ET tube over it into the trachea in case intubation difficulties occur.
- Stethoscope to identity breath sounds as part of the confirmation of successful intubation.
- Tape or ties to secure the ET tube when intubation has been confirmed by the presence of end-tidal CO_2, bilateral chest movement, and auscultation.

Patient preparation

- Explanation of the procedure, any questions answered, and reassurance given.
- Location of the cricoid cartilage by the anaesthetic assistant. If in any doubt the assistant must confirm with the anaesthetist that the cricoid cartilage has been successfully identified.
- Check that the patient is positioned appropriately at the head end of a tipping trolley or operating table.

- Optimal positioning of the patient's pillow under the head, neck, and just under the shoulders sufficiently to allow the patient to adopt the 'sniffing the morning air' position with their neck flexed and head extended.

Procedure

- Preoxygenation for a minimum of 3 minutes with 100% O_2.
- The application of gentle cricoid pressure (approx 10N).
- Administration of the anaesthetic induction agent.
- Full application of cricoid pressure : Initially 10–20 N then 30–40N.
- Administration of suxamethonium.
- No mask ventilation to avoid gastric insufflation, which would increase the risk of gastric reflux and aspiration.
- Wait for the muscle fasciculations to cease.
- Laryngoscopy and intubation with the ET tube cuff immediately inflated.
- The positioning of the ET tube within the trachea is confirmed by the presence of an end-tidal CO_2 trace, bilateral chest movement, and auscultation.
- Cricoid pressure is only released when the anaesthetist confirms that it is safe to do so.
- *Emergence from anaesthesia also presents the same risk of aspiration as induction of anaesthesia.*

At the end of surgery the following precautions are necessary:
- Administration of 100% O_2.
- Reversal of neuromuscular blockade.
- Patient positioned on their side on a tipping trolley, bed, or operating table.
- Extubation only when the patient is fully awake and able to remove the ET tube themselves.

Cricoid pressure or Sellick's manoeuvre

The cricoid cartilage is the only tracheal ring which is a complete circle. It is located immediately below the thyroid cartilage or 'Adams apple'. Cricoid pressure is applied: firstly by stabilising the patient's trachea between the assistant's thumb and middle finger, then secondly by using the index finger to apply posterior pressure to the cricoid cartilage. The amount of pressure required to compress the oesophagus against spines is significant, approximately 30N or 3kg of pressure. The circular cricoid cartilage compresses the oesophagus between itself and the vertebral bodies that are located behind it, thus preventing passive regurgitation of gastric contents.

It must be stressed that cricoid pressure must be released if the patient actively vomits to avoid the risk of oesophageal rupture.

References and further reading

Allman KG and Wilson IH (eds) (2006). *Oxford Handbook of Anaesthesia* (2nd edn). Oxford University Press: Oxford.

Royal College of Nursing (2005). *Perioperative fasting in adults and children: an RCN guideline for the multidisciplinary team*. RCN: London.

Sellick BA (1961). Cricoid pressure to control regurgitation of stomach contents during induction of anaesthesia. *Lancet* **2**, 404–6.

Failed intubation/failed ventilation

The seriousness of the failed intubation cannot be over emphasised but deaths occur when there is a failure to oxygenate a patient as a result of a failure to ventilate. Simple bag and mask hand ventilation will keep patients alive when difficulties with intubation are experienced.

Unanticipated airway difficulties can be categorised as follows:
• Difficult or failed intubation.
• Difficult or failed ventilation.
• Both of these.

Management

The management of airway difficulties can be divided up into four stages.
• *Initial intubation attempt:* when the initial intubation attempt fails then it is important to optimise anaesthesia, the patient position, and the equipment being used. Then to employ external manipulation of the larynx with the help of the assistant and to use a bougie
• *Secondary intubation attempt:* if the patient can be adequately ventilated by hand then an LMA or i-gel could be inserted and these could buy some time; but if intubation is required, then either another attempt is made with more equipment or more experienced staff, or an ILMA could be inserted and an ET tube passed through it.
• *If initial and secondary intubation attempts fail:* ventilation must be maintained with either a bag and mask technique or an LMA/PLMA. Consultation with the surgical team must then decide whether to proceed with surgery or to postpone it and wake the patient.
• *The 'can't intubate/can't ventilate' scenario:* if this scenario occurs then the only option remaining is the use of an invasive tracheal cricothyroidotomy to establish a route through which the patient's lungs may be oxygenated.

The role of the anaesthetic practitioner

• Keep calm and stay and assist the anaesthetist.
• Request the help of another senior anaesthetist.
• Assist with 2-person bag and mask hand ventilation.
• Check the patient's position and after discussion reposition the pillow if needed.
• Ensure that all patients monitoring continues to give accurate recordings.
• Request that the difficult intubation equipment be brought into the anaesthetic room immediately.
• This should contain ILMAs, PLMAs in a full range of sizes; a short-handled laryngoscope; McCoy laryngoscope blades (sizes 3 and 4); a range of bougies including extra long and hollow bougies through which the patient can be ventilated; stylets and guides wires over which an ET tube may be passed; ET tubes, standard and reinforced in a range of sizes from 5mm up; emergency cricothyroidotomy kit; and jet ventilation device. A fibreoptic bronchoscope needs to be brought as soon as possible.

Responsibilities of the anaesthetic practitioner

The anaesthetic practitioner must:
- Be able to locate the operating department's difficult intubation equipment, to fit it together, and understand how it works.
- Regularly check, if available, the jet ventilation equipment and be able to connect it to the anaesthetic machine and make sure that there are no missing parts.
- Be familiar with the latest guidelines for the management of failed intubation and ventilation. Display them prominently in the clinical areas.
- Use date expired equipment for the training of new staff.
- Share experiences and reflections with colleagues learning from the available expertise.

Rescue techniques for the 'can't intubate, can't ventilate' (CICV) situation

The Difficult Airway Society (DAS) develops and provides national guidelines for the management of the difficult airway.[1] The DAS CICV guidelines are illustrated in Fig. 10.2.

CICV is a life-threatening emergency, one which all anaesthetic practitioners must consider and understand. Thankfully, greater than 90% of cases can be resolved with 2-person hand ventilation or with the insertion of an LMA, ILMA, or PLMA. But on the rare occasions when these measures fail an invasive cricothyroidotomy is a life-saving measure. When the decision is made to undertake a cricothyroidotomy then speed will be essential to prevent brain damage from hypoxia and the anaesthetic practitioner will need to remain calm.

References and further reading

1. Difficult Airway Society (2007). *'Can't intubate, can't ventilate'* Available at: ⌨ http://www.das.uk.com/files/cvci-Jul04-A4.pdf

Allman KG and Wilson IH (eds) (2006). *Oxford Handbook of Anaesthesia* (2nd edn). Oxford University Press: Oxford.

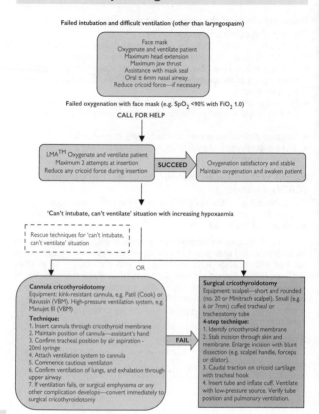

Fig. 10.2 Rescue techniques for the CICV situation. Reproduced and adapted with permission from Difficult Airway Society (2007). *Can't intubate, can't ventilate*. Available at: 🖥 http://www.das.uk.com/files/cvci-Jul04-A4.pdf

Complications associated with anaesthesia

Acid aspiration syndrome

Aspiration is the act of foreign materials inhaled into the lungs. Mortality figures can be as high as 60%.

- When consciousness is lost, the patient with stomach contents may regurgitate gastric material via the oesophagus; this may be aspirated into the lungs causing a severe pneumonitis (inflammation of the lungs) usually called 'aspiration pneumonitis'.
- This is especially severe, and often fatal, if the gastric contents are acidic (pH <2.5).
- As little as 30mL will cause a severe reaction.
- When solid foods are aspirated complete obstruction of the airway may occur.
- Normally the specialised junction between the oesophagus and the stomach—the oesophagogastric junction—acts as a sphincter to prevent material returning to the oesophagus after entering the stomach.
- When the conscious level is depressed this junction works less efficiently and if the intragastric pressure within the stomach is greater than the closing pressure of the sphincter then regurgitation will occur.
- Regurgitation, which is the flow of stomach content back in to the mouth, is the main course of acid aspiration syndrome during anaesthesia.
- Regurgitation is different from vomiting as regurgitation is a passive act and requires no muscle tone and occurs because of reduced or altered levels of consciousness.
- Vomiting is active and requires muscle tone therefore normal or near normal levels of consciousness.
- The aspiration of gastric acid into the lungs followed by bronchospasm, pulmonary oedema, and hypoxia is also referred to as Mendelson's syndrome.
- Aspiration of gastric acid into the lungs then alters the pathology in the lungs, consisting of chemical tracheobronchitis and pneumonia.
- Aspiration of foreign substances into the lungs can also predispose to bacterial pneumonia.
- Acid aspiration is just as likely to happen at induction as extubation and the outcomes can vary from benign consequences to acute respiratory failure leading to death (Table 11.1).

For obstetric anaesthesia patients, 30mL of 0.3 molar sodium citrate is normally given prophylactically. Elective patients thought to be at risk of aspiration are routinely prescribed metoclopramide and ranitidine prior to their anaesthetic. For these patient groups a RSI is part of the routine anaesthesia. Cricoid pressure is used as a preventative measure against regurgitation.

Early signs and symptoms

- Cyanosis.
- Tachycardia.
- Hypotension.
- Bucking of patient.
- Massive pulmonary oedema.
- Bronchospasm.
- Coughing.

Later signs and symptoms

- Reduced arterial oxygenation.
- Increased pulmonary artery pressure.
- Reduced compliance of the lungs.
- Chest x-ray can show pulmonary oedema though this will not necessary diagnose the extent of the pulmonary damage accurately.
- Cardiac failure.

Immediate patient management

- Call for help.
- Place the patient in a head-down position.
- Tilt the patient's head to the side; this enables any foreign material in the mouth to drain away from the patient.
- Aspirate content from the mouth.
- Bronchial aspiration and lavage.

Therapeutic management

- Corticosteroids.
- Ventilation.
- Fluid management.
- Bronchodilators, diuretics, etc.
- Physiotherapy.
- Treatment for complications as they arise.
- Prophylactic antibiotics are not usually given routinely (unless infected material aspirated) but they may be required for subsequent secondary infections.[1]

Table 11.1 Risk factors associated with aspiration[1]

Obstetric anaesthesia	Full stomach / delayed emptying
History of reflux /hiatus hernia	Diabetes mellitus
Raised intragastric pressure	Topically anaesthetised airway
Recent trauma	Oesophageal strictures
Perioperative opiates	Oesophageal incompetence

Reference

1. McIndoe A (2006). Anaesthetic emergencies. In Allman KG and Wilson IH (eds) *Oxford Handbook of Anaesthesia* (2nd edn). Oxford University Press: Oxford.

Further reading

Adams AP and Cashman JN (1991). *Anaesthesia, analgesia and intensive care*. Edward Arnold: London.

Simpson PJ and Popart MT (2002). *Understanding anaesthesia* (4th edn). Butterworth-Heinemann: Oxford.

Smith B, Rawlings P, Wicker P, et al. (2007). *Core topics in operating department practice: anaesthesia and critical care*. Cambridge University Press: Cambridge.

Vanner R. (2004). Preventing regurgitation and aspiration. *The Journal of Anaesthesia and Intensive Care Medicine* 5(9) p.293–7.

Anaphylaxis

- Anaphylaxis is a local or systemic hypersensitivity response to a foreign substance (allergen) that causes the release of histamine from mast cells and basophils.
- This process commonly follows previous sensitisation to the allergen (immunoglobulin (IgE) -mediated response), although in the clinically identical anaphylactoid response, this may not be the case.
- The topical response to an allergen is normally limited to a rash (urticaria) and itching (pruritus), whereas the systemic response causes smooth muscle constriction, vasodilation, and capillary leakage.
- This in turn may cause bronchospasm, nausea and diarrhoea, swelling of the face and upper airway (angioedema), and distributive shock, which may be severe and life threatening.
- These responses may take from between a few minutes to an hour to present from the time of contact, and symptoms may recur up to 24 hours after the initial response.

Common allergens found in the operating department

- Latex.
- Antibiotics.
- Muscle relaxants.
- Anaesthetic induction agents.
- Egg lecithin found in propofol.
- Colloid infusions.
- Blood products.

Management

- Treatment should follow the ABCDE approach as advocated by the Resuscitation Council.[1]
- When possible, contact with the suspected allergen (e.g. blood transfusion) should be terminated immediately.
- Where there is airway involvement it is imperative that this is managed promptly as complete airway obstruction may develop.
- IM injection of 500mcg 1:1000 adrenaline (epinephrine) is the first-line drug of choice, though smaller aliquots (e.g. 50–100mcg of 1:10000 solution) of this may be given IV under expert supervision providing full cardiovascular monitoring is employed and resuscitation equipment is at hand.
- Additional salbutamol (nebulised or IV) may be required to combat bronchospasm.
- An anti-histamine (e.g. chlorphenamine) should also be given, along with an anti-inflammatory (e.g. hydrocortisone), and IV infusion of crystalloid solution commenced to support the victim's circulation.
- Following severe reactions, observation of the victim should be continued for 24 hours to exclude recurrence.
- Blood is usually taken at specified intervals following anaphylaxis to test for serum tryptase and mast cell histamine.
- Patch tests should be conducted at an allergy clinic to identify the offending allergen and the victim encouraged to wear an appropriate medic-alert bracelet.

Reference

1. Resusitation Council (UK) (2008). *Emergency treatment of anaphylactic reactions: guidelines for healthcare providers.* Available at: ▣ http://www.resus.org.uk/pages/reaction.pdf

Further reading

Allman KG and Wilson IH (eds) (2006). *Oxford Handbook of Anaesthesia* (2nd edn). Oxford University Press: Oxford.

Marieb EN and Hoehn K (2007). *Human anatomy and physiology* (7th edn). Benjamim Cummings: San Francisco.

Awareness under general anaesthesia

Depth of anaesthesia is very difficult to measure as it depends on various factors including drug concentrations and effects, influence of noxious stimuli, and fluid volume. Anaesthetists strive to deliver the perfect balanced anaesthesia to all patients based on the 'triad' of anaesthesia, narcosis, relaxation, and analgesics; due to their experience and knowledge of pharmacodynamics and pharmacokinetics the overall outcome is that patients are anaesthetised safely and they do not experience any problems or awareness. Agarwal and Griffiths define anaesthesia as a 'lack of response and recall to noxious stimuli' and cite five stages of awareness: [1]

- Conscious awareness, spontaneous or prompted recall—explicit recall.
- Conscious awareness with amnesia.
- Dreaming.
- Unconscious recall with amnesia—implicit recall.
- No awareness or recall.

Awareness during anaesthesia

Ong states that the first case of awareness after the clinical use of a muscle relaxant was in the late 1950s when the use of d-tubocurare was common. [2] Previously, with the use of single agents—e.g. ether—the depth of anaesthesia was enough to keep the patient motionless, thus awareness was not recognised.

Patients who recalled awareness frequently had the same comment that they could feel the surgeon 'cutting them' but they were unable to shout or move to attract the surgeon's attention. [2] The occasions when awareness has occurred is identified by Ong[2] as follows:

- Difficult intubation: level of anaesthesia is not maintained.
- Major trauma, critically ill patients: lower concentration of the volatile agent is delivered because of the difficulty of maintaining cardiovascular stability.
- Caesarean section: awareness occurs because in order to avoid large amounts of drugs getting to the fetus across the placenta, the dose/concentration of drugs given to the mother is reduced.
- Cardiac surgery: when the anaesthetic is altered to facilitate cardiopulmonary bypass.
- Under-dosage of IV anaesthetic agent during total IV anaesthesia.
- Unfamiliarity of new drugs.
- Unintentional pressing of O_2 flush during general anaesthesia: lowering the intended concentration of the anaesthesia.
- Individual variations in the requirement of anaesthesia.

Monitoring depth of anaesthesia

- For a number of years anaesthetists have sought a monitor that could effectively measure the depth of anaesthesia.
- Current assessment includes the provision of a balanced anaesthetic in addition to monitoring the patient's vital signs: pulse, BP, skin tone, sweating, and lacrimation.
- Some patients with neuropathy will not react as predicted.
- In the late 1960s and early 1970s general anaesthesia for obstetric surgery was associated with a very high incidence of explicit recall. [3]

- This was due to the fact that lower doses of thiopental were used and volatile agents avoided.[4]
- With modern anaesthesia techniques and the reduced of general anaesthesia in obstetric surgery awareness can be reduced.[3]
- Several commercial devices exist to measure cerebral activity and gauge depth of anaesthesia e.g. bispectral index monitoring. However, none have so far been proven to reduce the incidence of awareness.

References

1. Agarwal M and Griffiths R (2004). Monitoring the depth of anaesthesia. *Anaesthesia and Intensive Care Medicine* **5**(10), 343–4.

2. Ong BC (1998). Awareness. In Hwang NC (ed) *Anaesthesia: A Practical Handbook*. Oxford University Press: Singapore.

3. Banks A and Levy D (2007). Maintenance of anaesthesia. *Anaesthesia and Intensive Care Medicine* **8**(8), 317–19.

4. Choi D (2004) General anaesthesia for operative obstetrics. *Anaesthesia and Intensive Care Medicine* **5**(8), 264–5.

Further reading

Allman KG and Wilson IH (eds) (2006). *Oxford Handbook of Anaesthesia* (2nd edn). Oxford University Press: Oxford.

Davey A and Diba A (eds) (2005). *Ward's anaesthetic Equipment*.Elsevier Saunders: Philadelphia.

Thompson R and Severn A (2007). Maintenance of anaesthesia. *Anaesthesia and Intensive Care Medicine* **8**(9), 373–8.

High spinal

Dijkema *et al.* define a high/total spinal as a local anaesthetic depression of the cervical spinal cord and the brainstem.[1] It may follow excessive spread of an intrathecal injection of local anaesthetic, or inadvertent spinal injection of an epidural dose of local anaesthetic. It may also occur as a complication of some regional anaesthestheic blocks, e.g. interscalene blocks on the shoulder or retrobulbar blocks on the eye. It occurs because the needle accidentally ends up within a sheath surrounding the nerve which allows local anaesthetic to pass back along the nerve into the CSF.

Influencing factors

- This is most common when an epidural solution (of local anaesthetic) is inadvertently given into the CSF while attempting epidural anaesthesia.
- Positioning of the patient is an important factor with all spinal and epidural anaesthesia. If a patient is placed in a head down position (Trendelenburg position) after the spinal or epidural is performed, especially when using hyperbaric solutions, this could also reproduce the same complication resulting in a high spinal block.
- It is also important to remember that positioning can still affect the block to extend some 20 minutes after the spinal or epidural has been performed.[2]
- The dose, volume, and barbaricity of the local anaesthetic can also have an effect on the level of the spinal anaesthesia.
- The technique can be another influencing factor e.g. type of needle, site of injection, direction of needle, velocity of injection.
- Most spinal and epidural anaesthesia aim to give a maximum upper level block in the region of T10 (nipple level). Anything above this level can produce symptoms that are at least unpleasant and at worst can result in cardiac arrest.

Early signs and symptoms

- Early warning signs would be numbness and tingling in the little fingers and weakness in the hands and arms. This is an indication that the block has reached the cervico-thoracic junction.
- Agitation.
- Difficulty breathing, dyspnoea. The patient will start to complain that they cannot take deep breaths.
- Husky voice. As the phrenic nerves become involved the patient will start to speak quieter until this eventually becomes a whisper.

Late signs and symptoms

- If the spinal/epidural solution dissipates as high as the cranial subarachnoid space 'not only are respiratory muscles paralysed, but also the patient loses use of the cranial nerves'[3] therefore this can progress to:
- Hypotension
- Bradycardia
- Unconsciousness.

- If the solution raises still further then this might enter the fourth ventricle paralysing the respiratory and vasomotor centres resulting in cardiorespiratory arrest.[3]

When experiencing the onset of a high spinal patients very often display increased anxiety. It is absolutely imperative that a member of the perioperative team provides psychological support to the patient at this point. Call for help as extra pairs of hands could be useful.

Treatment
- Ventilation and protection against aspiration.
- Maintaining the BP, both by physical elevation of the legs and administration of IV fluids.
- Use of vasopressor drugs.
- For obstetric patients, left uterine displacement is also advised to improve circulation due to caval compression and to preserve uteroplacental perfusion.[4]
- It must also be remembered that this condition is self limiting in the respect that the symptoms will dissipate with the potency of the local anaesthetic.

References

1. Dijkema LM and Haisma HJ (2002). Case report—Total spinal anaesthesia. *Update in Anaesthesia* **14**, 14. Available at: ⬛ www.nda.ox.ac.uk/wfsa/html/u14/u1414_01.htm#tpf

2. Casey WF (2000). Spinal anaesthesia: a practical guide. *Update in Anaesthesia* **12**, 8. Available at: ⬛ www.nda.ox.ac.uk/wfsa/html/u14/u1414_01.htm#tpm

3. Simpson PJ, Popat MT (2002). *Understanding anaesthesia* (4th edn). Butterworth-Heinemann: Oxford.

4. Braveman FR (2006). *Obstetric and gynaecological anaesthesia*. Mosby: Philadelphia.

Further reading

Adams AP and Cashman JN (1991). *Anaesthesia, analgesia and intensive care*. Edward Arnold: London.

Allman KG and Wilson IH (eds) (2006). *Oxford Handbook of Anaesthesia* (2nd edn). Oxford University Press: Oxford.

Yentis S, May A, and Malhotra S (2007). *Analgesia, anaesthesia and pregnancy: a practical guide*. Cambridge University Press: Cambridge.

Malignant hyperpyrexia

Incidence

- Malignant hyperpyrexia/hyperthermia (MH) is a hereditary condition that results in contracture of the muscle and creates a disruption to metabolic functions during general anesthesia.
- It is a rare syndrome that occurs in genetically pre-disposed patients who are exposed to MH-triggering agents used during general anaesthesia.
- It results in a series of biochemical changes triggered by volatile anaesthetic inhalation agents and suxamethonium, which alters the calcium ion movement within the sarcoplasmic reticulum of muscle cells during muscle contraction.
- This condition affects 1:100,000 of the population with MH episodes reported to be 1:12,000 paediatric and 1:40,000 adult anaesthetic procedures.[1]

Diagnosis

Consider MH if:
- Unexplained, unexpected increase in end tidal CO_2 together with:
- Unexplained, unexpected tachycardia together with:
- Unexplained, unexpected increase in O_2 consumption.
- Muscle spasm/rigidity after suxamethonium.
- Rapidly rising body core temperature—rises by 0.6°C (1.0°F) per minute.

Patient management

Immediate management:
- Call for help.
- Remove all trigger agents.
- Turn off vaporisers.
- Increase O_2 to 100%.
- Transfer to vaporiser-free anaesthetic machine and new breathing circuit.
- Hyperventilate.
- Maintain anaesthesia with IV agents .
- Administer dantrolene (2–3mg/kg IV initially and then 1mg/kg at 10-minute intervals).
- Abandon surgery if feasible.
- Use active body cooling but avoid vasoconstriction (convert active warming devices to active cooling, give cold IV fluids, cold peritoneal lavage, extracorporeal heat exchange).[2]

Patient monitoring should include:
- ECG.
- SpO_2.
- End-tidal CO_2
- Invasive arterial BP.
- CVP.
- Core and peripheral temperature.
- Urine output and pH.

- Arterial blood gases.
- Potassium.
- Haematocrit.
- Platelets.
- Clotting indices.
- Creatine.

Later management
- Transfer to ITU.
- Administer diuretic to avoid obstructive renal failure.
- Repeat arterial blood gases.
- Refer to National Screening Unit at St. James University Hospital, Leeds.
- Screen the patient's family in a specialised centre.

Management for future surgery
- Oral dantrolene preoperatively.
- Vapour-free anaesthetic machine and circuit.
- Propofol and opioid infusions.
- Temperature monitoring.
- Consider local or regional anaesthesia.

References and further reading

Association of Anaesthetists of Great Britain and Ireland (2007). *Guidelines for the Management of a Malignant Hyperthermia Crisis*. AAGBI: London.

Allman KG and Wilson IH (eds) (2006). *Oxford Handbook of Anaesthesia* (2nd edn). Oxford University Press: Oxford.

British Malignant Hyperthermia Association (BMHA). Available at: 🖥 www.bmha.co.uk/index.html

Respiratory arrest

Respiratory arrest, the *cessation of spontaneous respiratory effort* (see Box 11.1), is a common temporary side effect of general anaesthesia but may also be seen as a result of critical illness, drug overdose, or trauma. Respiratory arrest leads to a generalised hypoxia and hypercarbia (CO_2 retention) and causes an increase in anaerobic metabolism, contributing to a mixed metabolic and respiratory acidosis. Respiratory arrest may be preceded by a period of respiratory failure (failure *of the respiratory system to enable a suitable exchange of gases between the outside air and the patient's cells*[1]). If not recognised and managed appropriately, respiratory arrest will almost invariably lead to cardiac arrest.

Box 11.1 Mechanism of normal respiration

Normal respiration requires stimulation of the diaphragm and intercostal muscles (via the phrenic and intercostal nerves) to inspire air through the upper and lower airways into the alveoli (alveolar ventilation), where gases (O_2 and CO_2) are exchanged across the alveolar walls to and from the circulation by way of the capillary network of the pulmonary circulation. Expiration is normally passive, utilising the elastic recoil of the thoracic cage, thereby allowing the release of excess CO_2 to the atmosphere. The respiratory centre, located in the medulla oblongata, governs the rate and depth of respiration in response to the levels of CO_2 detected in blood. In chronic respiratory disease, the body will compensate for chronically high levels of CO_2 by responding instead to abnormal levels of O_2 (hypoxic drive). Effective elimination of CO_2 through respiration is integral to the homeostatic mechanism of acid–base balance.

Treatment

Treatment should be both supportive and definitive, and follow the ABCDE principles to *treat first that which kills first*:

- **A (airway)**: *assess* that the patient's airway is patent and free of foreign bodies and excessive secretions; *ensure* that the patient's airway remains open and clear using suction and *airway manoeuvres* (🕮 see A: airway, p.554) and adjuncts, including ET tubes or surgical airways, as required.
- **B (breathing)**: *assess* the patient's breathing: is it normal (regular, symmetrical, suitable depth), noisy (wheezy, snoring, or crowing), or absent? Noise on inspiration normally indicates partial upper airway obstruction (e.g. presence of foreign body, loss of protective airway reflexes, spasm of vocal cords (laryngospasm) etc.); noise on expiration indicates partial lower airway obstruction (e.g. bronchospasm); silence indicates either complete airway obstruction or respiratory arrest; *ensure* the patient's respiration is sufficient to prevent hypoxia and hypercarbia; artificial ventilation with high–flow O_2 using either a mechanical ventilator or a self–inflating resuscitation bag, or equivalent, may be required to achieve this. NB O_2 therapy is mandatory in all cases of respiratory insufficiency. If *tension pneumothorax* is suspected, needle thoracocentesis (🕮 see B: breathing, p.556) must be performed

immediately; in *bronchospasm*, nebulized bronchodilators (e.g. *salbutamol*) and anti–cholinergics (e.g. *ipratropium*) may be required, while in *laryngospasm*, positive end expiratory pressure ventilation (PEEP) and small doses of suxamethonium may be required to facilitate adequate ventilation. Continuous pulse oximetry and end–tidal CO_2 monitoring (in the anaesthetised patient), along with repeated blood gas analysis (in the critically ill patient) should be employed to monitor the effectiveness of ventilation.

- *C (circulation):* assess patient's circulation by monitoring pulse, capillary refill, BP, ECG, and urine output; in high–dependency areas invasive techniques may also be employed; *ensure* adequacy of the patient's circulation by securing IV access and administering boluses of crystalloid fluid as required (NB beware of fluid overload, especially in the young and old, and those with pre–existing heart conditions); in high dependency areas, *inotropes* may be utilised to support the cardiovascular system.
- *D (disability):* assess the patient's level of consciousness; confusion, aggression or coma may all be signs of cerebral hypoxia.
- *E (exposure):* assess and identify the underlying cause using the patient's clinical notes and previous history; *initiate* appropriate treatment e.g. surgical intervention, drug antagonists (*naloxone (opioids), flumazenil (benzodiazepines), neostigmine/glycopyrronium (muscle relaxants)* etc.), antibiotics etc.

Causes of respiratory arrest

See Table 11.2.

Table 11.2 Classification of causes of respiratory failure and arrest

Causes	Examples
Respiratory drive dysfunction	• Drugs e.g. anaesthetic agents, alcohol, opioids, sedatives, tranquillisers • Trauma to brain, spinal cord • Breath holding (especially in neonates) and sleep apnoea
Impaired function of the chest and lungs	• Obstruction e.g. by tongue, foreign bodies, tumours, excessive secretions • Trauma to airway (e.g. burns), or thoracic cage (flail chest etc) or soft tissues (pneumothorax, tension pneumothorax, haemothorax etc. • Pulmonary oedema e.g. due to gastric aspiration, fluid overload, cardiac or liver failure • Bronchospasm, laryngospasm • Infections and other disease processes e.g. pneumonia, COPD • Skeletal abnormality e.g. scoliosis; • Muscle weakness brought on by disease (e.g. myasthenia gravis) or fatigue (especially in acute episodes of asthma and COPD) or drugs (muscle relaxants) • Gastric/abdominal distension and diaphragmatic splinting • Pain following trauma, surgery etc.
Failure of circulatory gas transport mechanisms	• Hypovolaemia • Circulatory failure • Anaemia • Poisoning e.g. carbon monoxide, cyanide

Reference

1. Sue DY and Lewis DA (2002). Respiratory failure. In Bongard FS, Sue DY (eds) *Current critical care diagnosis & treatment.* Lange Medical Books/McGraw Hill: New York.

Further reading

Davies NJH and Cashman JD (2005). *Lee's Synopsis of Anaesthesia.* Butterworth-Heinemann: Oxford.

Resuscitation Council (UK) (2006). *Advanced Life Support Providers Manual.* London: Resuscitation Council (UK).

Suxamethonium apnoea

Incidence

Suxamethonium (scoline) apnoea is a rare condition that occurs due to an inability to break down the drug suxamethonium. As a result of this, the muscle relaxant effects of the drug last far longer than usual (several hours rather than a few minutes). The enzyme responsible for breaking down suxamethonium is plasma cholinesterase.

This condition can be inherited or appear spontaneously in a person with no family history. In cases where suxamethonium apnoea is inherited the level of plasma cholinesterase is reduced whereas in the acquired condition the level of plasma cholinesterase is normal but its activity is reduced.

Suxamethonium
- Suxamethonium is a depolarising, fast acting muscle relaxant and its main use in anaesthesia is to allow the rapid intubation of the trachea.
- Suxamethonium depolarises skeletal muscle and lasts for approximately 2–6 minutes imitating acetylcholine at the neuromuscular junction where it binds to the postsynaptic membrane.
- As it binds non-competitively at the junction it cannot be reversed by other drugs.

Inherited suxamethonium apnoea
- It is important to identify the possibility of atypical pseudocholinesterase (suxamethonium apnoea) as a genetically inherited condition so a comprehensive family history should be sought.
- Preoperative screening for cholinesterase activity is advised if the patient or a close relative has experienced prolonged paralysis after surgery that required ventilatory support for a significant length of time.
- The action of suxamethonium in inherited incidences can be increased from a few minutes to 2 hours or more.

Acquired suxamethonium apnoea
- Plasma cholinesterase is normal in patients with acquired incidence but has reduced activity.
- Acquired incidences in situations such as pregnancy, liver and renal disease, or if the patient may be taking medicines such as methotrexate, the action of suxamethonium can be increased by minutes as opposed to hours.

Diagnosis

Once suxamethonium has been administered, further muscle relaxants should be avoided until muscle tone returns or if there is a delay in breathing. Look for signs of awareness in an unexpectedly muscle-relaxed patient. Diagnosis can be confirmed by the use of a nerve stimulator to determine the level of neuromuscular transmission.

Patient management

If diagnosis is confirmed:
- Maintain anaesthesia.
- Maintain ventilation.
- Monitor neuromuscular transmission with nerve stimulator—if nerve stimulator is unavailable, maintain anaesthesia and ventilation and breathing becomes spontaneous.
- Transfer to intensive care unit until metabolism is complete and the patient breathes spontaneously.
- Extubate awake—when the patient is able to obey commands.
- Conduct family studies to determine exposure.

References and further reading

Allman KG and Wilson IH (eds) (2006). *Oxford Handbook of Anaesthesia* (2nd edn). Oxford University Press: Oxford.

Martyn J and Marcel D (2006). Succinylcholine: new insights into mechanisms of action of an old drug. *Anesthesiology* **104**(4), 663–4.

Rees J (2005). Suxamethonium apnoea. *Update in Anaesthesia*, **19**, Article 16. Available at: www.nda.ox.ac.uk/wfsa/html/u19/u1916_01.htm

Specialist anaesthesia

Obstetric anaesthesia

The aim of anaesthesia for Caesarean section or any surgery whilst pregnant is that it should be safe for both the mother and the foetus. The obstetric theatre must always be prepared for immediate use if required and the following points observed:

- Theatre temperature should be between 22–24°C.
- Anaesthetic machine checked and intubation equipment ready.
- Difficult intubation equipment available.
- Spinal/epidural equipment ready.
- IV fluids prepared.
- Many obstetric theatres have pre drawn-up induction drugs prepared daily and stored in theatre for expediency.
- ECG, BP, pulse oximeter, capnograph, and gas analyser.

Physiological changes significant to anaesthesia

Circulatory and respiratory changes provide for the metabolic needs of the fetus and mother.

Cardiovascular changes

- Increase in cardiac output.
- Increase in blood flow to many organs, biggest being to the uterus.
- Increase in plasma volume causing haemodilution—fall in haemoglobin leading to anaemia.
- Decrease in BP during first trimester.

Pre-eclampsia

- Causes problems with circulation which normally show up as high BP, protein in the urine, and swelling
- Can become serious and affect other systems such as the liver, brain, lungs, or clotting system.
- Haemolysis elevated liver enzymes low platelet count (HELLP) is considered a variant of pre-eclampsia and can be life threatening.

Aorto-caval compression

During pregnancy some women feel faint when lying supine due to the vena cava, and sometimes the aorta, being occluded. A collateral system of veins reaches the heart instead but if this pathway is not effective the heart is deprived of venous return, output is not maintained, and BP drops. It must be anticipated in all pregnant patients over 20 weeks and avoided by uterine displacement. This is done simply by placing a wedge under the patient's right hip causing a tilt to the left and thus preventing the compression.

Respiratory changes

- Increase in tidal volume due to increased levels of progesterone which has a stimulant effect on the respiratory centre and also an elevated diaphragm from the growing uterus.
- Rapid falls in O_2 saturation on induction of general anaesthetic due to:
  - Increased O_2 consumption.
  - Decreased cardiac output.
  - Decrease in functional residual capacity.
  - MAC values decrease in pregnancy increasing susceptibility to anaesthetic agents.

General anaesthesia

The placental barrier is readily crossed by most pharmacological agents used in anaesthesia and may have a potential effect on the foetus. It is fair to assume that all pregnant patients are at risk of inhalation of gastric contents due to regurgitation as a result of:

- 'Big bump': uterus compresses the stomach against the diaphragm.
- Heartburn: due to incompetence of lower oesophageal sphincter.
- Full stomach: due to delayed gastric emptying.

Post-delivery it can take up to 6 weeks for changes to revert back.

Prophylaxis and prevention

Raise the pH of gastric contents by administering alkali sodium citrate and block secretion of acid by administering H_2 antagonist. Antacids may also be given with regional anaesthesia as it may need to be converted to general anaesthesia.

Rapid sequence induction

- Patient on tilting trolley.
- Intubation equipment ready and to hand—consider smaller ET tubes and avoid nasal intubation as the respiratory mucous membrane becomes vascular and oedematous.
- Suction available.
- 100% preoxygenation for 3 minutes.
- Application of cricoid pressure.
- Intubation and inflation of cuff on ET tube.
- Check correct placement of tube.
- Release cricoid pressure on instruction of anaesthetist.

Risk of difficult intubation

- Full dentition, crowns.
- Laryngeal oedema.
- Large breasts, use polio blade.
- Tilted on their side.

Regional anaesthesia (spinal/epidural)

Benefit of potentially having partner present in theatre and able to start bonding with the baby straight away.

Consider

- Epidural may already be in place and just need topping up.
- Preload with IV fluids as risk of hypotension.
- IV ephedrine prepared.
- May be difficult for mother to get or keep in position for insertion.

Non-obstetric surgery for the pregnant patient

- Only emergency surgery should be performed.
- Local anaesthesia should be considered.
- General anaesthesia in 1st trimester should avoid N_2O.
- General anaesthesia in 2nd and 3rd trimester.
  - Avoid aorto-caval compression.
  - RSI.
- Avoid hypotension.
- Equipment available in case of need for emergency Caesarean section.

Paediatric and neonatal anaesthesia

Paediatric anaesthesia includes patients from the premature neonate to adolescents (Table 12.1).[1]

Table 12.1 Definitions of paediatric patients[1]

Neonate	First 44 weeks of post-conceptual age
Premature infant	<37 weeks' gestational age
Infant	Babies from 1–12 months old
SGA	Small for gestational age
Low birth weight	<2.5kg

Preoperative management

- Pre-assessment should involve the parents (carers) and children who are given the opportunity to ask questions.
- A designated paediatric intensive care unit (PICU) should be available for children who require intensive care following surgery.
- Day care surgery should be considered for surgical procedures that are neither complex nor prolonged.
- Preterm or ex-preterm neonates should not be considered for day case surgery unless they are medically fit and healthy and have reached 60 weeks' post-conceptual age.[2]
- Infants with a history of chronic lung disease or 'apnoea' should be managed in a centre equipped with facilities for postoperative ventilation.[2]
- Parents/carers should be kept informed of their child's progress, especially if there is an unexpected delay in theatre.

Anaesthetic management

- Paediatric anaesthesia services must be consultant led.
- Paediatric resuscitation equipment must be available and staff must regularly update their knowledge and competence in paediatric life support.
- Parental presence in the anaesthetic room should be encouraged.
- IV induction:
  - According to anaesthetist's preference, IV cannula should be introduced when the child is sitting on a parent's lap with his/her view obstructed.
  - Induction of anaesthesia with propofol.
  - Thiopental for neonates.
- Gas induction by sevoflurane is recommended whilst the child is sitting on a parent/carer's lap.
- It may not be possible to attach all monitoring before induction of paediatric patients.[3]
- Monitoring of paediatric patients should include BP, temperature probes, pulse oximetry, and ECG for all patients.
- A defibrillator and resuscitation drugs and equipment must be available wherever children are anaesthetised.

- Anaesthetic machines should incorporate ventilators, which have controls and bellows permitting their use over the entire age range together with the facility to provide pressure controlled ventilation.[2]
- Volumetric infusion pumps should be used for IV fluids.
- The size of the ET tube used for paediatric anaesthesia is important; an ET tube that is too large will exert pressure on the internal surface of the cricoid cartilage resulting in oedema which could lead to airway obstruction when the tube is removed (Table 12.2).[4]
- An uncuffed ET tube is recommended for use in children under 10 years old as it provides a larger internal diameter compared with a cuffed tube.[4]
- ET tube should be secured in place.

Table 12.2 Internal diameter of ET tube related to age[4]

Premature	2.5–3.0 mm
Neonate–6 months	3.0–3.5 mm
6 months–1 year	3.5–4.0 mm
1–2 years	4.0–5.0 mm
> 2 years—use the formula	4+ (age/4)

Thermoregulation

- Paediatric patients, particularly neonates, are prone to heat loss.
- The operating theatre should be warmed up to 26°C prior to surgery.
- A paediatric patient's head should be covered with a cap or gamgee.
- Gamgee can also be used to cover other parts of the patient's body to maintain heat.
- Utilise active warming devices and warm all fluids.

Postoperative management

- Recovery of a paediatric patient should be on a one-to-one basis.
- Apnoea is a common postoperative complication in neonates who are pre-term so provide apnoea monitoring equipment.
- Administer O_2 postoperatively if tolerated.
- Allow parents into recovery as soon as airway is maintained.
- Monitor SpO_2, pulse, and respiratory rate.
- Analgesia can include: NSAIDs and paracetamol; caudal analgesia; nurse-controlled analgesia (NCA) or patient controlled analgesia (PCA) for severe pain.

References

1. Berg S (2006). Paediatric and neonatal anaesthesia. In Allman KG and Wilson IH (eds) *Oxford Handbook of Anaesthesia* (2nd edn). Oxford University Press: Oxford.

2. Royal College of Anaesthetists (2004). *Guidelines for the Provision of Anaesthetic Service: Paediatric anaesthetic services*. RCoA: London.

3. Association of Anaesthetists of Great Britain and Ireland (2007). *Recommendation for standards of monitoring during anaesthesia and recovery* (4th edn). AAGBI: London.

4. Rusy L, Usaleva E (1998) Paediatric anaesthesia review. *Update in Anaesthesia* **8**, 2. Available at: www.nda.ox.ac.uk/wfsa/html/u08/u08_003.htm

Ear, nose, and throat anaesthesia

The procedures undertaken within this specialty often require specific tracheal tubes and interventions.

Procedures may include:
- Myringotomy.
- Mastoidectomy.
- Nasal polypectomy.
- Septoplasty.
- Tonsillectomy.
- Tracheostomy.

General considerations
- Shared airway between the surgeon and anaesthetist.
- Position of patient—extended breathing circuits may be required.
- Head ring or other suitable device should be available to aid positioning.
- Potentially difficult intubation.
- Protection of patient's eyes.
- Warming equipment for longer procedures.
- LMAs may be used.
- Mini-Trach should be available.
- Ear surgery.
- Surgeon may require patient to be hypotensive to produce a bloodless surgical field, therefore consider the need for invasive BP monitoring.
- N_2O diffuses into middle ear with the potential to displace surgical grafts; its use should therefore be avoided in middle ear surgery.

Nasal surgery
- Oral preformed tube (e.g. Ring, Adair, and Elwyn (RAE) to face away from site of surgery.
- Preformed shape fits over mouth without kinking.
- Throat pack to absorb secretions—insertion and removal must be recorded.

Tonsillectomy
- Oral preformed tube to allow surgical access.
- RAE tubes available uncuffed for paediatric patients.
- Theoretical risk of CJD from instrumentation[1]– refer to hospital policy.
- Lateral position with slight head down tilt prior to extubation.

Microlaryngoscopy/direct laryngoscopy
- Microlaryngoscopy tube (MLT), available in internal diameter sizes 5, 5.5, and 6. Allows surgeon maximum access.
- It is important not to cut tube length as it is longer by design to allow nasal intubation if necessary. Also gives greater length outside the mouth to allow circuit to be attached at a safe distance.
- Cuff size is bigger than a standard tracheal tube of the same internal diameter size to facilitate an adequate seal in an adult trachea.

Laser surgery

- Laser resistant tube required to prevent potential ignition of tube.
- Laser-Flex tube® (Mallinkrodt) consists of a stainless steel body which protects the tube against CO_2 laser beams.
- Tube has two cuffs which are inflated with sterile saline. This reduces the risk of an air-filled cuff igniting if hit by the laser.
- Some hospitals use methylene blue to inflate cuffs so surgeon is alerted to a ruptured cuff.
- The presence of two cuffs ensures a tracheal seal in the event of damage to one.
- Laser precautions to be followed, including protective spectacles and warning sign on all entrance doors.
- Ensure the patient's eyes are protected.

Laryngectomy

- Standard or reinforced tracheal tube initially.
- The laryngectomy tube is inserted after the larynx has been removed and when a tracheal stoma has been fashioned.
- When surgeon is ready to insert the laryngectomy/tracheostomy tube communication must be of paramount importance.
- Surgeon visually locates tracheal tube and withdraws it to just above incision. This allows the tube to be re-inserted should airway problems occur.
- Laryngectomy tubes e.g. Laryngoflex® (sizes 7, 8 & 9) and Montandon® (sizes 6, 7, 8, 9 &10) have the advantage of allowing the breathing circuit to be attached further from the surgical field, therefore improving access.
- If laryngectomy tube used, this will be changed to a tracheostomy tube at the end of surgery, as a shorter tube will reduce both the dead space and the risk of dislodging the tube.

Reference

1. Department of Health (2001). *Risk assessment for the transmission of vCJD: a modelling approach and numerical scenarios.* DH: London.

Further reading

Aitkenhead AR, Rowbotham DJ, and Smith G (2001). *Textbook of anaesthesia* (4th edn). Churchill Livingstone: Edinburgh.

Barash PG, Cullen BF, and Stoelting RK (2006). *Handbook of clinical anaesthesia* (5th edn). Lippincott, Williams & Wilkins: Philadelphia.

Neurosurgical anaesthesia

The RCoA state that an anaesthetic clinical service should provide:[1]
- Anaesthesia for neurosurgery including intracranial, complex spinal, and associated surgery.
- Anaesthesia for neuroradiology including diagnostic and interventional procedures.
- Neurocritical care including pre- and postoperative management of complex elective cases and the management of critically ill patients, e.g. severe head injury, intracranial haemorrhage, severe neurological disease, and those who develop systemic complications secondary to their neurological condition.

Anaesthesia for many neurosurgical factors has common factors; the greatest of which is the prevention of a rise in intracranial pressure.[2] Neuroanaesthesia for children should include shared responsibility between neuroanaesthetists and paediatric anaesthetists.[1]

Examples of neurosurgical procedures[3]
- Cerebral aneurysm repair.
- Craniotomy.
- Awake craniotomy.
- Posterior fossa surgery.
- Ventriculo-peritoneal shunt.
- Laminectomy.
- Pituitary surgery.
- Evacuation of traumatic intracranial haematoma.

Preoperative management
- Pre-admission clinics for elective neurosurgery should be available.
- Assessment for signs of raised intracranial pressure (ICP).
- Assess neurological observations.
- Sedative drugs in patients with raised ICP should be avoided.
- Prophylactic VTE therapy.
- Urinary catheter for surgical procedures of long duration.

Anaesthetic management
- The incidence of difficult intubation in neurosurgical units carrying out complex cervical spinal surgery is high.
- Difficult airway management equipment must be available.
- Patient monitoring should include:
  - ECG, SpO$_2$, naso-pharyngeal temperature.
  - CVP and arterial line for invasive BP monitoring for major neurosurgical procedures.
- Preoxygenate for at least 3 minutes.
- Hypertension and tachycardia should be avoided.
- Propofol or thiopental for IV induction administered slowly is recommended with vecuronium as a muscle relaxant.
- Avoid suxamethonium as it raises ICP—only use for RSI in emergency surgery where a full stomach is possible i.e. head injury.

- An armoured ET tube should be use for intubation and secured well.
- Transfer patient from operating theatre table to bed with care to avoid excess movement.
- Patient positions can vary for neurosurgery, so it is essential that all monitoring and ventilatory support are secured.

Signs of raised ICP

- Deterioration of levels of consciousness.
- Changes in breathing pattern or respiratory rate.
- Dilated pupil.
- Decreased movement of one side.
- If any of these signs occur, call the anaesthetist and neurosurgeon immediately!

Postoperative management

- Neurological observations.
- Hypotension decreases cerebral blood flow and may cause hypoxia and fitting.
- Ondine's curse, a complication of neurosurgery, can result from severe brain or spinal trauma; patients can forget to breathe or suffer respiratory arrest so re-intubation and ventilation may be necessary.
- Analgesia ± anti-emetic therapy.
- Some patients will be transferred immediately to ITU.
- For transfer to intensive care unit—O_2, ventilatory support, continuous monitoring, drug infusion pumps, anaesthetic assistance for emergencies, and resuscitation drugs.

References and further reading

1. Royal College of Anaesthetists (2004). *Guidelines for the Provision of Anaesthetic Service: Neuro anaesthesia and neuro critical care.* RCoA: London.

2. Simpson PJ and Popat M (2002). *Understanding anaesthesia* (4th edn). Butterworth-Heinemann: Oxford.

3. Clayton T and Manara A (2006). Neurosurgery. In Allman KG and Wilson IH (eds) *Oxford Handbook of Anaesthesia* (2nd edn). Oxford University Press: Oxford.

Association of Anaesthetists of Great Britain and Ireland (2007). *Recommendation for standards of monitoring during anaesthesia and recovery* (4th edn). AAGBI: London.

Dickenson A (2003). Complications of neurosurgery and spinal surgery. In Leaper DJ and Peel ALG (eds) *Handbook of Postoperative Complications.* Oxford University Press: Oxford.

Hatfield A and Tronson M (2001). *The Complete Recovery Room Book* (3rd edn). Oxford University Press: Oxford.

NICE Guidance: Nervous system surgery. Available at: ▣ www.nice.org.uk/guidance/index.jsp?action=byTopic&o=7606

Ophthalmic anaesthesia

Most cataract surgery is performed on an elderly population with 80% of patients being over the age of 70 years. 57% of these also have concurrent medical problems. Resuscitation equipment must be readily available.

Types of anaesthetic

General

- Pre-disposing factors: include age (child), dementia, severe anxiety, surgical duration, local anaesthetic sensitivity.
- Usually spontaneously breathing using LMA. Follow minimum monitoring guidelines,
- Total IV infusion (TIVA): used for induction and maintenance in most cases.
- Tape/protect non-surgical eye where appropriate.

Local

- Topical: provided by the application of local analgesic eye drops. Short acting, but useful for minor operations on the conjunctiva and cornea. Also required prior to sub-Tenon/peribulbar procedures.
- Surface analgesia: local infiltration of local anaesthetic is used to good effect for operations on the eyelids.
- Sub-Tenon injection: a technique where the local anaesthetic is deposited underneath the Tenon's capsule, using a special cannula introduced through a small incision in the conjunctiva.
- Peribulbar infiltration: rarely used now due to risk of nerve damage.

Sharp needle-based local anaesthetic blocks should be performed or directly supervised by anaesthetist or surgeon who has been specifically trained.

IV sedation should only be administered under the supervision of an anaesthetist, who must have sole responsibility to that list.

Anaesthetic equipment required

- Operating table, trolley, or reclining chair.
- Baseline observation recording—heart rate, O_2 sats, BP.
- Monitoring in accordance with local policy for general anaesthetic.
- Prescribed topical drugs (sterile) tetracaine.
- Sterile gloves.
- Needles, syringes—assorted.
- IV access—anaesthetist preference.

For anaesthetic

- Sub-Tenon cannula.
- Lid retractor—speculum.
- Forceps—Morefields.
- Scissor—Westcott.
- Aqueous povidone iodine,® or chlorhexidine—must be aqueous not alcoholic.

Within theatre

- Rubens pillow.
- Pillow under knees.

- Heal supports.
- Theatre practitioner or theatre assistant to hold the patient's hand, or patient alert method in place.
- Piped air supply (under drapes) nasal specs can be used for O_2 if required/prescribed.

Other factors for consideration

Raising intraocular pressure

- Suxamethonium raises intraocular pressure by the contraction of muscles surrounding orbit.
- Coughing, vomiting, and head-down tilt also raise pressures.

Oculocardiac reflex

- Squint surgery inevitably involves some form of traction on the extraocular eye muscles. This may cause cardiac arrhythmias including bradycardia or even asystole.

Anaesthesia for burns surgery

A major burn is defined as a burn covering 25% or more of total body surface area. However, any injury over more than 10% should be treated similarly.[1]

Rapid assessment is vital as swelling may develop around the airway in the hours after injury and require intubation. An assessment must be made to identify if the airway is compromised or is at risk of compromise:

- Preoperative assessment of the patient is vital and should include the history and events following the injury.
- It is essential to maintain safety for the individual undergoing treatment; protect vascular access and make appropriate and informed airway care decisions.[1]

The depth of the burn is important for the planning of treatment and can be classified as shown in Box 12.1.

Box 12.1 Classification of burns[2]

Erythema (1°): not included in the estimate of the burned area; it will not be blistered but may be painful and usually heals without treatment.

Superficial partial thickness (2°), deep partial thickness (2°), and full thickness (3°) areas are included in the estimate of the burned area. The difference between superficial and deep is that superficial partial thickness burns are more likely to heal without scarring. Under-resuscitation can cause deterioration of burned areas to a more severe grade.

Complex burns are inevitably included in the estimate of the burned area and involve destruction of tissues deep to the skin such as tendon muscle, and bone. Other complex burns include burns to the face, airway and perineum.

Anaesthetic considerations

Burns or plastics procedures can take many hours and every attempt should be made to ensure the environment is suitable to the needs of patients with burns. Burns patients are susceptible to heat and fluid loss, infection and airway difficulties, and require specialist pain control.

Monitoring

- Patients undergoing extensive burns or microvascular surgical procedures require invasive monitoring during resuscitation, surgery and intensive care.[3]
- Arterial lines should be inserted in unconscious patients and patients with major burns and/or inhalational injury.[4]
- Vascular access may be compromised by the burn.

Airway
- Difficult airway equipment must be available where burns patients are treated.
- Patient's airway may be compromised by the oedema of the burn and crystalloid resuscitation—also check mouth and lips.
- Airway difficulties can worsen as the injury matures by scarring and contracture and can render conventional laryngoscopy impossible.
- Blind intubation techniques or awake intubation may also be necessary.

Anaesthesia
- Gas inductions and spontaneous breathing techniques may be considered with the use of an LMA or fibre optic aided intubation.
- Caution should be applied with the use of suxamethonium as it can exaggerate hyperkalaemia.[2]
- Consider regional blockade with local anaesthesia for patients undergoing microvascular surgery.

Fluid management
- Fluid should be warmed to ensure that the development of hypothermia does not complicate clotting function or cause inappropriate vasoconstriction.
- Signs of inadequate fluid administration include oliguria, haemoconcentration, and hypotension.
- Fluid resuscitation may be performed to:
  - Preserve life.
  - Maintain organ function.
  - Ameliorate the injury.
  - Restrict surgery to necessity and functional restoration.
  - Limit psychological damage.[2]

Postoperative management
- If surgery is prolonged, postoperative ventilation may be considered.
- Both acute and chronic pain services will be needed to facilitate optimal pain management.[3]
- Repeated anaesthetic input may be required for debridement and dressings until stable wound coverage and healing is obtained.

References

1. Hettiaratchy S and Papini R (2004). Initial management of a major burn. *British Medical Journal.* **328**, 1555–7.

2. Milne M (2003). The Burn Injury. *Update in Anaesthesia* **16**, 13. Available at: 🖳 www.nda.ox.ac.uk/wfsa/html/u16/u1613_01.htm

3. Royal College of Anaesthetists (2004). *Guidelines for the Provision of Anaesthetic Services: Burns and plastics anaesthesia.* RCoA: London.

4. Nolan J (2006). *The critically ill patient.* In Allman KG and Wilson IH (eds) *Oxford Handbook of Anaesthesia* (2nd edn). Oxford University Press: Oxford.

Anaesthesia for plastic surgery

The range and complexity of anaesthesia during plastic/reconstruction surgery can involve routine and extensive surgical procedures (see Box 12.2 for some examples).[1]

Operative procedures can last many hours, may involve significant blood loss, and can require the presence of more than one anaesthetist.[2]

A burns and plastics service will require provision of anaesthesia for a diverse range of surgical procedures in both emergency and elective situations.[2] Appropriate postoperative care and/or critical care facilities may be required for patients requiring the following procedures:
- Surgery for minor and major hand injuries:
  - Replantation following traumatic amputations.
  - Minor and routine cosmetic surgery.
  - Dressing changes.
- Complex surgical procedures such as surgery for:
  - Head and neck cancers.
  - Microvascular techniques.
  - Breast reconstructive surgery.

Box 12.2 Examples of procedures requiring plastic/ reconstructive surgery[1]

- Breast augmentation.
- Breast reduction.
- Gynaecomastia.
- Insertion of tissue expander.
- Liposuction.
- Correction of prominent ears.
- Free-flap surgery.
- Skin grafting.
- Cranio-facial reconstruction.
- Abdominoplasty

Anaesthetic considerations
- Difficult airway equipment must be available in any area where plastic surgery is performed.
- Patient's airway may be compromised in the case of head and neck surgery and consideration should be given to the shared airway.
- Blind intubation techniques or awake intubation may also be necessary.
- Patients undergoing microvascular surgical procedures may require invasive monitoring.[2]
- Consider regional blockade with local anaesthesia for patients undergoing microvascular surgery.
- If the operating site is extensive, difficulties may arise with heat conservation, patient monitoring, and vascular access.[1]
- If surgery is prolonged, postoperative ventilation may be considered; additional considerations should be given to:
  - Vascular access.

- Blood loss.
- Fluid balance.
- Thermoregulation.
- Patient positioning.
- VTE prophylaxis.
- Eye care.
- ET cuff pressure.[1]
- Both acute and chronic pain services will be needed to facilitate optimal pain management.[2]
- A smooth emergence from anaesthesia is recommended by Warwick[1] to avoid tension on suture lines, which may increase bleeding and the formation of a haematoma.
- Ensure effective postoperative analgesia.

References and further reading

1. Warwick J (2006). Plastic surgery. In Allman KG and Wilson IH (eds) *Oxford Handbook of Anaesthesia* (2nd edn). Oxford University Press: Oxford.

2. Royal College of Anaesthetists (2004). *Guidelines for the Provision of Anaesthetic Services: Burns and plastics anaesthesia.* RCoA: London.

Association of Anaesthetists of Great Britain and Ireland (2007). *Recommendation for standards of monitoring during anaesthesia and recovery* (4th edn). AAGBI: London.

Humzah D (2003). Complications of plastic surgery. In Leaper DJ and Peel ALG (eds) *Handbook of Postoperative Complications.* Oxford University Press: Oxford.

Nolan J (2006). The critically ill patient. In Allman KG and Wilson IH (eds) *Oxford Handbook of Anaesthesia* (2nd edn). Oxford University Press: Oxford.

Cardiac anaesthesia

Cardiac surgery can be divided into closed heart procedures and open heart procedures (see Box 12.3 for some examples). Simpson and Popat state that the heart and lungs function normally during closed heart procedures, whereas during open heart procedures, blood to the heart and lungs is diverted or bypassed 'to an extracorporeal circuit comprising a pump and gas exchanger and allowing arrest of lung ventilation and heart beat'.[1]

> **Box 12.3 Examples of cardiac surgical procedures[2]**
> - Coronary artery bypass graft
> - Aortic valve replacement
> - Mitral valve replacement
> - Pulmonary thromboembolectomy
> - Implantable defibrillators
> - Thoracic aortic aneurysm surgery

Preoperative management

- Comprehensive pre assessment should to include 12-lead ECG.
- Assessment of airway.
- Smoking cessation and preoperative physiotherapy is recommended prior to elective cardiac surgery to optimise lung function.
- Dental check for patients with valvar disease and who are at risk of infective endocarditis.
- Diuretic drugs should continue until the day of surgery.
- Digoxin should be discontinued 36–48 hours preoperatively.[1]

> 'The aim of induction of anaesthesia for cardiac surgery is to produce unconsciousness while maintaining a stable cardiovascular system in which myocardial oxygen demand is minimised and myocardial oxygen supply is maximised.'[1]

Anaesthetic management

- Ensure a defibrillator and resuscitation drugs are available in the anaesthetic room.
- Patient monitoring should include:
  - 5-lead ECG.
  - SpO_2.
  - CVP.
  - Naso-pharyngeal temperature following induction of anaesthesia.
  - Arterial line for invasive BP monitoring.
- Preoxygenate for at least 3 minutes.
- Prophylactic antibiotic therapy for some procedures.
- Hypertension and tachycardia should be avoided.

Cardiopulmonary bypass

- Cardiopulmonary bypass is the joint responsibility of surgeons, anaesthetists, and clinical perfusionists but the safety of the cardiopulmonary bypass remains the primary responsibility of the perfusionist who must be present at all times.

- Only an accredited clinical perfusionist registered with the College of Clinical Perfusion Scientists of Great Britain and Ireland can undertake or supervise the conduct of cardiopulmonary bypass.
- Anti-coagulant therapy prior to commencement of bypass.
- Once bypass has commenced, the ventilator should be turned off and IV anaesthesia administered.
- Blood gases and activated clotting time should be checked every 30 minutes.[2]
- It is sometimes necessary to lower the patients' temperature.

'Cardiopulmonary bypass replaces the function of the heart and lungs while the heart is arrested, allowing for a bloodless and stable surgical field'.[1]

Postoperative management
- Patients are usually transferred immediately to ITU.
- Adequate postoperative analgesia and physiotherapy is recommended to reduce the incidence of respiratory dysfunction and aid mobilisation.
- O_2 that is warmed and humidified should be administered postoperatively.
- Close observation of the patient is essential to monitor signs of complications.
- For transfer to ITU:
  - O_2.
  - Ventilatory support.
  - Continuous monitoring (ECG, SpO_2, BP).
  - Drug infusion pumps.
  - Anaesthetic assistance for emergencies.
  - Sedative, analgesic, and resuscitation drugs.

References and further reading
1. Simpson PJ and Popart MT (2002). *Understanding anaesthesia* (4th edn). Butterworth-Heinemann: Oxford.

2. Sinclair M, Evans R (2006) Cardiac surgery. In Allman KG and Wilson IH (eds) *Oxford Handbook of Anaesthesia* (2nd edn). Oxford University Press: Oxford.

Association of Anaesthetists of Great Britain and Ireland (2007). *Recommendation for standards of monitoring during anaesthesia and recovery* (4th edn). AAGBI: London.

Munsch C and Guerrero R (2003). Complications after cardiopulmonary surgery. In Leaper DJ and Peel ALG (eds) *Handbook of Postoperative Complications*. Oxford University Press, Oxford.

Nicholls A, Wilson I (2000). *Perioperative medicine: managing surgical patients with medical problems.* Oxford University Press: Oxford.

Nolan J (2006) The critically ill patient. In Allman KG and Wilson IH (eds) *Oxford Handbook of Anaesthesia* (2nd edn). Oxford University Press: Oxford.

Royal College of Anaesthetists (2004). *Guidelines for the Provision of Anaesthetic Services.* RCoA: London.

Society of Clinical Perfusion Scientists of Great Britain & Ireland, Association of Cardiothoracic Anaesthetists, Society for Cardiothoracic Surgery in Great Britain & Ireland (2007). *Recommendations for Standards of Monitoring during Cardiopulmonary Bypass.* Available at: ▣ www.sopgbi.org

The Society of Clinical Perfusion Scientists of Great Britain and Ireland. Available at: ▣ www.scps.org.uk/perfusionists.html

Thoracic anaesthesia

Patients presenting for thoracic surgery can have limited respiratory reserve and pulmonary function.[1] Sanders explains that 'successful thoracic anaesthesia requires the ability to control ventilation of both lungs independently, skilled management of the shared lung and airway and a clear understanding of planned surgery'.[2] See Box 12.4 for examples of procedures.

Box 12.4 Examples of thoracic surgical procedures[2]

- Oesophagectomy.
- Thoracotomy.
- Thymectomy.
- Pneumonectomy.
- Pleurectomy.
- Mediastinoscopy.
- Mediastinotomy.
- Lobectomy.
- Rigid bronchoscopy and stent insertion.
- Lung volume reduction and bulletectomy.
- Repair of broncho-pleural fistula.
- Wedge resection of lung.
- Lung biopsy.

Anaesthetic management

- Comprehensive pre assessment should include:
  - Past medical history including cardiac events.
  - Assessment of cardiorespiratory reserve.
  - Observe colour, signs of cyanosis, breathlessness.
  - Monitor vital signs including non-invasive BP.
  - 12-lead ECG.
- Assessment of airway.
- Smoking cessation and preoperative physiotherapy is recommended prior to elective thoracic surgery to optimise lung function.

One-lung ventilation

- Double-lumen endobronchial tubes (DLTs) are recommended for intubation.
- A left DLT is advocated for surgery on the right lung.
- A right DLT is advocated for surgery on the left lung.
- Confirmation should be sought to assess the position of a DLT.
- Two-lung ventilation should be recommenced slowly following surgery except where a pneumonectomy has been performed.[1]

Postoperative management

- Postoperative ventilation should be avoided due to excess stress on pulmonary suture lines.
- Adequate postoperative analgesia and physiotherapy is recommended to reduce the incidence of respiratory dysfunction and aid mobilisation.
- O_2 that is warmed and humidified should be administered postoperatively.

- *Close observation of the patient is essential to monitor signs of complications.[1] These can include:*
  - Bleeding.
  - Cardiac arrhythmias.
  - Pulmonary oedema.
  - Retention of secretions.
  - Basal atelectasis/consolidation.
- A thoracic epidural should be considered for postoperative analgesia.
- For transfer to ITU:
  - O_2.
  - Ventilatory support.
  - Continuous monitoring (ECG, SpO_2, BP).
  - Drug infusion pumps.
  - Assistance for emergencies.
  - Sedative, analgesic and resuscitation drugs.

Intrapleural drainage

Indications for use

- To allow the lung to re-inflate.
- To facilitate drainage of air, blood, and fluid from the pleural space.

Care of chest drains

- Patients should be monitored closely for any change in respiratory and cardiovascular status. This includes SpO_2, respiratory rate and pattern, colour, unequal chest movement, blood gases, BP, and heart rate.
- Ensure patient comfort with upright positioning.
- The drain and drain tubing must remain secure at all times.
- The drain must be well positioned—observe for kinks.
- Clamps must be available close to the patient in case of accidental disconnection.
- The drain must remain below the chest—volume and output must be recorded on a fluid balance chart.

If a drain becomes disconnected

- Call for medical assistance.
- Reconnect the drain immediately.
- Encourage coughing to dispel air.
- Arrange for chest x-ray to assess changes in condition.

References and further reading

1. Faber P and Klein AA (2008). Theoretical and practical aspects of anaesthesia for thoracic surgery. *Journal of Perioperative Practice* **18**(3), 121–9.

2. Sanders D (2006). *Thoracic surgery.* In Allman KG and Wilson IH (eds) *Oxford Handbook of Anaesthesia* (2nd edn). Oxford University Press: Oxford.

Association of Anaesthetists of Great Britain and Ireland (2007). *Recommendation for standards of monitoring during anaesthesia and recovery* (4th edn). AAGBI: London.

MacKenzie E and Maguire J (2004). Intrapleural drainage. In Dougherty L and Lister S (eds). *The Royal Marsden Hospital Manual of Clinical Nursing Procedures* (6th edn). Blackwell Publishing: Oxford.

Pudner R (2005). *Nursing the surgical patient* (2nd edn). Elsevier: Edinburgh.

Royal College of Anaesthetists (2004). *Guidelines for the Provision of Anaesthetic Services.* RCoA: London.

Principles of day surgery

The AAGBI[1] emphasise that a condition of day surgery is that pain, nausea and vomiting must be controlled and that day case anaesthesia and surgery must be based on proven patient safety and quality of care. Examples of procedures suitable for day surgery are identified in Table 12.3.

Anaesthetic management

- The anaesthetic technique should induce minimum stress and maximum comfort for the patient.
- Premedication is not recommended except in exceptional circumstances.
- Many anaesthetists advocate propofol-based techniques, due to their beneficial reduction of PONV.[2]
- Prophylactic anti-emetic therapy should only be considered in patients with a history of perioperative PONV and some surgical procedures; this might include laparoscopic sterilisation, laparoscopic cholecystectomy and tonsillectomy.[1]
- General anaesthesia and regional anaesthesia are suitable for day surgery.
- If regional anaesthesia is employed, the patient should be placed at the beginning of the operating theatre list to allow time for the anaesthetic to 'wear off'.
- Caution should be employed if considering femoral nerve blocks in adults; this is due to potential mobility difficulties if sensation is not re-gained prior to discharge.[4]

Anaesthetic technique

- Consider total IV anaesthesia with propofol and incremental doses of fentanyl (without N_2O).[4]
- LMA is recommended where possible in place of intubation.
- Consideration must be given to prevention and treatment of PONV and pain management.
- Consider low dose spinal anaesthesia for patients who would normally be excluded for general anaesthetic.
- Fine bore pencil-point needles reduce the incidence of a post dural-puncture headache.
- If a patient experiences 'no demonstrable block', the British Association of Day Surgery (BADS)[5] advise that the spinal anaesthetic can be repeated or converted to a general anaesthetic.
- The advantages of spinal anaesthesia include:[5]
  - Fewer problems with respiratory function and airway management.
  - Patients may observe surgery and discuss options with the surgeon.
  - Reduction in perioperative venous thrombo-embolic disease.
  - Reduced incidence of PONV.
  - Immediate return to normal oral intake—particularly for patients with diabetes.
  - NSAIDs as an adjunct to anaesthesia should be considered.
  - Morphine can be administered postoperatively if required.

Reasons why a patients' hospital stay might be extended are identified by Davies[4] in Box 12.5.

Table 12.3 Procedures suitable for day surgery[2,3]

General surgery	Orthopaedic	Gynae	ENT
Laparoscopic cholecystectomy	Arthroscopy ± menisectomy	Termination of pregnancy	Tonsillectomy Adenoidectomy
Haemorrhoidectomy	Manipulations	D&C	Myringotomy
Orchidopexy Circumcision	Removal of metalware	Hysteroscopy	Sub mucous resection
Varicose vein stripping or ligation	Change of plaster	Laparoscopy	Reduction of nasal fracture
Inguinal hernia repair	Release of trigger thumb	Vaginoscopy	Fracture of nasal bones
Excision of breast lump	Tenotomy		Antral washouts

Box 12.5 Reasons for extended hospital stay[4]

- Post-operative complications—unexpected.
- Unexpected extensive surgery.
- Inadequate social circumstances.
- Patient does not meet discharge criteria prior to unit closing.
- Uncontrolled pain.
- Uncontrolled nausea and vomiting.

References and further reading

1. Association of Anaesthetists of Great Britain and Ireland (2005). *Day surgery*. AAGBI: London.

2. British Association of Day Surgery (2006). *BADS directory of procedures*. BADS: London.

3. Royal College of Nursing (2004). *Day surgery information: selection criteria and suitable procedures*. RCN: London.

4. Davies P (2006). Day surgery. In Allman KG and Wilson IH (eds) *Oxford Handbook of Anaesthesia* (2nd edn). Oxford University Press: Oxford.

5. British Association of Day Surgery (2004). *Spinal anaesthesia in day surgery*. BADS: London.

Royal College of Anaesthetists (2004). *Guidelines for the Provision of Anaesthetic Services*. RCoA: London.

Section 4
Intraoperative care

Decontamination and sterilisation

Overview

Decontamination

Decontamination refers to the pre-sterilisation process of reusable surgical and anaesthetic instruments which may be performed manually or by machine or, more usually, both. Used instruments are inspected for visible soil and may be manually brushed or washed. Delicate instruments and those with lumens may be decontaminated in an ultrasonic washer. Most instruments are washed in the washer/decontaminator machine which works much like a dishwasher which would take approximately 1 hour. The purpose of decontamination is to make the instruments safe for the packing staff to handle during the packing process.

Sterilisation

There are nine types of sterilisation available, most of which are generally not offered in the hospital setting—steam, ethylene oxide, dry heat, microwaves, formaldehyde gas, hydrogen peroxide plasma, ozone gas, chemical solutions, and ionising radiation. Only the ones that are either used or commonly encountered will be considered here. To be considered sterile all micro-organisms and bacterial spores should be destroyed. Bacterial spores are the most resistant of all living organisms as they are able to withstand external destructive agents. Packaging is required to indicate that the item within the package is sterile by use of a marker that will have changed colour (e.g. autoclave tape), what method of sterilisation has been used, the date of sterilisation, and the expiry date, which is when the product can no longer be guaranteed as sterile.

Steam

This is used in an autoclave with pressure greater than atmospheric to increase the temperature to achieve thermal destruction. The heated, pressurised steam must penetrate to reach the items to be sterilised. During the main sterilisation cycle the time that the steam is in contact with the instrument will depend on the temperature the autoclave reaches. At 130°C it is 3 minutes while at 120°C it is 15 minutes. At the end of the cycle, re-evaporation of water condensate must effectively dry contents of the load to maintain sterility. This method of sterilisation is suitable for metal (stainless steel) instruments that are reusable and are designed to withstand the extreme temperature and is available in most UK hospitals.

Ethylene oxide (EO)

This is suitable for heat or moisture sensitive items. EO gas must have direct contact with the organisms on, or in, the item. EO gas is highly inflammable and has to be contained within an explosion-proof chamber. It is also toxic and takes longer than steam sterilisation, typically 16–18 hours for a cycle. EO is used commercially and in certain hospitals in the UK.

Ionising radiation

This is the most effective form of sterilisation but is only available for commercial use. The process uses beta particles and gamma rays and takes between 10–20 hours depending on the strength of the radiation source.

Instrument management

Checking and packing

After decontamination the instruments pass into a strictly controlled clean packing environment, sometimes referred to as 'the clean room'. The instruments will usually have been through the washing process in their sets to simplify the checking and packing process. They are then placed onto a prepared instrument tray ready for packaging prior to sterilisation and at this time are inspected for any damage or wear which are removed and replaced.

Before the tray is finally packed up, the instrument set is checked by the packer and another member of staff against the tray list, and any instrument(s) missing are noted on both the packed list and ideally on the outside of the instrument tray. The instrument trays are packed as dictated by the type of instruments and the local requirements to protect them. The tray is wrapped in a protective sheet made of a single use non-woven textile in such a way that enables it to be opened without contaminating the inner part of the tray. Some specialist instruments may be packed in a rigid metal container which is designed to withstand the heat of the autoclave while others may be individually wrapped in heat-sealed pouch packaging.

Reusable instruments

The process described for checking and packing will relate to instruments that are designed to be used a number of times. They are made of stainless steel to the highest standard so that they can withstand the autoclave process. Whilst there is not a maximum number of times they can be used they do require checking each time they are re-processed and maintained as required. There have been products, such as electro-surgical pens with their accompanying electrical lead, that have a finite life and should only be processed a number of times (typically 50). These products should have a record card with them that is marked off after each use until the item reaches the maximum number after which it is discarded.

Single use items

These are produced commercially and may range from large anastomosis guns to small items such as skin marking pens. They often contain plastic material and are usually sterilised using irradiation. They should not be re-sterilised unless the manufacturer has instructed that it is safe to do so and they must also state how reprocessing should be conducted including the method to be used and how long the item can be regarded as sterile and safe to use. Any sterile processing unit or individual re-sterilising an item that is designed for single use will assume the manufacturer's liability for the sterility and safety of the item when in use.

As a general rule practitioners should observe the maxim that if you want a reusable item then buy one that is designed to be reused.

Instrument tracking

In the modern era this has become an important issue for the protection of patients and to source any processing issues in the event of surgical site infections so that action can be taken should such an outbreak occur. Instrument sets and sundries should have a unique number to identify them which is placed on the outer wrap or the packaging. This is normally provided as a readable bar code that can be read by a laser scanner in much the same way as products in a supermarket. This system will identify the instrument or the set and will typically be scanned at various stages of the cycle so that the item can be located. It will also indicate the decontamination and sterilisation cycles that the item has been through as well as the surgical cases that it has used in.

There are also marking systems that can be used to place a unique code on the instrument, whether part of an instrument set or a sundry, itself so that if it becomes separated from the packaging it or is taken out of service to go for servicing or repair can still be traced until it is taken out of commission entirely.

Thermoregulation

Overview

The skin maintains the body's normothermic state that is at a temperature of 37°C. As the body temperature increases, the peripheral blood vessels dilate allowing more blood to circulate near the surface. If the body temperature drops then the body will attempt to self-regulate by decreasing the flow of blood near to the surface to conserve internal heat. The loss of heat or the ability to produce heat may directly affect the patient's physiological response to surgery. During surgery the loss of heat is primarily the result of

- Exposure to the physical environment.
- The surgical incision.
- The immobility of the patient.
- The effect of any existing co-existing circulatory conditions.

📖 See also Heat and humans, p.170.

Other causes of hypothermia

Contributory factors that will add to inadvertent hypothermia include:

- Exposure of the skin or body cavities to cool ambient room air or drafts due to operating theatre ventilation air changes.
- Patients undergoing longer surgery will be more susceptible to hypothermia as will those that undergo irrigation of body cavities with unwarmed fluids.

Adverse effects of hypothermia

It has been shown that inadvertent hypothermia:

- Increases postoperative discomfort.
- Increases the chance of bleeding.
- Increases the incidence of ischemia and tachycardia.
- Can cause impaired wound healing.
- Can increase the risk of wound infection which may result in a longer stay in hospital.[1]

Reference

Fecteau D (1999). Patient and environmental safety. In Meeker MH and Rothcock JC (eds) *Alexander's Care of the patient in surgery*. Mosby: St Louis, MO.

Vulnerable patient groups

Older patients

While all patients are potentially susceptible to hypothermia during surgery, older patients are more vulnerable due to the aging process—their metabolic rate is reduced which means they are prone to be more sensitive to cold.

- They have decreased ability to regulate their temperature and they tend to have a lower core temperature.
- The efficiency of the shivering response also reduces the ability to overcome a loss of temperature.

Paediatric patients

Like older adults, babies and children are also susceptible to heat loss during anaesthesia and surgery and will become hypothermic more quickly than adults. Babies and children will lose body heat in the same way and for the same reasons as adults, but are more at risk for the following reasons:

- In paediatric patients, the head represents a far larger fraction of the total surface area of their body. As the skull and scalp are thin, this allows further loss of heat.
- Because cutaneous heat loss is roughly proportional to surface area it is relatively easy for infants and children to lose large amounts of heat from the skin surface.[1]

Reference

Sesser DI (2000). Perioperative heat balance. *Anesthesiology* **92**, 578 –96.

Warming devices and techniques

It is advisable to maintain the patient's body heat which can be helped by keeping the patient warm preoperatively. It is better to prevent heat loss than treat a hypothermic patient.

Preoperatively

- Check patient's temperature.
- Where possible, use forced-air warmer for 30 minutes to pre-warm the patient.

Intraoperatively

Techniques to reduce the inadvertent hypothermia include:

- Use blankets to maintain heat pre- and postoperatively.
- Minimise exposure until access is required.
- Increase the anaesthetic room and operating theatre temperature.
- Warm IV and irrigation fluids.
- Use a forced-air warming device during induction of anaesthesia and intraoperatively in accordance with the manufacturer's instructions.
- Monitor and record the patient's temperature throughout the perioperative process.
- Burns are potential complication if warming devices are used inappropriately particularly in patients that have vascular impairment.

Postoperatively

- Apply all the pre- and intraoperative measures where possible.
- Avoid the use of excessive layers of ordinary blankets which may cause restriction of movement and respiration and cause discomfort.
- Avoid disturbing the closest layer to patient's skin as this will result in further heat loss.
- Do not allow the patient to leave the recovery room until normothermic.

Further reading

National Collaborating Centre for Nursing and Supportive care (commissioned by NICE) (2008). *The management of inadvertent perioperative hypothermia in adults.* Available at: http://www. gserve.nice.org.uk/nicemedia/pdf/CG65Guidance.pdf or by writing to National Institute for Health and Clinical Excellence, MidCity Place, 71 High Holborn, London, WC1V 6NA

Chapter 15

Patient skin preparation

Surgical site infection

Surgical site infections (SSIs) are one of the commonest healthcare-associated infections. As well as causing distress to patients they are estimated to cost the NHS in excess of 1 billion pounds each year.[1] The incidence of SSI is around 2–5% of patients[2] though this may be underestimated due to a lack of good postoperative surveillance data.

SSIs are classified by their location and can be superficial incisional, deep incisional, or organ/space. The Centres for Disease Control provides detailed definitions for each classification of SSI.[3] A general definition is that a SSI occurs within 30 days of surgery (1 year if there is an implant), exudes pus, swabs positive for organisms, and shows one of the following: pain, localised swelling, redness, or heat. Patients who are immuno-compromised may not produce pus, swelling, or redness due to diminished white blood cells but may exhibit fever or pain at the infection site.

Bacterial sources for SSIs

Most SSIs arise from bacteria, predominantly *Staphylococcus aureus*, entering the wound during the operative phase. The sources of these bacteria are the operating room environment, operating room staff and the surgical team, the surgical procedure, and the patient.

Risk factors for acquiring a SSI

Several factors affect the risk of patients acquiring a SSI. These relate to bacterial exposure during surgery and the body's ability to fight and overcome the infection. For example, during long surgical procedures there is more opportunity for bacteria from the surgical team and the theatre environment to enter the incision site. Hypothermic patients will have reduced blood supply to the incision site and therefore the cellular response will be reduced.

The following factors affect the risk of patients developing a SSI[4]
- Patient's overall state of health
- BMI.
- Surgical wound classification—📖 see Surgical wound classification, p.261.
- Surgery lasting longer than 1 hour.
- Pre-existing local or systemic infection.
- Hypothermia.
- Poor tissue perfusion—diabetes, vascular disease, hypotensive anaesthesia, hypothermia.
- Poor nutrition—low albumin, trace element deficiencies.

Each patient's risk of developing a SSI can be calculated by using a risk score. The most widely used risk tool is the National Nosocomial Infections Surveillance (NNIS) score. This is calculated from the patient's ASA classification, wound class, and duration of operation.[5]

Surgical wound classification

Surgical wounds are classified as clean, clean contaminated, contaminated, and dirty. Each category is associated with an increasing risk for developing a SSI.

- *Clean*: an uninfected surgical wound where the respiratory, GI, and genitourinary tracts are not incised.
- *Clean contaminated*: surgery where the respiratory, GI, and genitourinary tracts are incised under controlled conditions with minimal spillage.
- *Contaminated*: infected wounds (without pus) or recently traumatised wounds, or with a major spillage from the GI or genitourinary tracts.
- *Dirty/infected*: surgery in infected wounds with pus or involving trauma wounds more than 4 hours old.

Practices to reduce SSI

Practices are undertaken to reduce the opportunity for bacteria to be transferred to the surgical site, multiply, and cause infections. Common practices include the following;

- Environmental:
  - Theatre layout design.
  - Minimal traffic through theatres.
  - Laminar flow.
- Theatre personnel and the surgical team:
  - Surgical attirè.
  - Surgical hand antisepsis.
  - Aseptic techniques.
- Patient preparation:
  - Antiseptic skin preparation.
  - Preoperative hair removal.
  - Total body washing.
- Surgical techniques:
  - Intra-operative antibiotics.
  - Minimally invasive surgery.
  - Shorter procedures.
  - Surgical drapes.
  - Single use items.

References

1. Department of Health (2007). *Summary of the preliminary results of third prevalence survey of healthcare-associated infections in acute hospitals.* Available at: 🖳 www.dh.gov.uk

2. National Audit Office (2004). *Improving patient care by reducing the risk of hospital acquired infection. Report by the Comptroller and Auditor General HC 876 Session 20032004.* The Stationery Office: London.

3. Mangram A, Horan T, Pearson M, *et al.* (1999). Guideline for prevention of surgical site infection. *Infection Control and Hospital Epidemiology* **20** (4), 247–78.

4. Gottrup F, Melling A, and Hollander DA (2005). *An overview of surgical site infections: aetiology, incidence and risk factors.* Available at: 🖳 www.worldwidewounds.com/2005/september/Gottrup/Surgical-Site-Infections-Overview.html

5. National Nosocomial Infections Surveillance (2002). National Nosocomial Infections Surveillance System report. *American Journal of Infection Control* **30** (8), 458–75.

Antiseptic skin preparation

Skin is covered by two types of organisms; transient and resident. Resident organisms are the organisms which are normally found on an individual's skin and can include S. epidermidis and cornyeforms. Resident organisms can vary between individuals. For example, around 30% of people are colonised by S. aureus. Transient organisms are transferred to the surface of the skin through contact with a source. These organisms are not normally resident on the patient's skin and may include S. aureus, enterococci, clostridia, and Pseudomonas. These organisms temporarily contaminate the skin but can be removed through simple hand washing. Resident organisms are harder to remove.

During surgery, transient and resident organisms can enter the incision site where they multiply and cause SSIs. Preoperative patient skin preparation involves using antiseptics and mechanical friction to remove transient organisms, reduce the number of resident organisms, and inhibit organism re-growth.

Antiseptic solutions

An ideal antiseptic agent should have the following properties:
- A broad range of activity against Gram negative and Gram positive bacteria, viruses, and fungi.
- Fast acting.
- Have a residual effect.
- Not be inactivated by organic material.
- Non-irritant.
- Safe to use.

In the UK, the commonest antiseptic agents are povidone iodine and chlorhexidine gluconate in either alcohol or aqueous preparations. It should be noted that alcohol itself is an antiseptic. Choosing which solution to use depends on the area to be incised and the condition of the patient's skin. The most effective solution combines the widespread and persistent activity of chlorhexidine gluconate with the rapid kill of an alcohol solution.

Alcohol

Alcohol is effective against a wide range of Gram positive and Gram negative bacteria, mycobacterium tuberculosis, and many fungi and viruses. Compared with other common antiseptic products alcohol is associated with the most rapid and greatest reduction in microbial count, but it does not remove dirt and is not sporicidal. Alcohols have little or no residual effect but are very fast acting.

Povidone iodine[1]

Povidone iodine is effective against a wide range of Gram positive and Gram negative bacteria, Mycobacterium tuberculosis, fungi, and viruses. It is a combination of polyvinylpyrrolidone (povidone) and iodine. Povidone prolongs the activity of iodine by releasing it slowly. Iodophors rapidly reduce transient and resident bacteria but have little residual effect. Iodine is inactivated by organic materials such as blood.

1 Note that povidone iodine concentrates in breast milk and should be used with caution in nursing mothers.

Chlorhexidine gluconate (CHG)

CHG is effective against a wide range of Gram positive and Gram negative bacteria, lipophilic viruses, and yeasts. It binds to the outermost layer of skin which results in a persistent activity. Repeated exposure can lead to a cumulative effect where both transient and resident organisms are reduced. CHG is effective in the presence of blood.

Further reading

Edwards P, Lipp A, and Holmes A (2007). Preoperative skin antiseptics for preventing surgical wound infections after clean surgery. *The Cochrane Database of Systematic Reviews*, Issue 4.

Joint Formulary Committee (2007). *BNF 54th edition*. BMJ Publishing Group Ltd. and RPS Publishing: London

Applying antiseptic solutions

Applying antiseptic solution to the patient's skin immediately before surgery is commonly referred to as 'prepping' the patient. See p. 265 for information regarding the application of specific solutions.

Prepping the patient's skin

- Before applying an antiseptic solution the patient's skin should be assessed to identify any abrasions or rashes which should be documented.
- The patient's skin should be clean before applying antiseptic solution as alcohol does not remove dirt and iodine is inactivated by organic material such as blood.
- Most antiseptic solutions are available in multi-use bottles and single-use sachets. Bottles are used more commonly though studies have shown bacteria growing on the inside of bottles.
- Once opened, a bottle of antiseptic solution should be labelled with the date. The length of time an open bottle can be kept varies between solutions; therefore refer to manufacturers instructions for this specific information. Bottles should not be refilled to allow tracking in the event of an infection outbreak.
- Try to keep the patient as warm as possible during skin preparation to enhance recovery and reduce SSIs. Most manufacturers advise storing antiseptic solutions at 25°C.
- Skin preparation is usually carried out by a member of the scrub team using an aseptic technique.
- The antiseptic solution can be applied with sterile swabs or sponges specifically manufactured for this process. The swabs and sponges are held with sterile forceps. If swabs are used for prepping then they should be included in the swab count. ('One-step' prepping systems are also available where a sterile swab is attached to a sterile applicator containing a measured dose of antiseptic solution.)
- The skin should be rubbed gently with the swab to generate the mechanical friction required for cleaning without traumatising the skin. Special care is needed when prepping skin near malignant cells to prevent dislodging cells.
- The area of skin to be prepped should extend beyond the intended incision site. It must allow for the incision to be extended during surgery, any drains to be sited, and accommodate drapes slipping during the procedure.
- Swabbing should begin at the incision site and move outwards. The principle is to move from 'clean to dirty'. Do not move a swab from an outer area back to the incision site as this may re- introduce bacteria.
- When a contaminated area is to be prepped the surrounding clean skin should be prepped first. Heavily contaminated areas such as the perineum should be prepped last. This prevents spreading bacteria from dirty areas to clean areas.
- Isolate stoma sites. For example, these can be covered with sterile waterproof dressings.
- Do not dip a used swab back into the pot of antiseptic solution—use a fresh swab for each application.

- Do not allow solutions to pool as this can cause skin irritation and may facilitate a burn injury. Solutions should not come into contact with diathermy plates.
- Solutions should be in contact with the skin as long as possible to allow maximum antiseptic effect. Povidone iodine should be in contact with the skin for at least 2 minutes as iodine is released slowly from its povidone carrier.
- Alcohol based solutions should be allowed to air dry completely before draping commences.
- Povidone iodine does not need to be rinsed off. This removes the active component of the antiseptic. Early preparations of iodine, before povidone iodine, were highly irritant if left in contact with the skin and had to be rinsed.
- The following information should be documented; condition of the skin, antiseptic solution used, reactions to the solution and post operative skin assessment.

Indications, cautions, and contra indications

Solutions containing alcohol can cause drying and should not be applied to mucous membranes or sensitive skin, such as dry 'papery' skin in older patients. Iodine can cross mucous membranes. CHG 0.5% in cetrimide 0.015% is a possible alternative for prepping mucous membranes.

Iodine may be absorbed and it should be used with caution in patients who are pregnant, breastfeeding, or have renal impairment. Iodine is contraindicated in neonates and should not be used regularly for patients with thyroid disorders. If iodine is used on large wounds it may cause metabolic acidosis, hypernatraemia, and impaired renal function. Iodine and chlorhexidine may cause corneal damage if in contact with eyes. Chlorhexidine should not be applied to the middle ear as it can cause functional impairment.

When preparing graft sites, colourless solutions should be used to allow the vascularity of the skin to be observed.

Further reading

Association of perioperative Reistered Nurses (2006). *Standards, Recommended Practices and Guidelines*. AORN Publications: Denver, CO.

Association for Perioperative Practice (2007). *Standards and Recommendations for Safe Perioperative Practice*. AfPP: Harrogate.

Preoperative hair removal

Hair is removed from the area surrounding the intended surgical site as its presence can interfere with the exposure of the incision, suturing, and the application of adhesive drapes and dressings. In addition, hair is perceived to be unclean and its removal is thought to reduce the risk of SSIs. However, hair removal can cause microscopic cuts and abrasions to skin which can become colonised and result in infections.

There are three methods of hair removal; shaving, clipping, and depilatory creams. Patients should be made aware if hair is to be removed as this may cause some distress.

Shaving

This method uses a sharp blade within the head of a razor, which is drawn over the patient's skin to cut hair close to the surface of the skin. Of the three hair removal methods, razors cause most damage to skin and patients shaved with a razor have the highest risk of developing SSIs.

Clippers

Clippers use fine teeth to cut the hair close to the patient's skin leaving short stubble of around 1mm in length. The heads of clippers should be disposed of or sterilised between patients to minimise the risk of cross infection.

Depilatory creams

Depilatory creams use chemicals to dissolve the hair itself. This is a slower process than shaving or clipping as the cream has to remain in contact with hair for between 5–20 minutes. In addition, there is a risk of irritant or allergic reactions to the cream and patch tests should be carried out 24 hours in advance.

Recommended method of hair removal

- Only remove hair when absolutely necessary.
- If removing hair, use clippers or cream as these cause fewer SSIs than razors.
- When using clippers or razors, hair should be removed as close to the start of the surgical procedure as possible to minimise the amount of time organisms have to colonise any cuts.
- When using cream it is acceptable to remove hair the day before surgery. Patch tests should be carried out 24 hours before hair is removed.
- If hair is being removed at home using cream this is likely to be carried out by the patient or their carer.
- If hair is being removed in the hospital by razor or clipper there is no evidence to show who is the best person to do this.
- Hair should not be removed in the operating theatre as loose hair may contaminate the sterile field.

Further reading

Tanner J, Moncaster K, and Woodings D (2006). Preoperative hair removal to reduce surgical site infection. *The Cochrane Database of Systematic Reviews*, Issue 2.

Total body washing

One factor which influences the risk of acquiring a SSI is the patient's bacterial burden, or the amount of bacteria on the patient's skin. Transient and resident bacteria from patients' skin can enter the surgical site where the bacteria then multiply and cause infections. The purpose of a preoperative body washing regimen is to make the skin as clean as possible by reducing transient and resident bacteria, therefore reducing the risk of SSI.

Though there is clear evidence that antiseptic solutions reduce bacteria on skin, evidence of the impact of total body washing in reducing SSIs is inconclusive. Several studies have shown mixed results and a Cochrane systematic review of total body washing to reduce SSI found no clear evidence.[1] However, there are good quality studies[2] which show the effectiveness of total body washing in eliminating meticillin resistant *Staphylococcus aureus* (MRSA) in patients prior to admission as part of a screening programme. Total body washing is also known as preoperative bathing or showering, or topical eradication.

MRSA screening

Some hospitals screen all elective surgical patients for MRSA prior to admission. Ideally, screening is carried out at least 2 weeks before the admission date to allow for results to be processed and treatment to be completed. Swabs are usually taken from the nose, perineum, wound sites if present, urine if the patient is catheterised, and sputum if there is a productive cough. Patients who are MRSA postive will be prescribed a total body washing regimen, such as the one described next. Following completion of the body washing regimen, patients should be tested again for MRSA.

In hospitals with screening programmes, non-elective patients may commence total body washing prophylactically on admission to hospital until rapid screening swab results can be obtained.

Total body washing method of application

There is limited evidence to show the most effective method of body washing to reduce SSI. Current practices range from a single bath or shower with antiseptic solution on the day of surgery to repeated applications in the week before surgery. Body washing protocols to eradicate MRSA, such as the one described here, are more intensive.

- Patients commence body washing 1 week before surgery or immediately after receiving positive identification from an MRSA screening programme.
- The body washing programme lasts 5 consecutive days.
- Patients wash once daily with an antiseptic solution, for example triclosan or CHG.
- Hair should be washed with antiseptic solution a minimum of two times during the 5-day period.
- Mupirocin should be applied to the anterior nares three times daily for 5 days as the nose is a common site for harbouring MRSA.

Special instructions

- Patients who show signs of a urinary tract infection and whose urine has tested positive for MRSA can be prescribed systemic antibiotics.
- Total body washing regimens to eradicate MRSA are generally limited to two courses as patients may become resistant to mupirocin.
- Patients with MRSA positive sputum do not routinely require treatment unless the chest infection is causing an acute illness.

References

1. Webster J and Osborne S (2007). Preoperative bathing or showering with skin antiseptics to prevent surgical site infection. *The Cochrane Database of Systematic Reviews*, Issue 4.

2. Nixon M, Jackson B, Varghese P, *et al.* (2006). Methicillin-resistant *Staphylococcus aureus* on orthopaedic wards. *Journal of Bone and Joint Surgery* **88**(6), 812–17.

Operating theatre practice

Theatre preparation: heating, lighting, and humidity

Heating

There is no ideal temperature for an operating theatre that will be correct in all circumstances as it will depend on the type of surgery undertaken. For example, when operating on babies or young children the temperature will often be higher to assist in the maintaining the patient's core temperature, while in theatres carrying out cardiac surgery the temperature may be low to aid in the cooling of the patient. Consideration must also be made for the elderly patient and those undergoing procedures under local or regional anaesthesia. The use of warming equipment to maintain the body temperature of the patient will usually mean that the ambient air temperature is less of a consideration and so can be set at a more comfortable working temperature for staff.

The ambient temperature will often be a level that is comfortable for the staff in which to work. The scrub team in particular may request that the temperature is low as they are wearing more protective clothing and are often standing under operating lights which emit heat. The wall-mounted control panel is used to select the desired room temperature. A general principle would be to adjust the temperature using small increments so that a general comfort level is achieved. Many modern operating theatres have a 'setback' control for the ventilation unit that can be used when the theatre is not in use so that the number of air changes within the theatre is reduced, thereby cutting back on electricity consumption. The ventilation system should be placed on to the full setting prior to commencing the operating list in accordance with local guidelines and the manufacturer's instructions.

Ventilation systems:
• Change the air at least fifteen times an hour.
• Cause a positive air pressure within the theatre.
• Force air in from the ceiling and out through exhaust panels.
• Provide a unidirectional airflow to reduce the risk airborne contamination.

Lighting

Generally lighting will be set to full for 'open' operations while some cases, particularly those which telescopes, microscopes, cameras, and monitors are utilised, may require some of the lighting to be reduced to aid the surgeon's view of the surgical field. The positioning of the operating theatre light is crucial, particularly in surgery in deep cavities of the body. Several centres now have operating theatre lamps with handles which can be sterilised, enabling the surgical team to place the light in the best position to view the surgical field. Where circulating staff are required to position operating lamps, it is advisable for novice staff to familiarise themselves with equipment during a time that no patient is in the operating theatre.

Humidity

Along with temperature controls many theatre departments have a wall-mounted control panel that controls the atmospheric humidity. This should be set to a level not in excess of 60% or below 30% as this will minimise static electricity and reduce the potential for bacterial growth, while a higher rate could result in condensation of ambient moisture which may result in damp materials.

Cleaning of the operating theatre

At the end of a day or session the operating theatre must be cleaned in readiness for the following session; this is termed terminal cleaning and practice will vary between departments. All operating theatre departments will have policies for the cleaning process, the basic principles of which are;

• Furniture to be cleaned with an approved disinfectant.
• Wheel and casters cleaned and any debris removed.
• Horizontal surfaces are cleaned.
• The floor is wet-scrubbed once the furniture is removed.
• The furniture is replaced once the floor is dry.

The theatre may also be cleaned between cases as required, using a mop to clean spillage onto the floor. The used mop head should be dealt with in accordance with the local cleaning policy. Damp dusting of horizontal surfaces using the approved disinfectant prior to the commencement of the day's operating list may also be carried out to reduce the viable bacterial contamination.

The management of surgical equipment

The amount of surgical equipment that is not used directly on patients has increased greatly as surgery has developed over recent times. The type of equipment that might commonly be found in operating theatre departments may include:

- Stack systems containing audio equipment, light source, monitor, and insufflator.
- Microscopes.
- Irrigation equipment.
- Specialist drilling equipment.
- Cell salvage machine.

As new equipment is purchased, storage space will need to be found to accommodate it when it is not in use in order that it is protected from damage. Staff need to be familiar with the set-up and use of specialist equipment and it may prove necessary to restrict the number of staff that may use the equipment to those that are conversant with it, to minimise damage caused by misuse which may prove expense to repair. Consideration should be given to the provision of regular updates for staff which can be provided by company representatives or staff that are familiar with the equipment. This should include how to set up, use, clean, and store the equipment. Maintenance contracts should also be in place for essential equipment with a specialist contractor.

Further reading

Phillips N (2007). *Berry and Kohn's Operating Room Technique*. Mosby: St Louis, MO.

Correct site surgery

- Wrong site surgery is an endemic problem in modern healthcare systems. Complexity in delivery of surgical healthcare results in regular reports of operations on the wrong site or patient.
- The requirement to operate on the correct patient, on the correct side, and the correct procedure is unquestionable. There are reports internationally identifying that the numbers of wrong site surgical procedures are increasing.[1]
- Work in the US has indicated that wrong site surgery will happen once every 5–10 years in an organisation or 1 in every 113 000 cases. The most common root causes associated with wrong site surgery are not following procedures and communication.[2]
- Anecdotal evidence from wrong site surgical events in the UK suggests that many incidents could have been avoided if patients had been correctly marked in some cases, and the team had stopped prior to surgery to confirm the procedure in a majority of cases.
- There are many underlying issues which contribute to wrong site surgery; the nature of the surgery itself (emergency, trauma, and orthopaedics[2]), the misidentification of surgical site in the medical records and, more commonly, on the operating list, and the lack of consistent marking practices both between teams in the same hospital as well as between hospitals.
- Various international agencies have proposed strategies for tackling wrong site surgery, including the WHO with the *Safe Surgery Saves Lives* checklist.[3]
- In the UK this work has been driven jointly by the National Patient Safety Agency (NPSA) and the RCS, with the release of guidance to the NHS in March 2005. In 2008–2010 the WHO 'High 5s' patient safety solution work will pilot in the UK[4] and provide standing operating procedures (SOPs) to promote correct site surgery.

Aims of care

To eliminate incidents of wrong site surgery by:
- Instigating a preoperative verification process ensuring that:
  - The mark should only be applied after checking the relevant and reliable documentation, e.g. medical notes, x-rays.
  - The patient should only be marked by a qualified person who will be present during the surgical procedure, e.g. surgeon, registrar.
  - Using only one way to mark patients who are having unilateral surgery, i.e. with an arrow.
  - Only mark patients with an indelible surgical skin marker.
  - The arrow should be visible after surgical preparation solutions have been applied.
  - The arrow should be visible after the surgical drapes have been applied.
  - Once the mark has been applied the surgical site verification form should be signed.

- The presence of a mark should be confirmed at various stages of the patient's journey to theatre; prior to leaving the ward, during the 'sign in' process prior to anaesthesia, and finally during the 'time out' prior to the surgical incision.[3] Each verification process should be recorded.
- Prior to the surgical incision the whole team should pause and verbally confirm they have the correct patient, for the correct procedure, on the correct side.
- Exceptions: life threatening emergencies, neonates, and dental surgery.

References

1. National Patient Safety Agency (2005). *Correct Site Surgery*. Available at: ▣ http://www.npsa.nhs. uk/patientsafety/alerts-and-directives/alerts/correct-site-surgery/

2. Joint Commission on the Accreditation of Healthcare Organizations (2007). Available at: ▣ http://www.jointcommission.org/NR/rdonlyres/3CD55986-387C-4071-8D32-1982EC928280/0/07_financial.pdf

3. World Health Organization (2008). *Safe Surgery Saves Lives*. Available at: ▣ http://www.who. int/patientsafety/challenge/safe.surgery/en/

4. World Health Organization (2008). *Action on Patient Safety – High 5s*. Available at: ▣ http:// www.who.int/patientsafety/solutions/high5s/project_plan/en/index.html

Further reading

Advisory Pennsylvania Patient Safety Authority (2007). Doing the 'right' things to correct wrong site surgery. *Patient Safety Advisory* **4**(2), 29–45.

Kwaan MR, Studdert DM, Zinner MJ, et al. (2006). Incidence, patterns, and prevention of wrong site surgery. *Archives of Surgery* **141**(4), 353–7.

Maintaining a sterile field

Definition
The sterile field refers to the area around the surgical site that has been prepared by cleansing with an antimicrobial agent and surrounded with sterile drapes, which separate it from the rest of the patient's body. This is called 'prepping and draping'. The sterile field also includes all furniture covered with sterile drapes, such as the instrument table and the scrub team who are covered in sterile garb.

Purpose
The purpose of creating and maintaining a sterile field is to protect the patient's wound from microbial contamination during surgery, and to isolate the operative site from the surrounding, unsterile environment.

Principles
- All items used in a sterile field must be sterile. This includes drapes, instrument trays, sponges, swabs, and basins.
- Items of doubtful sterility are considered unsterile. This includes packaged items that may have been dropped on the floor or when the integrity of the packaging material is in doubt.
- All surgical personnel scrubbed for the case (the scrub team) are gowned and gloved. Gowns are considered sterile in front from chest level to the sterile field, sleeves from 5cm (2 inches) above the elbow to the stockinette cuff. Once sterile personnel are gowned and gloved, they keep their hands in sight at all times, and at or above waist level or the level of the sterile field.
- Sterile drapes are used to create a sterile field. Once placed, sterile drapes are not moved.
- Tables (once draped) are sterile only at the table level. The edges and sides of the drapes extending below table level are considered contaminated. This rule applies to the operating table edge, once the patient has been prepped and draped.
- Any item falling below the edge is considered contaminated.
- Sterile personnel touch only sterile items or areas; unsterile personnel touch only unsterile items or areas. Members of the scrub team maintain contact with the sterile field by means of sterile gowns and gloves.
- Items must be dispensed to the sterile field by methods that preserve sterility. The edges of anything that enclose sterile contents are considered unsterile; thus the circulating practitioner must ensure when opening sterile packages that a margin of safety is maintained. For example, the flaps on peel packages should be pulled back not torn, and the contents offered to the scrub practitioner for removal, and not flipped onto the instrument table.
- Unsterile personnel avoid reaching over the sterile field. The unsterile circulating practitioner never reaches over a sterile field to transfer an item. For example, the scrub practitioner sets basins or medicine cups to be filled at the edge of the sterile table, and the circulating practitioner stands at least 30cm (12 inches) away from the edge of the table to fill them. This distance applies to any part of the sterile field.

- The scrub team keeps well within the sterile field or area. They do not walk around or go outside of the operating room, and they keep movement to a minimum to avoid contamination of sterile items.
- Movement of the scrub team is from sterile area to sterile area, keeping a wide margin of safety when passing an unsterile area. They pass each other back-to-back and turn their backs to an unsterile area or person when passing.
- Unsterile personnel avoid the sterile field and maintain awareness of sterile, unsterile, clean and contaminated areas and their proximity to each.
- When a sterile area is permeated it is considered contaminated. Strike-through, the soaking of moisture from an unsterile layer or area to a sterile layer, or vice versa, breaches the integrity of the sterile field, contaminating it. If solution soaks through a sterile drape to an unsterile area, the wet area must be covered with impervious, sterile drapes or towels.
- Every sterile field must be continuously monitored. Someone must remain in the operating room at all times during set up of the sterile field and thereafter, until the surgical procedure is completed.
- The sterile field is created as close as possible to the time of use. Sterile instrument tables are set up immediately prior to the surgical procedure. There is no period of time wherein the table is considered sterile or unsterile and the potential degree of contamination is proportionate to the length of time that sterile items are exposed to the environment. Tables containing sterile items should not be covered; it is impossible to uncover them without risk of contamination.
- Micro-organisms must be kept to an irreducible minimum. Sterile technique at the surgical site is an ideal to be approached; it is not an absolute. This is because it is not possible to eliminate all micro-organisms from the environment. However, strict application of the measures described here and the exercise of one's surgical conscience are crucial; there is no place for compromise of sterility in the operating room.

Scrubbing up

Introduction

The patient's surgical outcome is influenced by the establishment and maintenance of an aseptic environment. The wearing of appropriate attire in the operating suite is one of a series of aseptic environmental control measures, which includes scrubbing, gowning, and gloving.

Purpose

All personnel who work in the semi-restricted or restricted areas of the operating suite must wear theatre attire, which consists of a two-piece pantsuit, head covering, and shoe covers, as appropriate. These items provide an effective barrier that prevents the dissemination of micro-organisms shed continuously from the skin and hair of everyone from entering the patient's body. Theatre attire also protects staff from patients' blood and body fluids. Additionally, members of the scrub team wear a mask, protective eyewear, and don sterile gowns and gloves. This is necessary because they are part of the sterile field.

Using masks and protective eyewear

Prior to scrubbing, members of the scrub team must remove all jewellery and cover their mouth and nose with a single, disposable surgical mask, which conforms to their facial contours and fits closely. Effectively worn, masks will filter inhalations and exhalations, and prevent droplets from the wearer's mouth and nasopharynx contaminating the wound. Eyewear such as goggles or eyeglasses which incorporate top and side shields must also be worn. Alternatives include a combination surgical mask with a visor eye shield or chin-length face shield. Eyewear is worn to protect the wearer from hazardous substances such as blood and body fluids.

Scrubbing, gowning, and gloving

Before donning a sterile gown and gloves, members of the scrub team must complete a surgical hand wash (called the surgical scrub). Its purpose is to remove as many micro-organisms as possible from the hands and arms by a combination of mechanical washing and the use of chemical antiseptic solutions. A standardised procedure is recommended. The first scrub of the day is 5 minutes long; all scrubs thereafter should be 3 minutes.

Scrubbing up

• Lay a sterile gown pack on a dressing trolley and open it to expose the contents without touching them, or the inner surface of the wrapping. This becomes a sterile field.

• Peel open the glove packaging and keeping the inside package sterile, tip the inner packet containing the gloves onto the sterile field. Repeat adding a second, smaller pair of gloves.

• Adjust running water to a comfortable temperature; open a disposable sterile brush, and wet hands and arms to above the elbow. Thereafter, keep the hands above elbow level.

• Clean the nails using the supplied nail pick then discard.

- Wash both hands and up to elbows for 1–2 minutes systematically using a circular motion. The time needed will depend on the degree of soil and the effectiveness of the cleansing agent/recommended antimicrobial solution used.
- Rinse from fingertips to elbows in one direction only.
- Apply further antimicrobial solution and over 3 minutes scrub the nails, all sides of the digits, the palms,, and the back of hands. Use a circular motion to scrub up the arms to elbow.
- Rinse off thoroughly, carefully pick up sterile towel from gown trolley and dry first one hand then arm with one half of the towel, then repeat on the other hand/arm with second half of towel.

Gowning

- Pick up gown at top, shake gently to open out without touching anything and then slip arms in, shrugging gown onto shoulders. Keep hands enclosed in ribbed cuffs while the circulating practitioner ties up gown at the back.

Gloving

- Pick up left glove (of the larger pair) and lay on left hand, thumb to thumb, with glove fingers pointing to elbow. Slip thumb of right hand under cuff of the glove and stretch glove up and over fingers of the left hand and pull on. The cuff of the glove should cover the ribbed cuff of the gown.
- With the gloved hand, remove the right glove from wrapper by placing the left hand inside the folded glove cuff. Repeat the procedure as for the left glove.
- Tug on the sleeves of the gown to adjust gloves for good fit, and then don the second, smaller pair of gloves.
- Hand the tag-enclosed end of the gown's back tie to the circulating member of staff then make a ¾ turn to the left. Retrieve the back tie carefully by pulling it out of the tag held by the circulating practitioner then tie it to the other back tie, which has been secured to the front of the gown throughout.

Notes

- A plastic waterproof apron must be worn under the sterile gown unless an impervious gown is used.
- Artificial nails have been linked to the transmission of bacteria or fungi and are best avoided.
- The use of powder-free or latex-free gloves is recommended.
- At all times, scrub personnel must keep their gloved hands above waist level and close to the upper, gowned body.

Draping of the patient

Introduction

To create a sterile field, sterile sheets and towels—known as surgical drapes—are strategically placed to isolate the operative site from the remainder of the patient's body. Once placed, they provide a sterile surface on which sterile items such as instruments, sponges, swabs, other sterile equipment, and the gloved hands of the scrub team can rest. Surgical drapes are not placed until the patient's skin has been cleansed with an appropriate antimicrobial solution. Draping materials are chosen to create and maintain an effective barrier that eliminates the passage of micro-organisms between sterile and non-sterile areas. To be effective they must be blood and aqueous fluid-resistant, lint-free, antistatic, and penetrable by steam or gas for sterilisation purposes. They must also be resistant to tearing, sufficiently porous to eliminate heat build-up, flame resistant, and free of toxic ingredients such as non-fast dyes.

Draping materials are folded and packaged so scrub personnel can handle them easily and safely; large drapes are fan-folded, rolled, or otherwise folded in a way which assists with their subsequent placement on the patient. Large drapes may be fenestrated (have an opening) that, when placed, exposes the incision area. Smaller drapes such as chest sheets, towels, and so forth may be used to 'square drape' a small operative site; they are packaged folded in halves or quarters. Many procedures utilise custom packs. These are sterile, pre-packaged, procedure-specific packs which contain all the draping requirements—and often other disposable items, such as sponges and Ray-Tec® swabs—required for a given surgical intervention such as a joint replacement or a Caesarean section. The drapes in these packs are often custom-designed.

Types of drapes

Surgical drapes can be reusable, disposable, or reposable; additionally, there are plastic incisional drapes.

- Reusable drapes: these are made of 100%, tightly woven cotton. They are permeable to fluid so a moisture repellent plastic drape is placed on the patient first. They require sterilised towel clips (ball and socket type) to hold them in place, once they've been laid on the patient. Their use is decreasing because of costs associated with laundering and processing them.
- Disposable drapes: these are soft, lightweight, moisture-resistant, and made of antistatic material. They are produced, pre-packaged, and sterilised commercially, and are discarded after one use. They are designed to adhere to the patient's skin, once positioned, and do not require the use of towel clips.
- Reposable drapes: these are drapes which are designed for limited reuse and theoretically combine the advantages of reusable drapes (environmentally friendly) with the advantages of disposables (superior quality).
- Plastic incisional drapes: these are transparent, self-adherent drapes designed to cover the operative site itself, providing a complete seal between the incision and wound and the skin in the immediate vicinity. They facilitate the draping of irregular body surfaces such as joints.

Procedure

- Drapes should be handled as little as possible.
- The scrub practitioner protects their gown and gloves by cuffing the drapes over their hands and holding drapes close to body.
- Scrub personnel should carry the folded drape to the operative site, unfold, and then place it.
- Care must be taken to maintain the appropriate distance from non-sterile areas to avoid contamination of scrub gown (30cm or 12 inches).
- The operative site must always be dry.
- Once placed, drapes should not be removed.
- If drapes fall before or during placement they are discarded.
- If a drape is contaminated or its sterility in question, it is discarded.
- Drapes are applied from sterile area to unsterile area, and the area nearest the scrub person is draped first. Scrub personnel should not reach across or over an unsterile area to drape—they walk around the operating table. Sterile drapes are not passed from one scrubbed person to another across an unsterile surface.
- Drapes should not be flipped, fanned, or shaken. Rapid drape movements create air currents on which dust can migrate. Shaking drapes causes uncontrollable movement and exposes the drape to potential, unseen contamination.
- The area of the incision site is draped first, followed by the peripheral or other areas.
- A drape should never be pulled from an unsterile area to a sterile one.

Role of circulating practitioner

Introduction

The circulating practitioner is an integral member of the perioperative team and is vital to the smooth flow of activities before, during, and after the surgical procedure. The ability to multitask is necessary as the circulating practitioner must co-ordinate patient care, the activities in an operating room, other members of the surgical team, and documentation. The role also demands initiative and good anticipatory skills. The circulating practitioner, as patient advocate, plays a central role in protecting patients from a range of adverse events that may arise in a high-risk environment such as the operative room. The circulating practitioner assists with the preparation of the operating room ensuring all needed equipment, sterile instrumentation, and consumables are available preoperatively. S/he assists intraoperatively working with the scrub practitioner to set up the instrument table, helping with patient transfer to the operating table, managing surgical specimens and consumables, and completing perioperative documentation.

Activities associated with the circulating practitioner role

During the course of (most) surgical procedures, the circulating practitioner, in conjunction with other surgical team members, or alone, will undertake the following:
- Adhere to standard precautions and, when indicated, transmission-based precautions, at all times.
- Understand and apply the principles of aseptic technique.
- Be accountable for own actions and delegations.

Preoperatively
- Ensure the operating room is clean, has the necessary equipment, sterile instruments, and consumables such as sponges and Ray-Tec® swabs.
- Assist in the preparation of scrubbed surgical team members.
- Help the scrub practitioner prepare for the surgical intervention by opening and dispensing sterile supplies.
- Lifting a limb to assist with the application of antiseptic skin preparation. It is important that this is carried out in accordance with accepted lifting techniques to minimise the risk of injury to staff or patient.
- Shaving of the patient's incision site (☐ see Preoperative hair removal, p.266).
- In conjunction with the scrub practitioner ensure all accountable items are counted immediately before the procedure begins; at the commencement of the closure of the body cavity; and at the commencement of skin closure.
- Assist in ensuring the correct patient is admitted for the correct operation, at or on the correct site or side (which is marked, as appropriate).
- Establish that a valid consent has been obtained and that the patient understands the anticipated operation in broad terms.
- Ascertain the patient's fasting status, known allergies, pertinent medical history, and that any necessary preoperative preparation (e.g. bowel preparation) has been completed.
- Confirm patient details with the scrub practitioner.

- *Intraoperatively*
- Assist with the transfer of the patient, which must be properly co-ordinated by staff trained in techniques for safe patient transfer using appropriate lifting devices.
- Ensure the patient is correctly positioned for the anticipated procedure and that pressure areas are protected by the use of gel mattresses, pads, head rings, heel supports, padded boards, stirrups, and so on, as determined by the requirements of the surgical position and status of individual patient.
- If necessary, make sure the patient is secured to the operating table by a reusable belt or by sticking plaster tape, particularly if they are in a lateral position.
- Check if antiembolism stockings are in use and that they are correctly applied, especially those that are thigh length.
- If required, apply the leggings of the sequential calf compression device (SCD) (DVT prophylactic system) and activate it.
- Apply the disposable, electrosurgery return electrode (diathermy plate) to a clean, muscular, well-vascularised, hairless site on the patient's body. Connect it to the electrosurgical generator (diathermy machine).
- Connect and/or activate other equipment as necessary, such as suction devices, active diathermy electrode, operating lights, other light sources, and so on.
- Supply sterile consumables, additional instruments, and other items as required throughout the course of the procedure.
- Record any use of single instruments that are contaminated and subsequently cleaned and 'flash' sterilised in both the patient's medical record and the department's 'Flash' log.
- Maintain communication with and between the team members in the sterile field, and with other personnel in the perioperative unit/ operating department and beyond.
- Exercise a surgical conscience, recognising and correcting any breaks in aseptic technique throughout the case.
- Support and teach any health professional learners in the environment.
- Document all aspects of perioperative care in the patient's medical record including each of the three counts; position of patient; pressure relieving devices and DVT prophylaxis, if used; position of the diathermy plate; skin preparation solution used; the operation performed; specimens taken; any implants or prosthesis used; any drains in situ, and wound dressings applied.
- Assist with the transfer of the patient on completion of the operation ensuring the medical records, x-rays, and other imaging records (and if necessary, personal belongings) accompany the patient to the recovery unit.
- Oversee the cleaning of the operating theatre in accordance with unit policies and protocols, first ensuring all rubbish, clinical waste, sharps, and soiled linen are removed.
- Check all the requirements for the next case are available.

Opening of sterile packs

Introduction

Sterile packs are necessary in order to create and maintain a sterile field, and their use is one of a number of measures taken to protect the patient's wound from microbial contamination during surgery.

As their name suggests, sterile packs contain sterile items such as instruments, draping materials, consumables—e.g. sponges and Ray-Tec® swabs,—and other items such as kidney trays. These items may be packed singly or in a combination. For example, most operating departments have standardised instrument tray sets for major and minor procedures, and for each surgical specialty. Additionally, they have some surgical instruments packed singly. They also have standardised linen (or drape) bundles, as well as single drape packs; this is also true of bowl sets, kidney trays, and so forth. These items may be prepared by the operating department's theatre sterile supply unit (TSSU) or the hospital's central sterile supply department (CSSD). Increasingly, however, there is a trend towards the purchase of commercially-prepared sterile surgical packs. This is because of the escalating costs associated with 'in house' reprocessing of sterile supplies, necessitated by the need to meet exacting manufacturing standards for items of this nature. Note, some items, such as sponges and Ray-Tec® swabs, are almost always purchased from surgical supply companies, and are not prepared 'in house'. Increasingly, surgical supply companies are working with perioperative practitioners to design and manufacture customised sterile packs which contain the drapes and consumable requirements necessary for a given procedure, such as a craniotomy or joint replacement procedure.

Principles

Sterile packs are prepared and manufactured in such a way that they can be opened without touching and thereby contaminating their contents.

- Sterile packs should be opened as close to their time of use as possible.
- Each sterile pack is inspected to check for package integrity, and that the outer wrapping is clean, dry, and intact.
- Each pack is also examined closely to ensure that it has sterilisation process (chemical) indicator tape present, which identifies that it has been through a sterilising process, and one suited to the particular contents of the sterile pack.
- Sterile packs must not have exceeded their shelf life, which is both event-related and determined, in part, by the nature and type of packaging used.
- Any outer dust covers are removed before the pack is subsequently opened and offered to the scrub practitioner, or placed on a table top for opening. All heavy items such as instrument trays are placed on a suitable, dry surface.
- Once opened, the edges of a sterile pack are considered unsterile. The contents must be dispensed onto the sterile field in a manner that preserves their integrity, as well as the integrity of the sterile field.

- As the boundaries between sterile and unsterile are often intangible, 2.5cm (1 inch) is considered standard for wrapped packs, whereas the boundary on a wrapper used to drape a table is at the table edge.
- When opening a sterile pack, the top flap is opened first, away from the circulating practitioner (or non-scrub personnel) opening it. This is followed by opening each of the side flaps, then finally, opening the inside or proximal flap last. As each flap is opened out, it is grasped, pulled down, and held underneath by the hand holding the pack. This stops the flaps from dangling and contaminating other sterile items. The outer side of the wrapper also serves to cover the circulating practitioner's hand, further protecting the sterile contents.
- The item is then offered to the scrub person so it can be lifted straight up and away from its wrapper.
- On peel-pack pouches, the inner edge of the heat seal is the edge of the sterile boundary. Peel packs should be pulled back evenly, by grasping each edge of the pouch or package top and peeling away smoothly. These packs should not be torn open.
- Peel-pack contents can be retrieved by the scrub practitioner as already described (lifted straight up) or they can be flipped onto the sterile field by the non-scrubbed person. They should not be allowed to slide over the edge of the pack.
- When opening large sterile packs—e.g. packs of drapes—they should be laid on the instrument table because, when opened, the outer wrapper subsequently forms the first sterile covering for the instrument table. When opening the cover of the pack, the hands of the circulating practitioner are kept under the folded pack cuff, thereby protecting the inner, sterile contents, as the practitioner draws the cover back over the table exposing the contents.
- When opening items the hand and arm motions of the circulating practitioner are always from unsterile to sterile objects.
- If the sterility of the item is in doubt, it should be discarded.

Movement within the theatre

Introduction

A further aspect of perioperative care aimed at keeping the patient free from infection is related to movement within the operating theatre, which is a restricted area. Traffic within and out of the operating theatre must be kept to a minimum and only essential personnel should be allowed inside the theatre. This is because the amount of activity in the room increases as the number of persons present increases. In turn, this heightens the potential for contamination as a result of additional shedding and air turbulence that carries micro-organisms with it onto the sterile field and the patient's wound. Like many aspects of surgical aseptic technique, the following principles and actions are predicated on the premise that most infections are caused by microorganisms exogenous to the surgical patient's body.

Principles

- The doors of the operating theatre should be kept closed at all times except when it is necessary to provide a passage for the patient, perioperative personnel involved in the particular procedure, and required supplies and equipment. This ensures the higher positive air pressure in the theatre remains so, and is not allowed to equalise to the lower (or negative) air pressure beyond the theatre, mixing the clean theatre air with that from outer, less clean areas, as well as increasing turbulence.
- Clean and sterile supplies should be separated from contaminated items by time, space, or traffic patterns.
- Movement of personnel within the theatre should be kept to a minimum.
- All members of the surgical team must understand which areas within the theatre are considered sterile and which are considered unsterile, and maintain a continual awareness of them.
- Sterile individuals touch only sterile items or areas; unsterile personnel touch only unsterile items and areas.
- Movement within and around the sterile field must not contaminate the field.
- Scrubbed personnel must guard the sterile field and prevent unsterile items from contaminating the field, or the individuals themselves.
- The circulating practitioner must monitor movement within the theatre and be vigilant for, and address, breaks in aseptic technique.
- Unsterile personnel must not touch or lean over a sterile field.
- Sterile personnel must stay close to the sterile field. If they change position, they turn face-to-face, or back-to-back, while maintaining a safe distance between themselves and other objects.
- The circulating practitioner and other non-sterile personnel face the sterile field when approaching it.
- Unsterile personnel never walk between two sterile fields.
- The circulating practitioner maintains a minimum distance of 30 cm (12 inches) from the sterile field.
- If a solution must be poured into a sterile receptacle on the sterile table, the scrub practitioner holds the receptacle away from the table, or places it near the edge of the waterproof-draped table.

Communication with the surgical team

Introduction

Good communication is fundamental to the effective management and functioning of the operating department. It involves the exchange of information between patients and staff, between individuals and teams, and within and beyond the operating department. It is necessary for successful interpersonal relationships and to clarify actions. It is effective when the receiver of a message interprets it in the way the sender intended. Communication can be:

- *Verbal:* the most frequently used form of communication.
- *Non-verbal:* such as the use of body language.
- *Written:* for example, the patient's medical record; perioperative care plans; theatre department policy manuals.
- *Electronic:* increasingly information such as laboratory results, personal (email) communication, and digital imaging (to name but a few) is conveyed this way.

Effective communication is also critical to the formation of functional teams, such as the surgical team. Within the team there must be a shared understanding of the nature and manner of all communication; a shared language; and a commitment to direct and open verbal (and other) interactions. Communication skills can be learned and staff should be supported to access appropriate education, such is the significance of good communication in the operating department.

Coordinating the operating list

The coordination of the operating list is a crucial activity in the operating department, it involves virtually all perioperative (and other) personnel, and other departments within the hospital, and it can be a complex and fraught task. It is also a shared one. While the details may vary from hospital to hospital (indeed, it may differ within the same organisation, if the latter has more than one operating department), it involves a number of key personnel. For example, the operating department manager (or the floor co-ordinator), a senior anaesthetist/anaesthetic representative, and a member of the surgical staff would be the minimal number of personnel involved in coordinating an operating list. They will be assisted in this endeavour by administrative staff, such as operating department clerks, admissions or outpatient department staff, or the hospital's bed manager. Ideally, elective surgical lists are determined 2 weeks (or more) ahead of the scheduled day of surgery, and patients on the relevant waiting list are contacted. At this time, they are given the date of surgery and other information pertinent to their procedure. Alternatively, the decision to add patients' names to any given surgical list may be determined during their visit to a pre-admission or preoperative clinic, or following a visit to their surgeon. Once an operating list has been compiled and distributed to all stakeholders, it forms an important part of the operating department's records.

- It needs to be printed and posted in several places within the operating department the night before the intended surgical list is to occur.

- Every operating theatre should have its own copy as should each surgical ward, the anaesthetic and surgical departments, the perioperative unit, pathology, x-ray and imaging departments, and any other pertinent departments.
- Any changes to the list must be determined in a collaborative fashion, by the theatre co-ordinator in conjunction with relevant anaesthetic and surgical personnel. These changes should then be relayed promptly to all key personnel and departments, as well as to the staff in the affected operating room, and the patient(s) concerned, and/or their carers.
- Changes must be noted in the operating department's permanent records.
- There must be a written policy and clear set of guidelines which spell out the manner in which patients will be sent for and by whom, so they are transferred to the operating department in a timely fashion.
- Patients should not be called to the operating department too soon, resulting in them having an excessive wait prior to surgery.
- If patients have pre-medication drugs ordered by the anaesthetist, which are to be given on a phone order from the department, there must be clear guidelines/clinical protocol for this, particularly if peroperative staff are expected to make the phone call, authorising the dispensation of the ordered drugs.
- Recovery room personnel should ensure that ward staff are notified of the admission of patients immediately following surgery; additionally, they should alert ward staff before transferring the patient back to the ward.

Specimens

Introduction

During the course of many surgical interventions samples of the patient's tissue (specimens) are removed for histopathological and other forms of examination. Occasionally, the removal of tissue samples is the main or sole purpose of the surgical procedure. The removal of tissue samples may be invasive and involve the use of local, regional, or general anaesthesia. Correct handling, labelling, and transportation to the laboratory are crucial. Loss of specimens or damage due to incorrect handling, or delay in transporting them, can result in misdiagnosis or patients requiring further surgery to acquire additional specimens for pathology. Alternatively, patients may receive inappropriate or delayed treatment, as a diagnosis cannot always be confirmed in the absence of pathology testing. When a sample of tissue or fluid is removed for pathology, it is referred to as a *biopsy*. In contrast, when all tissue is removed during a surgical procedure, for example, gastrectomy, these tissues are referred to as *surgical specimens* and they are sent to the pathology laboratory for verification of diagnosis.

Specimen types and tests

Specimens can be categorised into several types:

Fluid, such as:

- Exudates.
- CSF.
- Cell washings.
- Urine.
- Fluid from cysts or abscesses.
- Blood.
- Bone marrow.
- Amniotic fluid.
- Semen.

Tests performed on fluid specimens include bacteriology, virology, cytology, cell counts, grouping (blood), and genetic studies.

Tissue, such as:

- Solid organ biopsy.
- Margin of a malignant lesion.
- Suspicious lesion or growth.
- Skin.
- Breast tissue/mass.
- Brushings from respiratory or urinary tracts.
- Bone.
- Muscle.
- Ova.
- Calculi, such as gallstones.

Tests performed on tissue specimens include histopathological examination of frozen and permanent sections, hormonal assays, and tissue typing (for donor compatibility).

Non-biological, such as:

- Foreign bodies—fish bones; glass fragments.
- Projectiles from a crime scene—bullet.
- Explanted items—orthopaedic screws, plates.
- Retained surgical swabs.
- Clothing from accident or crime victims—underclothes of rape victim.

There are no 'tests' for non-biological material, normally.

Principles

- It is the responsibility of the circulating practitioner to identify, document, and properly care for specimens collected during the course of a surgical procedure.
- Standard and transmission-based precautions should be used to protect individuals handling specimens. Labels should identify the need for precautions as well as the presence of biohazardous material.
- Each specimen must be labelled with the correct (and full) patient's name and medical record number, as well as the specific origin, type, and nature of the specimen. If indicated, the theatre location and phone number should also be included.
- The surgeon must supply clear, descriptive information about the specimen and the circulating practitioner should 'repeat-back' this information.
- The specimen details are documented in the patient's medical record; additionally, all specimen details should be entered into the department's specimens' record.
- Specimens should be prepared and cared for in accordance with the specific protocols established by the receiving laboratory.
- As a general rule specimens should be handled in ways which preserve their integrity, be kept moist, and be transported to the laboratory as soon as possible.
- Formalin is frequently used to preserve specimens that are not taken to the laboratory immediately. Formaldehyde should be handled cautiously to avoid exposure, as it is a hazardous substance which causes watery eyes and respiratory irritation.
- When tissue identification or determination of malignancy is needed immediately—that is, a result is required intraoperatively—specimens are taken for a 'frozen section' examination. Such tissue samples are placed in a specimen container, kept dry, and then transported directly to the laboratory. Here they are fast-frozen, sliced, stained, and examined under a microscope immediately. The examining pathologist then phones the operating theatre and conveys the results of the examination to the circulating practitioner.
- If the circulating practitioner receives the phone report, it is imperative that s/he 'reads-back' the test result to the pathologist to verify them, before informing the surgical team of the results.

Infection control and prevention

Surgical site infection (SSI) is the commonest form of hospital-acquired infection in surgical patients with approximately 10% of patients in the UK and 38% of patients in the US acquiring an SSI).[1,2] Patients have a right to be protected from preventable infection and practitioners have a duty to safeguard the well-being of their patients. Control of infection in the perioperative area is of paramount importance. Recommendations for standard precautions are intended primarily for the care of patients in acute hospitals. However, the principles should be applied in any setting where patient care is undertaken.

Best practice recommends that all patients are treated as potentially infected. *Universal Precautions* have been replaced by *Standard Infection Control Precautions*. 'Standard Infection Control Precautions' is the term used to describe the approach to infection control which offers protection to individuals whether or not they carry a known infection risk.[3,4] Standard Infection Control Precautions assess the activity to be performed rather than the individual receiving care.

The precautions constitute a single set of recommendations to be used for the care of all patients regardless of their infection state when exposed to:
• Blood.
• Excretions: e.g. urine, faeces, vomit, but not sweat.
• Secretions: e.g. mucous, seminal fluid, vaginal fluid, lactations, saliva, and sputum.
• Other body fluids: such as serum, lymph fluid, and CSF.
• Non-intact skin.
• Mucous membranes.
• Care must be taken with *all* body fluids to avoid skin, mucous membrane, and environmental contamination.

Nine elements of Standard Infection Control Precautions have been compiled principally based on Garner's guidance.[5] This is the primary strategy for the control and prevention of nosocomial infection.
• Hand hygiene.
• Use of personal protective equipment.
• Prevent occupational exposure to infection.
• Manage blood and body fluid spillage.
• Decontamination of patient care equipment.
• Environmental hygiene.
• Safe use and disposal of waste and sharps.
• Safe disposal of used linen.
• Provide care in the most appropriate place.

Transmission-based Precautions is a second tier of guidelines designed only for the care of specified patients with documented or suspected infection or colonisation with highly transmissible or epidemiologically significant pathogens for which *additional precautions* are necessary to interrupt transmission.[4]

- Airborne precautions: patients with tuberculosis (TB), measles or varicella (chickenpox)
- Droplet precautions: patients with respiratory illness
- Contact precautions: patients with GI/enteric infection e.g., hepatitis A, shigellosis, *Escherichia coli*, *Clostridium difficile*.

Recommendations include:

Airborne precautions

- Respiratory protection.
- Allowing appropriate ventilation air changes in the operating theatre following surgery.

Droplet precautions

- Mask wearing when within 3 feet (~90cm) of patients.
- Use of mask for patients during transfer.

Contact precautions

- Wearing gloves when touching the patient.
- Washing hands after removal of gloves.
- Gowning.
- Dedicated equipment if possible.
- Cleaning and disinfecting common equipment.

References

1. NINSS (2001). *Surveillance of Surgical Infection in English Hospitals 1997-2001*. Public Health Laboratory Service: London.

2. Mangram AJ, Horan TC, Pearson ML, *et al.* (1999). Guideline for prevention of surgical site infection. *Infection Control and Hospital Epidemiology* **20**(4), 247–78.

3. Beesley J and Pirie S. (2005). *Standards and Recommendations for Safe Perioperative Practice*, p115. National Association of Theatre Nurses: Harrogate.

4. Gruendemann BJ and Mangum SS (2001). *Infection Prevention in Surgical Settings*, p.319. Saunders: New York.

5. Garner J (1996). Guideline for isolation precautions. *Infection Control and Hospital Epidemiology* **17**(1), 54–80.

Common infection control terms

- *Antiseptic:* a chemical solution which will reduce and prevent growth of micro-organisms on skin.
- *Bacteraemia:* bacteria in the blood stream.
- *Bactericidal:* causing the destruction of bacteria.
- *Bacteristatic:* causing the inhibition of bacterial growth.
- *Colonisation:* the presence of microorganisms at a particular site without detrimental effect.
- *Cleaning:* the removal of foreign material e.g. soil, organic matter, and dust.
- *Chemical disinfectant:* a chemical solution which may be used to disinfect or sterilise items of equipment.
- *Contamination:* this occurs when either equipment or articles have been in contact with blood, body fluids, or pathological specimens.
- *Decontamination:* a procedure that removes the majority of harmful pathogenic organisms from objects and renders them safe to handle.
- *Disinfectant:* the removal or destruction of harmful micro-organisms but not bacterial spores.
- *Endogenous infection:* micro-organisms originating from the patient's own body which cause harm in another body site.
- *Exogenous infection:* micro-organisms originating from other people or inanimate objects which are spread by contact or airborne.
- *Flora:* micro-organisms resident in an environment or body site.
- *Incidence:* the number of new cases of a disease (or event) occurring in a specified time.
- *Infection:* the damaging of body tissue by micro-organisms or by poisonous substances released by the organism.
- *Immunity:* the activation of the body's response to infection.
- *Nosocomial infection:* infection acquired during hospitalisation, not present or incubating at time of admission to hospital.
- *Pathogen:* a micro-organism capable of causing disease.
- *Prevalence:* the ratio of the total number of individuals who have a disease at a particular time to the population at risk of having the disease.
- *Sepsis:* inflammation and/or pus formation at an infected site.
- *Septicaemia:* the multiplication of micro-organisms in the blood stream causing clinical signs of infection.
- *Sterilisation:* the complete destruction or removal of all living micro-organisms including bacterial spores.
- *Surveillance:* a system of collecting, tabulating, analysing, and reporting data on the occurrence of disease.
- *Virulence:* the degree of activity of pathogenic organism.

Handwashing

The spread of infection via hands is well established. The current spread of antibiotic-resistant organisms can be attributed, in part, to the failure of healthcare workers to wash their hands either as often or as efficiently as the situation requires. The importance of handwashing cannot be over emphasised.

Types of handwashing
- Social handwash.
- Antiseptic hand disinfection.
- Surgical scrub/antesepsis.

Routine handwashing removes most transient micro-organisms from soiled hands. Transient micro-organisms can be bacterial or viral. They are located on the surface of the skin and beneath the superficial cells of the stratum corneum. Any damaged skin, moisture, or ring wearing will increase the possibility of colonisation. Unlike resident flora, transient micro-organisms can be easily removed with handwashing and the risk from cross infection is immediately reduced.

Frequent handwashing and effective handwashing techniques are important in the prevention of nosocomial infection.

Surgical hand antisepsis is used to destroy transient microorganisms and to inhibit the growth of resident micro-organisms. This is routinely carried out before undertaking invasive procedures.

Purpose of surgical hand antisepsis
- Remove debris and transient organisms from nails, hands, and forearms.
- Reduce resident microbial count to a minimum.
- Inhibit growth of micro-organisms.
- Reduce numbers of micro-organisms on hands and reduce contamination of the operative site.

There are three types of antiseptic solution available for surgical hand antisepsis.
- Aqueous scrubs: water based solutions containing active ingredients e.g. CHG, povidone iodine.
- Alcohol rubs: alcohol-based solutions available in preparations of 60% to 90%, e.g. ethanol, isopropanol.
- Alcohol rubs containing additional active ingredients: alcohol-based solutions which contain an additional active ingredient such as CHG.

Active ingredients can be added to water to make aqueous scrubs or added to alcohol to make alcohol rubs with additional active ingredients.
- Iodophors.
- Biguanides.
- Phenolic compounds.

There is evidence from studies in favour of both scrubs and rubs as forms of antisepsis.

Variables associated with hand antisepsis
- Selection of antiseptic agent.
- Pre-antisepsis handwash.
- Duration of process.
- Use of brushes/sponges/nail picks.

Guidelines for hand antisepsis
Numerous organisations provide guidelines for hand antisepsis with variations in their recommendations.
- Centers for Disease Control.[1]
- Association of periOperative Registered Nurses.[2]
- Association for Perioperative Practice.[3]
- Australian College of Operating Room Nurses.[4]

References

1. Mangram AJ, Horan TC, Pearson ML, *et al.* (1999). Guideline for prevention of surgical site infection. *Infection Control and Hospital Epidemiology* **20**(4), 247–78.

2. Association of periOperative Nurses (2004). *Standards, Recommended Practices and Guidelines.* AORN Publishing: Denver, CO.

3. Beesley J and Pirie S. (2005). *Standards and Recommendations for Safe Perioperative Practice.* National Association of Theatre Nurses: Harrogate.

4. Australian College of Operating Room Nurses (2004). *Standards for Perioperative Nursing.* ACORN Ltd.: Australia.

Further reading

Gruendemann BJ and Mangum SS (2001). *Infection Prevention in Surgical Settings* p.111. Saunders: New York.

Tanner J, Swarbrook S, and Stuart J (2008). Surgical hand antisepsis to reduce surgical site infection. *Cochrane Database of Systematic Reviews. Issue 1.*

Management of a patient with an infection

It is good practice to maintain universal precautions since a patient may have an undiagnosed infection. This will include the use of facial/eye protection, procedure gloves, and gowns to protect staff from being splashed with potentially infected bodily fluids.

Meticillin-resistant *Staphylococcus aureus* (MRSA)

MRSA has been responsible for outbreaks of infection in primary and secondary care. These organisms are not only resistant to all the beta lactams but also to many other antibiotics. It is often introduced into a setting by a colonised or infected patient or healthcare provider.

The main mode of transmission is via hands, usually the hands of healthcare workers.

Prevention—definition of MRSA carrier

Consider definite MRSA positive—isolate and screen:
• MRSA positive culture.
• MRSA clearance incomplete.
• MRSA past positive with an unhealed wound.

Consider probable MRSA positive—ideally isolate and screen:
• Transfers from other hospitals.
• Transfer from positive nursing/residential home.

Consider possible MRSA positive—screen on admission:
• Transfer from nursing/residential home.
• Past cleared positive.

Management
• Correct handwashing procedures.
• Removal of unnecessary equipment from theatre.
• Gowns and gloves worn by staff transferring.
• Traffic control.
• Barrier precautions—non-scrubbed surgical team.
• Contaminated instruments taken directly to 'sluice' area/utility room.
• Recover in PACU using dedicated equipment or in operating theatre.
• Shower and change of attire following procedure—surgical team.
• Operating theatre terminally cleaned.
• Operating theatre may be used immediately after cleaning.

Hepatitis B
• Hepatitis B (HBV) is also known as serum hepatitis and is easily transmitted percutaneously or permucosally through direct contact with blood and body fluids, needlestick/sharps injury, break in skin, or splash in eye, nose, or mouth.
• Hepatitis B has an incubation period of 6 weeks.
• Immunisation is recommended for all high-risk healthcare professionals.

Hepatitis C

- Hepatitis C (HCV) is also known as the silent killer and is usually transmitted through large or repeated exposure to blood.
- Hepatitis C often has no detectable symptoms.
- There is no vaccine for Hepatitis C.

Management of hepatitis B and C

- Use of gloves, gowns, masks, and eyewear.
- Non-sterile gloves readily available to prevent contact with blood or body fluids.
- Sharps safety to prevent injuries from needles, scalpels, and other sharp equipment.
- Double-gloving practice recommended.

Clostridium difficile (C. diff)

C. diff is a species of Gram positive, anaerobic spore-forming bacteria. It is the most significant cause of pseudomembraneous colitis, a severe infection of the colon, often after normal gut flora has been eradicated by the use of antibiotics. C. diff is acquired from contact with humans or objects harbouring the bacteria and occurs through ingestion.

Management

- Consider type of surgery planned and if surgery is necessary or can be postponed.
- Withdrawal of antibiotics. In many situations when antibiotics stopped then normal gut flora re-grows.
- Evaluate current treatment/period of treatment/effectiveness. Metronidazole first line treatment. If not working vancomycin, rifampicin, or teicoplanin.
- Non-sterile gloves readily available to prevent contact faeces.

Creutzfeldt–Jakob disease (CJD)

Spongiform encephalopathies or prion diseases are caused by prions which are composed mainly of protein and are highly resistant to inactivation by physico-chemical agents or normal sterilisation techniques. This means that there is the theoretical possibility of transmission of disease during invasive procedures.

There are three categories of CJD
- Sporadic.
- Genetic.
- Aquired.

Variant CJD (vCJD) is an acquired form of human prion disease associated with the consumption of bovine spongiform encephalopathy (BSE)-affected meat. It is rare; however, there are likely to an unquantifiable number of individuals in the population that will now be incubating the disease and will be undergoing surgery. All types of the disease are fatal and once symptoms develop lead to death within a few months. In order to manage the risk of spreading the disease it is necessary to establish which tissues will be operated on. These are divided into high, medium, or low.

- High risk includes: brain, spinal cord, and posterior eye.
- Medium risk includes: the anterior eye and olfactory epithelium.
- Low risk includes the remainder of the body tissues.

In vCJD cases lymphoid tissue is regarded as medium risk. It is advisable to utilise disposable instruments for a known vCJD patient; if it proves necessary to use reusable items these must either be sacrificed or quarantined.

There is thought to be a negligible risk of transmission of CJD prions during fibreoptic endoscopes, in particular gastroscopy, due to the proximity of the tonsils and lymphatic tissue in the gut. Any risk is thought to be from the contamination of biopsy forceps and the biopsy channel of the endoscope. Therefore, the taking of a biopsy on an infected patient should be only be considered if absolutely necessary since the instrument should be quarantined after use and disposable biopsy forceps are recommended.[1]

Management of patients infected should follow up-to-date local and national policy and guidelines. The issue of CJD management is under constant review.

Reference

1. Axon ATR, Beilenhoff U, Bramble MG, et al. (2001). Variant Creutzfeldt–Jakob disease (vCJD) and gastrointestinal endoscopy (ESG Guidelines). *Endoscopy* **33**(12), 1070–80.

Further reading

Gruendemann BJ and Mangum SS. (2001). *Infection Prevention in Surgical Settings*. Saunders: New York.

Health Protection Agency (2007). *Variant CJD and blood products*. Available at: 🖳 http://www.hpa.org.uk/webw/HPAweb&HPAwebStandard/HPAweb_C/1195733818681?p=1191942152861

Role of the scrub practitioner

The scrub practitioner, who may be a qualified nurse, operating department practitioner (ODP), or healthcare support worker (HCSW), is a member of the perioperative team, which also includes (but which is not exhaustive of) a surgeon, a surgical assistant, a circulating practitioner, an anaesthetist, and an anaesthetic practitioner. Depending on training, education, level of competency and experience, practitioners will perform in more than one role, e.g., the scrub practitioner will also practice in the circulating role, and the surgeon in the role of the surgeon's assistant.

The role of the scrub practitioner encompasses:

- Donning sterile surgical attire and any additional personal protective equipment (PPE) necessary for the procedure.
- Setting up the surgical instrument tray, including checking all instruments are present, clean, and in good working condition.
- Ensuring checks of all instruments, swabs, needles, blades, sutures, and any other sharps and accessories are correct and accounted for before, during (as necessary), and after the procedure, and that the surgeon is thus informed, therefore reducing the risk of retaining a foreign body.
- Maintaining a sterile operative field throughout the procedure to reduce the risk of SSI.
- Anticipating the surgeon's needs throughout the surgery therefore assisting in its facilitation.
- Ensuring that handling of instruments, sharps, and any associated equipment and accessories avoids injury to the surgical team and/or the patient.
- Ensuring that all medical device equipment, instruments, accessories, and equipment are used in accordance with the manufacturer's recommendations.
- Maintaining a safe operating room environment throughout the procedure.
- Maintaining an awareness of the risks and complications associated with the surgical practice, inclusive of the instrumentation and other equipment and accessories being used, example, e.g., patient positioning, diathermy, skin preparation solutions, and dressing products.
- Ensuring effective communications with the perioperative team, including checking the patient's identity, consent, allergies, skin integrity, proposed surgical procedure, and surgical site.
- Making sure that the patient's dignity is maintained by the whole perioperative team from entering the operating room to leaving the operating room.
- Ensuring that all specimens are handled, documented, and forwarded to the appropriate department in accordance with local policy.
- Accurately documenting the patient's care in accordance with local policy, inclusive of all instrument and product/implant traceability information.

- Disposing of all contaminated instrumentation, accessories, and associated equipment, including linen and PPE into the appropriate waste receptacles in accordance with local waste disposal guidelines for decontamination or incineration.
- Training and education.
- Adhering to local and national policies, procedures, guidelines, and recommendations in relation to perioperative practice.
- Practicing at all times within professional guidelines and legal boundaries.

Further reading

Association for Perioperative Practice (2007). *Standards and Recommendations for Safe Perioperative Practice*. AfPP: Harrogate.

Clarke P and Jones J (1998). *Bridgen's Operating Department Practice*. Churchill Livingstone: Edinburgh.

Wicker P and O'Neill J (2006). *Caring for the Perioperative Patient*. Blackwell Publishing: Oxford.

Woodhead K and Wicker P (2005). *A Textbook of Perioperative Care*. Elsevier Limited: Edinburgh.

Setting up of the surgical instrument tray

The majority of operating departments are supplied with sterile surgical instrument trays and supplementary instruments from a TSSU. Tray sets are usually standardised and named according to specialty and usage, e.g. laparotomy set. Instruments and tray sets should all have a system for tracking and tracing in compliance with decontamination guidelines.

Pre-set tray systems are either perforated or solid. Some trays are modified to house specialty-specific instruments, e.g. some orthopaedic sets. To maintain the sterility of the instruments, trays are often wrapped with a double lining of either reusable or disposable linen. The *outer layer* is non-sterile, and when opened reveals an inner sterile layer, which only the scrubbed practitioner handles. The outer layer is opened away from the body first then towards the body by the circulating practitioner, and the scrub practitioner opens the *inner sterile layer* in the opposite direction, towards the body first then away. If using a trolley set-up system, the trolley should be prepared with a double layer of drapes large enough to cover the surface and sides of the trolley.

The instrument set should be prepared as close to the time of the surgery as possible to maintain sterility. Each tray should have a checklist detailing all the instruments held on the tray. Each instrument should be checked against this list by the scrub and circulating practitioners before each procedure. Each instrument should be inspected to make sure it is in good working order, intact, and free from any contaminants such as dried blood and body tissues. Any instruments which are damaged or contaminated should be removed. If an instrument on the tray set is contaminated the entire tray should be discarded.

> Instruments are usually set on the tray in the order that they will be used and in groups of the same types of instruments.

Instruments with ringed handles should be kept together and aligned according to any curves or angles, for example, curved scissors should all point in the same direction. Instruments are laid out beside each other and not on top of each other, and fine instruments, for example micro-instruments should be treated with extra care. Any tip protectors should be removed. Any sharps should be protected at all times, and blades mounted onto the blade handle using an appropriate instrument, not fingers. Care should be taken to avoid metal-to-metal, as this can increase the chance of instrument damage.

To maintain sterility, neither the scrub nor circulating practitioner should lean over the instrument tray/trolley set. The circulating practitioner should hand over any supplementary instruments and other necessary sundries avoiding any contamination either of the tray or the contents of the pack. The outer wrapping of any sterile packs should be opened away from the body then secured allowing the scrub practitioner to take the contents without contamination. Supplementary packs should be presented from the side of the tray/trolley and not dropped onto the tray which may result in contaminating the tray, dropping the pack contents or displacement of tray instruments.

Sharps and heavy instruments should be passed to avoid piercing the tray linen and injury. The circulating practitioner should avoid splashes when pouring liquid solutions into tray pots presented by the scrub practitioner. Wet linen can affect the tray's sterility.

The scrub practitioner is responsible for the instrument tray, and once prepared should stay with it at all times.

Further reading

Association for Perioperative Practice (2007). *Standards and Recommendations for Safe Perioperative Practice.* AfPP: Harrogate.

Clarke P and Jones J (1998). *Bridgen's Operating Department Practice.* Churchill Livingstone: Edinburgh.

Phillips N (2007). *Berry and Kohn's Operating Room Technique* (11th edn). Mosby: St Louis, MO.

Taylor M and Campbell C (1999). Back to basics: introduction to instruments. *British Journal of Theatre Nursing* **9**(8), 369–71.

Woodhead K and Wicker P (2005). *A Textbook of Perioperative Care.* Elsevier Limited: Edinburgh.

Accountability of swabs, sharps, and instruments

The purpose of undertaking instrument and consumable counts is to reduce the risk of them being retained within the body. Retaining items within the body is considered preventable; therefore, if this occurs legal proceedings may result. If an item is retained within the body it is treated as a foreign body which can cause problems immediately or after a significant period of time; these can include wound infections, infections within body cavities, pain—including referred pain—bleeding, delays in wound healing, loss of anatomical structure function, and formation of abscesses, fistulae, and adhesions. Further surgery may be required to remove the foreign body and this may have its associated risks.

All of the surgical team is accountable for the surgical count; however it is the scrub practitioner who is responsible for implementing the checks of all items being used before, during, and after the surgical procedure, and generally undertakes these checks with the circulating practitioner. This includes checking (but is not exhaustive of), instruments (and any detachable parts including screws), swabs, sharps (needles, blades, sutures), clips, slings/sloops, tapes, cotton wool balls, pledgets, ribbon gauze, packs, patties, sponges, diathermy blades and tips.

If no scrub practitioner is required for the procedure, counts should be undertaken by the surgeon and the circulating practitioner.

All tray instruments are audibly and visually checked against the corresponding tray list and counted. Additional consumable items, such as swabs and sutures are visually checked and audibly counted. Consumable items are added onto the theatre wall-mounted swab board. If the count is interrupted for any reason, it should be restarted.

Counts are undertaken:

- At the beginning of surgery.
- As items are added during surgery.
- Before closing a cavity within a cavity.
- Before closing the wound/any deep incision.
- Before skin closure.
- If either the scrub or circulating practitioner is replaced during the surgical procedure.
- At any time the scrub practitioner feels it is appropriate to do so.

All counts must be signed for by two practitioners, one of whom must be registered. This is usually the scrub and circulating practitioners, whose names should be added to the theatre register and into the patient's intraoperative record. It is advocated that the two practitioners who undertake the initial count undertake all counts throughout the surgery. If either practitioner is replaced, their names should also be added into the theatre register and in the patient's intraoperative documentation.

All swabs and consumables such as patties, pledgets, and ribbon gauze should be packed and counted in 'fives', and to ensure easy identification at x-ray should they be retained, have an x-ray detectable band

Any bundle that does not contain 'five' should be immediately discarded. Items such as blades, sutures, and needles are counted in multiples of 'one'. Any instruments, blades, sutures, or needles which break during surgery should be accounted for and all parts returned. All items, inclusive of waste disposal bags and laundry, used during the surgical procedure should be kept in theatre until surgery is completed. These will be checked if an item goes missing.

> If in the case of life-threatening emergency it may not be possible to perform the count. In this situation, all packaging should be kept, and a count undertaken as soon as is realistically possible.

At every count performed during the procedure, the scrub practitioner should audibly inform the surgeon of the result, and this should be audibly acknowledged by the surgeon. If there is a discrepancy in the count the surgeon should be made aware straight away, as it is the surgeon's responsibility to decide whether to continue or stop until the missing item is found. If the surgical team are unable to find the lost item, an X-ray must be taken either before the patient leaves the operating room or before leaving the theatre suite. Any missing items which have not been found must be recorded in the patient's documentation and an incident form completed.

Further reading

Association for Perioperative Practice (2007). *Standards and Recommendations for Safe Perioperative Practice*. AfPP: Harrogate.

Association of Perioperative Registered Nurses (2008). *Perioperative Standards and Recommended Practices*. AORN: Denver, CO.

Brown J and Feather D (2005). Surgical equipment and materials left in patients. *British Journal of Perioperative Nursing* **15**(6), 259–65.

Bynom S (1998). Reflection – a lost swab. *British Journal of Theatre Nursing* **8**(5), 15–18.

Clarke P and Jones J (1998). *Bridgen's Operating Department Practice*. Churchill Livingstone: Edinburgh.

Phillips N (2007). *Berry and Kohn's Operating Room Technique* (11th edn). Mosby: St Louis, MO.

Taylor M and Campbell C (1999). Back to basics: introduction to instruments. *British Journal of Theatre Nursing* **9**(8), 369–71.

Wicker P and O'Neill J (2006). *Caring for the Perioperative Patient*. Blackwell Publishing Ltd.: Oxford.

Williams M, Clancy J, and McVicar A (2001). How do you keep your patients safe? *British Journal of Perioperative Nursing* **11**(3), 124–30.

Woodhead K and Wicker P (2005). *A Textbook of Perioperative Care*. Elsevier Limited: Edinburgh.

Administration of drugs during surgery

During 1995 and 2005, the American JCAHO cited by Gregory[1] reported that 10% of adverse incidents incurred by patients were drug-related; most of these errors happening as a result of poor communication followed by poor procedural compliance, and although less commonly reported in the literature, drug errors within perioperative practice do occur, with devastating results.[2]

UK Government legislation aims to reduce the incidence of drug errors and ultimately improve patient safety. This legislation includes the Medicines Act 1968 (relates to manufacturing supply, licensing, and sales), the Misuse of Drugs Act 1971 (particularly relates to controlled drugs), and the Misuse of Drugs Regulations 2001 (allows identified practitioners within their field of practice to possess, prescribe, and dispense controlled drugs). Guidance aimed at ensuring safer practices in drug administration is also offered from organisations such as the NMC and the AAGBI 2006.[3,4] There should be compliance with local policies and procedures, including guidance on ordering, receipt, storage, and management of controlled and emergency drugs, should further ensure good management in drug administration.

Drug errors can happen at any stage in the process from prescription to administration and some reasons offered for these errors include:
• Failure to cross-reference patient identity with the prescription.
• Illegible handwriting.
• Fatigue.
• Inaccuracies in the prescription dosage.
• Use of abbreviations in the prescription.
• Administration of the wrong drug.
• Discrepancies in the frequency of administration.
• Poor communication.
• Distractions.
• Missing/inaccurate documentation.
• Administration of drugs patient is known to be allergic to.
• Incorrect labelling.

Drugs within perioperative practice are not just restricted to traditional pharmaceuticals; they are developed from natural, synthetic, and semisynthetic sources and they come in a variety of different forms including liquids, gases, solids, powders, and creams/ointments. The types of drugs used include antibiotics, analgesics, opiates, gaseous agents (inhalations and IV agents), muscle relaxants, anti-coagulants, hormones, laxatives, thrombolytics, diuretics, and anti-emetics, and this list is not exhaustive.

Drugs are used locally (via the skin and/or mucous membranes) and systemically (via the digestive system, parenterally, intravenously, subcutaneously and/or through the peritoneal cavity) throughout all three phases of the patient's perioperative journey, for example:
• Preoperatively in an attempt to improve the patient's physical condition to promote a better clinical outcome during and post surgery, and/or immediately before surgery, e.g. to reduce anxiety and provide pain relief.

- Intraoperatively, which often includes some form of local, regional, or general anaesthetic (sometimes a combination of all three).
- Postoperatively, for example to reduce pain and control nausea.

Perioperative practitioners involved in the administration of drugs must ensure the right patient receives the right drug, at the right time, in the correct dosage, via the right route. Drugs should not be administered unless the dispensing practitioner has an underlying knowledge of the drug, the strength, its action, the route of administration, the side effects, and knows what to do if the wrong drug is administered or if the patient suffers an allergic reaction. Additional considerations are required for paediatrics; for example, the amount prescribed will depend on the child's body weight and/or the surface area, and the elderly, whose physical condition may, for example, affect the absorption rate.

Local departments should develop their own policies to ensure safe drug practices and to encompass incidences when drugs are prepared by one professional and administered by another, as is common practice during anaesthesia and during surgery, for example, the circulating practitioner prepares the medication, delivers it to the scrub practitioner who hands it to the surgeon to administer. Drugs administered in this way should always be verbally and visually checked to confirm the drug type, the dose, the strength, and the expiry date.

All drugs administered should be labelled correctly, and all drug packaging should stay in the operating room until surgery is complete.

All pharmaceutical preparations used should be clearly documented in the patient records, and any un-used medication disposed of appropriately.

References

1. Crum BSG (2006). Revised National Patient Safety Goal on Medication Handling. *AORN Journal* **83**(4), 955–7.

2. Wanzer MB (2006). Study of perioperative medication errors provides clues for improving care. *OR Manager* **22**(3), 8–9.

3. Nursing and Midwifery Council (2007). *Standards for Medicines Management.* NMC: London.

4. Association of Anaesthetists of Great Britain and Ireland (2006). *Controlled Drugs in Perioperative Care.* AAGBI: London.

Further reading

AORN Guidance Statement–Safe medication practices in perioperative practice settings. *AORN Journal* **79**(3), 674–6.

Phillips N (2007). *Berry and Kohn's Operating Room Technique* (11th edn). Mosby: St Louis, MO.

Wicker P and O'Neill J (2006). *Caring for the Perioperative Patient.* Blackwell Publishing: Oxford.

Handling of surgical instruments

The instruments used during surgery are classified according to what they will be used for, including:
- Cutting.
- Dissecting.
- Retracting.
- Grasping.
- Clamping.
- Aspirating.
- Probing.
- Measuring.
- Suturing.

The surgical team should know the instruments for the procedure being undertaken, including knowing the instrument's name and what it is used for.

Whether reusable or single-use instruments, to ensure instruments remain fully functioning and in optimum condition for use during surgery they must be handled correctly and with care. Incorrect usage of instruments usually occurs when the correct instrument is unavailable, which can be avoided if instrument sets are pre-selected appropriately for each procedure.

Appropriate instrument handling also helps to reduce the incidence of injury to the patient and/or the surgical team, including personal injury, and prolongs the life of the instrument.

All surgical instruments should be handled gently, particularly micro-instruments:
- Dropping should be avoided—any dropped instruments should not be returned to the surgical field or instrument tray.
- Heavier instruments should not be placed on top of more delicate instruments.
- Tips and sharps points should be protected with tip protectors, e.g., needles, scissors, and hooks.
- Instruments should be handled either individually or in groups of similar instruments, e.g., artery forceps, scissors.
- Care and attention should be given during the decontamination process, e.g., instruments should not be dropped into wash sinks.
- Used instruments should be sent to a sterile services decontamination unit for reprocessing inclusive of lubricating and drying. (Single-use instrumentation should be discarded in accordance with local and national decontamination guidelines, polices and procedures.)

Before use the scrub practitioner should ensure that all tray instrumentation and supplementary instrumentation is sterile. If the sterility is in question, the instrument should be discarded. This includes whether the instrumentation is still within its shelflife, that is, the length of time that the instrument is considered to be sterile.

Good practice in instrument handling involves:

- Passing decisively to the surgeon's operating hand (awareness should be given to whether the surgeon is right- or left-handed), in a manner that allows the surgeon to use immediately without the need for any adjustment. Instruments with curves should be handed over with the curve in the direction of the surgeon's palms. Instruments are often used in sequence, and appropriate to the site, for example, short instruments will be used for superficial wounds and longer instruments for deeper body cavities.
- Passing and returning sharps to the hand should be avoided—it is recommended that a 'no-touch' technique is used, for example, sharps instruments are placed into a container such as a kidney dish.
- Not placing or leaving instruments on the patient—this increases the risk of injury to the patient and/or surgical team and increases the potential for contamination. All instruments should be returned to the instrument trolley.
- Mounting all needles/sutures onto a needle holder before handing over to the surgeon.
- Checking all powered instruments, for example, saws and drills for function, and particular attention paid to accidental activation. When not being used, powered instruments should be kept in 'safe' mode.

Instruments should not be used if damaged. Prior to use and during reprocessing all instruments should be checked for any damage including cracks, chips, blunting, and alignment. When instruments become damaged they should be returned to the manufacturer for repair and/or replacement.

All surgical instrumentation should be stored in an area, which is clean, dust-free, and dry. Storage surfaces should be easy to clean with smooth surfaces. The store room temperature should remain between 22–24° and the humidity at approximately 35–68%.

Further reading

Association for Perioperative Practice (2007). *Standards and Recommendations for Safe Perioperative Practice*. AfPP: Harrogate.

Clarke P and Jones J (1998). *Bridgen's Operating Department Practice*. Churchill Livingstone: Edinburgh.

Phillips N (2007). *Berry and Kohn's Operating Room Technique* (11th edn). Mosby: St Louis, MO.

Management of sharps

Sharps can be defined as suture needles, scalpel blades, or any other sharp equipment/instrument with potential to cause injury. Suture needles and scalpel blades have been found to be the leading cause of percutaneous injury. Suture needles alone account for 50% of these injuries. Scalpel injuries have been found to occur most often while passing, disassembling or disposing of the blade.

Sharps safety is important to prevent injuries which risk the transmission of viruses such as HBV, HCV, and HIV.

• A local policy for handling and disposal of sharps should be in place.
• Sharps should not be passed hand to hand. A 'hands-free' technique should be employed when passing sharps. Consider the use of a 'neutral zone'.
• Disposal of sharps is the responsibility of the individual members of the perioperative team.
• An appropriate instrument/device should be used for removal of surgical blades.
• Needles should not be resheathed, bent, or broken before disposal.
• A disposable sharps pad should be used to contain sharps and disposed of safely at the end of a procedure.
• Sharps containers should be placed close to the point of use.
• Sharps containers must not be filled to more than three-quarters and should not contain any protruding sharps.
• Sharps containers should be stored off the floor.

Needlestick injury

A local policy for needlestick injuries should be in place. In the event of injury:

• Encourage bleeding.
• Wash under running water.
• Dry and apply a waterproof dressing.
• Consent must be obtained from the patient to obtain a sample of blood for storage and testing. Patients have the right to refuse this.
• The patient needs to be fully recovered from the effects of general anaesthesia before they are informed of the incident.
• An incident form should be completed.
• Infection Control Team and/or Occupational Health should be informed as soon as possible.
• Professional counselling and follow-up should be available.

References

Beesley J and Pirie S. (2005). *Standards and Recommendations for Safe Perioperative Practice*, pp.118–19. National Association of Theatre Nurses: Harrogate.

Gruendemann BJ and Mangum SS (2001). *Infection Prevention in Surgical Settings*, pp.334–6. Saunders: New York.

Wicker P and O'Neill J (2006). *Caring for the Perioperative Patient*, pp.163–7. Blackwell Publishing: Oxford.

Clinical waste

Clinical waste has been defined under the Controlled Waste Regulations as:[1]
- Human or animal tissue.
- Blood or other body fluids.
- Excretions.
- Drugs or pharmaceutical products.
- Swabs and dressing.
- Used sharps.

Clinical waste has been categorised as:
- Hospital waste.
- Medical waste.
- Infectious waste.
- Regulated medical waste.

Infectious waste has been defined as waste with a potential risk of causing infection during handling. Medical waste is a category of hospital waste. Infectious waste is a category of medical waste.

Infectious waste has been categorised as:
- Microbiological cultures.
- Pathological waste.
- Human blood and blood products.
- Used sharps.

All clinical waste must be managed safely and should be segregated for disposal, according to local policy. For this purpose, clinical waste has been further categorised as:
- Category A: identifiable human tissue, blood, surgical dressings, swabs, or soiled waste.
- Category B: contaminated sharp instruments, syringes, needles, or broken glass.
- Category C: potentially infected waste e.g. microbiological waste from pathology or other laboratories.
- Category D: pharmaceutical products.
- Category E: items used to dispose of urine, faeces, or other body fluid e.g. bedpans, incontinence pads, stoma bags, or urine bags.

DoH *Safe Management of Healthcare Waste* obliges organisations to segregate waste into specific colour-coded waste streams.[2] Waste should be segregated accordingly into colour-coded bags and containers.
- Yellow: category A waste requiring incineration.
- Yellow with black stripes: category E waste suitable for landfill sites.
- Blue/or blue writing: waste requiring autoclaving prior to disposal.
- Black: non-clinical and household waste and paper.
- Clear: return of instruments to sterile services.

Disposal of waste
- Waste bags should not be overfilled.
- Bags must be clearly labelled to indicate the department they came from.
- Waste should be collected promptly and stored securely while awaiting incineration.

- Waste container for storage of waste bags should be easy to clean.
- Spillages from bags should be dealt with immediately.
- Handwashing facilities should be available.
- Adequate provision of sharps' bins.

Sharps bins
- DoH guidance suggests the colour coding for sharps bins.[2]
- Orange lids: sharps not contaminated with medicinal products and/or fully discharged sharps.
- Yellow lids: partially discharged sharps contaminated with medicinal products other than cytotoxic or cytostatic medicines. Pharmaceutical products.
- Purple lids: sharps contaminated with cytotoxic or cytostatic medicinal products.
- Blue or green lids: pharmaceutical products. Although DoH guidance suggests that these should also be included in yellow containers.

References
1. HMSO (1992). *The Controlled Waste Regulations 1992: Environmental Protection (Statutory Instruments: 1992: 588).* Stationery Office Books: London.

2. Department of Health (2006). *Safe Management of Healthcare Waste.* 🖳 www.dh.gov.uk/en/Publication and statistics/Publications/PublicationsPolicyAndGuidance/DH_063274

Further reading
Beesley J and Pirie S (2005). *Standards and Recommendations for Safe Perioperative Practice,* pp.50–1. National Association of Theatre Nurses: Harrogate.

Hind M and Wicker P (eds.) (2000). *Principles of Perioperative Practice,* pp.26–7. Churchill Livingstone: London.

Gruendemann BJ and Mangum SS (2001). *Infection Prevention in Surgical Settings,* pp.111, 303–8. Saunders: New York.

Instrument trays

The patient's surgical outcome is dependent on the competence, knowledge, and skills in the application of aseptic technique of practitioners. The basic principles of aseptic technique promote a sterile field in which surgery may be safely performed. Competent preparation and use of equipment is a major investment.

- The type of instrument tray used for a procedure is influenced by the type of surgery to be performed.
- Surgical instruments must be prepared immediately prior to use.
- A designated area should be identified for the purpose of preparing instrument trays for a procedure.
- Equipment should be collected in advance.
- Instrument trays must be checked for sterility, integrity, packaging, and expiry date.
- Instrument trays should be covered with a minimum of two layers of sterile drapes.
- Items/instruments extending over the edge of the trolley are at risk of contamination.
- Instrument trays should be opened away from the body first then towards.
- Prepared instrument trays must be accompanied at all times.
- Staff should adhere to an agreed method of setting the instrument trolley. This facilitates continuity of care for patients and safety for staff if someone else was required to take over for any reason.
- Instruments must always be returned to the trolley when not in use.

Further reading

Beesley J and Pirie S. (2005). *Standards and Recommendations for Safe Perioperative Practice*, pp.138–40. National Association of Theatre Nurses: Harrogate.

Decontamination of equipment

Surgical equipment must be cleaned and decontaminated following use in preparation for storage and packaging or disinfection/sterilisation. Decontamination is necessary in order to render a reusable instrument safe for handling by staff and for use on patients.

Decontamination

Decontamination is the term used to describe the process of removing or reducing contamination from infectious organisms or any other harmful substances. Decontamination is the combination of cleaning, disinfection, and sterilisation.

Methods of decontamination

- *Cleaning* is the term used to describe the removal of visible dirt, soil, or organic matter from equipment. Cleaning does not infer killing of micro-organisms. Cleaning is necessary before disinfection or sterilisation. Failure to adequately clean instruments will render the disinfection or sterilisation process ineffective.
- *Disinfection* is the term used to describe a reduction of the number of vegative microorganisms and viruses to relatively safe levels.
- *Sterilisation* is the term used to describe the complete killing or removal of all micro-organisms including spores.

The cleaning and decontamination area must be separate from the sterilising and packing area.

Cleaning/decontamination process:
- Water.
- Mechanical action.
- Detergent or enzymatic products.

Selection of detergent

- Detergents should facilitate removal of debris without damaging instrument/equipment.
- Detergents should be low sudsing and rinse off without leaving any residue.
- An acidic detergent is preferable for the removal of inorganic debris e.g. urine.
- An alkaline detergent is preferable for the removal of organic debris e.g. blood and faeces.
- It is important to follow manufacturers' instructions.

Automated washers

Cleaning by machine is preferable to manual cleaning as it offers greater protection to the worker.
- Washer decontaminators.
- Washer decontaminator/disinfectors.

Ultrasonic cleaners

Ultrasonic cleaners may be used to clean and decontaminate instruments/equipment that may not tolerate the automated washer process.

Preparation of cleaned and decontaminated instruments

Cleaned and decontaminated instruments are safe to handle in preparation for storage and packaging or disinfection/sterilisation.

- Instruments must be inspected for cleanliness, functioning, defects, sharpness/blunting of cutting edges.
- Lubrication of moving parts is important; a water-based lubricant is recommended.
- Instruments must be dried before storage.

Further reading

Association of periOperative Nurses (2004). *Standards, Recommended Practices and Guidelines*. pp.283–8. AORN Publishing: Denver, CO.

Beesley J and Pirie S (2005). *Standards and Recommendations for Safe Perioperative Practice*, pp.169–79. National Association of Theatre Nurses: Harrogate.

Gruendemann BJ and Mangum SS (2001). *Infection Prevention in Surgical Settings*, pp.153–8. Saunders: New York.

Protective clothing and eye protection

The correct and appropriate use of protective clothing has taken on considerable importance in recent years with greater awareness of the risks posed by infectious patients to healthcare workers and the need to reduce transmission of infection from patient to patient.

Health and safety legislation indicates that protective clothing is worn appropriately and correctly to manage the risk of exposure to micro-organisms which may be hazardous to health.[1] The principles are underpinned by the Health and Safety at Work Act 1974 and legislation relating to PPE at work.[2]

Health care workers have a professional responsibility to ensure that protective clothing is worn appropriately. The NMC state that 'as a registered nurse or midwife, you are personally accountable for your practice. In caring for patients and clients, you must: 'act without delay if you believe that you or anyone else may be putting someone at risk'.[3]

The use of protective clothing in preventing cross-infection is extremely important given:
- The morbidity and mortality associated with hospital acquired infection.[4]
- The cost of treating hospital acquired infections.[5,6]
- The increasing problem of antibiotic resistant micro-organisms.[7]

The primary use of protective clothing in healthcare settings is:
- To protect the skin and mucous membranes of healthcare workers from exposure to blood/body fluids.
- To prevent contamination of clothing and to reduce the opportunity of the spread of organisms from patients/fomites to other patients or environments.

Gloves

The aim of gloves is to:
- Protect users' hands from becoming contaminated with organic matter and micro-organisms.
- Protect users' hands from exposure to certain chemicals that may adversely affect the condition of the skin.
- Minimise cross-infection by preventing the transfer of organisms from staff to patients and vice versa.

Glove use—undertake a risk assessment to determine whether gloves are required:
- Gloves are required for procedures involving contact with blood, body fluids, excretions and secretions, non-intact skin, or mucous membranes.
- Gloves must be changed between patient contacts and between separate procedures on the same patient.
- Change gloves if torn or punctured.
- Gloves are single-use and should never be washed or re-used.
- Plastic gloves should never be worn for clinical tasks.
- Hands should be decontaminated following the removal of gloves.

Gowns

Gowns principally perform two functions:
- Single-use fluid-repellent aprons protect the healthcare worker's clothing from contamination with blood, body fluids, or microorganisms.
- Sterile gowns protect the patients from hospital-acquired infections, usually worn by staff when performing invasive procedures e.g. surgery or the insertion of a central venous catheter.
- The wearing of sterile gowns is necessary in theatres or when performing aseptic invasive procedures in a clinical area.
- Gowns should be disposed of after use as clinical waste and hands decontaminated immediately.

Masks

- Historically, the principal function of a mask has been to:
- Protect patients from the potential shedding of microorganisms from staff.
- Protect the healthcare worker from potential exposure to microorganisms.

Masks should be:
- Worn for all procedures where there is a risk of blood, body fluids, secretions or excretions splashing into the mucous membranes (⌷ see Eye protection).
- Used as single-use items and disposed of immediately after removing.
- Changed if moist or wet.
- Appropriate for their purpose.
- Worn correctly.
- Close fitting.
- Handled as little as possible.
- Removed by untying and handled only by the ties as they may be heavily contaminated.
- Never worn loosely around the neck.

Eye protection

Eye protection is principally worn to protect the eyes of the healthcare worker from contamination with blood, body fluids, or chemicals.

Eye protection must be readily available in clinical areas where procedures likely to produce splashing are performed. The types commonly used in the health care setting are:
- Goggles.
- Visors.
- Face-shields—single-use surgical facemask with integral eyeshield.

Goggles/visor/face-shield should be worn:
- When splash or spray of blood/body fluids is likely.
- When dealing with chemicals.
- During aerosol prone procedures.

Goggles/visor/face-shield should:
- Be comfortable to wear.
- Fit correctly.
- Allow for clear uncompromised vision.

Multi-use goggles/visors should:
- Be cleaned with detergent and hot water and dried thoroughly after use.
- Be cleaned as above and the disinfected with 70% alcohol if contaminated with blood or body fluids.
- Be replaced when lenses become scratched/opaque or the elastic ceases to provide a correct fit.

Caps

Caps are principally worn:
- To reduce the dispersal of hair and skin.
- To protect the wearer from contamination from blood or body fluids.

References

1. Control of Substances Hazardous to Health. (COSHH) (Amendments) Act (1999). Health & Safety Executive: London.

2. Health and Safety Executive (1992). *Health and Safety at Work Act 1974.* HMSO: London.

3. Nursing and Midwifery Council (2008). *The Code: Standards of conduct, performance and ethics for nurses and midwives.* NMC: London.

4. Department of Health (1995). *Hospital Infection Control. Guidance on the Control of Infection in Hospitals.* DoH: London.

5. National Audit Office. (2000). *The Management and Control of Hospital Acquired Infection in Acute Trusts in England. HC 230 Session 1999-00.* National Audit Office: London.

6. Plowman R, Graves N, Griffin M, et al. (1999). *The socio-economic burden of hospital acquired infection.* Public Health Laboratory Service: London.

7. House of Lords Select Committee on Science and Technology (1998). *Resistance to antibiotics and other antimicrobial agents (7th report).* HMSO: London.

Further reading

Ayliffe GAJ, Fraise AP, Geddes AM, et al. (2000). *Control of Hospital Infection, a Practical Handbook* (4th edn). Arnold: London.

Damani NN (2003). *Manual of Infection Control Procedures* (2nd edn). Greenwich Medical Media: London.

Department of Health (1995). *Hospital Infection Control. Guidance on the Control of Infection in Hospitals.* DoH: London.

Health and Safety at Work Act (1974). Health Services Advisory Committee. The Stationery Office: London.

Horton R and Parker L (2002). *Informed Infection Control Practice* (2nd edn). Churchill Livingstone: London.

Infection Control Nurses Association (ICNA) (1999). *Glove Usage Guidelines.* ICNA: Bathgate, UK.

Infection Control Nurses Association (ICNA) (2002). *Protective Clothing, Principles and Guidance.* ICNA: Bathgate, UK.

McCulloch J (2000). *Infection Control, Science, Management and Practice.* Whurr: London.

Wilson J (2001). *Infection Control in Clinical Practice* (2nd edn). Balliere Tindall: London.

Patient positioning for surgery

Principles for selecting patient position

The selection of the position of the patient on the operating table will depend on the type of surgery that is to be undertaken, so that access to the part of the body is maximised for the surgeon while making it possible for the anaesthetist to deliver a safe anaesthetic and monitor the patient. Most important is that the patient is safe on the operating table and that no harm is done to them while they are moved on or off the operating table and positioned for the procedure.

It is useful when a patient is being positioned on the operating table in the operating theatre, for a member of staff, often the scrub practitioner, to coordinate the positioning by placing themselves where they can oversee the moving and positioning of the patient. The best place to stand is at the foot of the table. It is also important that the patient is positioned anatomically and that limbs in particular are placed in their natural position. This is very important for patients with contractions or deformities of their limbs which must be allowed to remain in their natural position. The same is true for the patient's body alignment, for example when the patient is placed in the supine position that they are laying in what looks like a comfortable sleeping position.

Whilst overseeing the transfer of the patient the scrub practitioner should also see that the patient is transferred safely, that the neck and head are supported, and that IVIs and other lines are safe.

Particular care must also be taken to protect pressure points such as elbows and heels with suitable padding, or pressure-relieving devices such as gel pads, or cushioning such as pillows. Care must also be taken to protect the eyes and consideration may be made by the use of padding where appropriate.

Practitioners should be aware that the positioning of the patient can have on BP, venous return, and ventilation.

Further reading

Turnbull D, Farid S, Hutchison S, *et al.* (2002). Calf compartment pressures in the Lloyd-Davies position: a cause for concern? *Anaesthesia* **57**(9), 905–8.

Supine and Trendelenberg positions

Supine

This is probably one of the most widely used and natural positions for the surgical patient and is suitable for many general surgical procedures such as laparotomy, vascular, or breast surgery. The patient is positioned on the operating table on their back with their arms extended on arm boards or alongside their body (Fig. 17.1). If arm boards are used the angle of the arms must not exceed 90° with the palms ideally tuned upwards. Hyperabduction of the arm may result in the stretching of the subclavian and axilliary blood vessels and stretching of the brachial plexus, ulner nerve, and superficial nerves of the arm. The head can be placed on a pillow and the knees are supported by padding. Padding is used to avoid damage caused by pressure to the heels, sacrum, and elbows, and all peripheral nerves such as the ulnar nerve at the elbow and the lateral nerve at the head of the fibula.

Trendelenburg position

This is a variation of the supine position as already described which involves the tilting of the table to a head-down angle of up to 40°. It is used for abdominal/pelvic gynaecological procedures and operations for varicose veins. Care must be taken to ensure that the patient does not slip headfirst down the table. This can be achieved by the use of an anti-slip mattress, or securing straps around the patient, or by the use of shoulder pads. In the Trendelenburg position BP can increase due to the pooling of blood in the upper torso. Care should be taken to return the patient to the supine position slowly to avoid a drop in BP.

The reverse Trendelenburg position is also utilised for head and neck procedures to promote venous drainage away from the operation site. The use of a footboard may be required in order to prevent the patient slipping feet first. In the reverse Trendelenburg there are considerations regarding BP:

- Diminished cardiac return resulting in diminished cardiac output.
- Decrease in brainstem perfusion due to gravity.
- Pooling of blood in lower extremities.
- Possibility of circulatory overload if returned to the supine position too quickly.

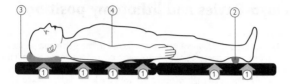

① Pressure points

② Ankle support prevents heel and calf pressure

③ Head support prevents neck hyperextension

④ Access to arm veins restricted:– Extension to cannula or abduct arm

Fig. 17.1 Supine position. Reproduced from Quick C, Thomas P, and Deakin P. *Principles of Surgical Management*, 2001, ISBN 9780192622303, with permission from Oxford University Press.

Lloyd-Davies and lithotomy positions

Lloyd-Davies

This position is used where access is required to the pelvis and perineum for colorectal, gynaecological, or urological operations and is a modification of the lithotomy position (Fig. 17.2). The legs are placed in the Lloyd-Davies stirrups at an angle of about 45° with the knee slightly flexed. Care must be taken when placing the legs in position, especially in older patients who may have arthritic problems with hips and knees. The placing should be coordinated with legs gently lifted at the same time and the anaesthetist informed that the legs are to be lifted. The end of the table is removed and often a tray is attached to the table in the space between the patient's legs for the placement of surgical instruments. The patient's bottom may also be placed on a pad to further aid access to the pelvic region and the table is usually tipped with the patient's head slightly down.

Great care needs to be taken to ensure that pressure areas and bony prominences are protected. If the patient is kept in this position for more than 4 hours the risk of compartment syndrome of the calves is increased[1] which can affect the patient's BP and may increase their postoperative pain and may result in significant permanent damage and morbidity.

Lithotomy

This is used for operations or examination of the perineum, vagina, or rectum. The patient is placed on the table with their buttocks placed at the lower break in the table with the feet placed in stirrups fixed to either side of the table taking care not to place them in an excessively high position (Fig. 17.3). The considerations are similar to those for the Lloyd-Davies position but since most procedures that utilise this position are usually shorter there are generally fewer complications.

Reference

Turnbull D, Farid S, Hutchison S, *et al.* (2002). Calf compartment pressures in the Lloyd-Davies position: a cause for concern? *Anaesthesia* **57**(9), 905–8.

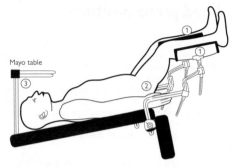

Mayo table

1. Pressure on calf may cause venous stasis or compartment syndrome
2. Better hip position but hip and femoral vessel injuries still possible
3. Anaesthetic access difficult

Fig. 17.2 Lloyd-Davis position. Reproduced from Quick C, Thomas P, and Deakin P. *Principles of Surgical Management*, 2001, ISBN 9780192622303 with permission from Oxford University Press.

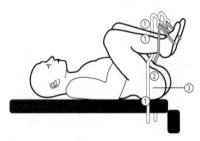

1. Danger of touching metal and causing diathermy burn
2. Femoral and obturator nerves in danger
3. Hip joint damage and vascular injury possible

Fig. 17.3 Lithotomy position. Reproduced from Quick C, Thomas P, and Deakin P. *Principles of Surgical Management*, 2001, ISBN 9780192622303 with permission from Oxford University Press.

Lateral and prone positions

Lateral

This position can be used for such procedures as hip arthroplasty, kidney surgery, and some chest operations. The patient will be anaesthetised in the supine position and then positioned onto their side using a suitable technique, utilising slide sheets and other positioning aids (Fig. 17.4). Care must be taken to position the downward shoulder slightly forward to relieve pressure on the brachial plexus while the lower arm can be flexed to rest beside the patient's head on a suitable arm board with a pad under the placed high in the axilla to relieve pressure on the brachial plexus and deltoid muscle. This will also help to prevent axilliary artery and vein obstruction.

The upper arm is placed on an adjustable arm rest with the neck not overly extended to avoid stretch damage to the brachial plexus. The patient may need to be secured in position to prevent them from rolling and a pillow or pad is placed between the legs to relieve the pressure of the upper leg and the lower legs which should be slightly flexed to aid stability. Special care must be taken to provide proper support for the head since necrosis of the ear can be caused by the pressure of the head which can be achieved by use of a soft pillow or a gel headrest.

Prone

This is used for procedures on the spine, neck, or the buttocks. Anaesthesia is induced with the patient in the supine position and then the patient rolled into their front (Fig. 17.5). Techniques to undertake the transfer onto the table should be developed locally and the use of slide sheets and other moving equipment can be useful to ensure staff and patient safety. The arms should be placed along the patient's side and not around the head. The head can be placed on a padded headrest or 'doughnut' and the eyes and nose protected. The lower limbs are supported under the knees and care taken to prevent pressure caused by the feet resting on the table mattress. A void below the abdomen should be made for the abdominal contents to avoid caval obstruction and hypotension. This can be achieved by use of pillows or a Montreal mattress.

Lateral +/-Break

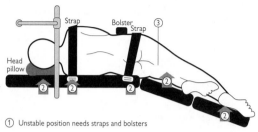

① Unstable position needs straps and bolsters

② Several pressure points

③ Need to separate legs with pillow

④ Needs careful positioning to avoid injury

⑤ Check for contact with metal and all pressure points padded

Fig. 17.4 Lateral position. Reproduced from Quick C, Thomas P, and Deakin P. *Principles of Surgical Management*, 2001, ISBN 9780192622303 with permission from Oxford University Press.

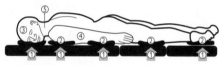

① Pressure points

② Position of padding to keep abdomen clear

③ Turn head to one side to avoid facial and eye congestion

④ Arm position important – see below

⑤ Armoured and secured tube needed

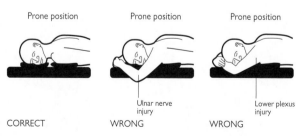

Prone position   Prone position   Prone position

CORRECT   WRONG   WRONG

Ulnar nerve injury

Lower plexus injury

Fig. 17.5 Prone position. Reproduced from Quick C, Thomas P, and Deakin P. *Principles of Surgical Management*, 2001, ISBN 9780192622303 with permission from Oxford University Press.

Wound management

Surgical incisions

A surgical incision is when an intentional cut or wound is made on the body usually involving a sharp instrument (scalpel or blade).

A badly placed incision can have a detrimental impact on the healing of the wound, causing haematomas, wound dehiscence (break down), and an increased risk of infections. Also, psychologically, an ugly, inappropriately large or disfiguring scar can influence the patient's perception of the surgery and impact their quality of life afterwards.

Criteria for placement of incision

A surgeon must take into account when determining the positioning of the incision:

- That it allows adequate access to the operative site.
- That the incision can be extended if more extensive surgery is required.
- The ease with which the wound can be closed and how secure the wound will be postoperatively.
- That it will provide the lowest postoperative complication rate.
- That it will reduce postoperative pain.
- That it will provide the most aesthetically acceptable appearance when healed.
- That an incision along a skin plane is less likely to result in problem scarring.

Further considerations

The surgeon must also consider the patient's:

- Medical status: e.g. diabetes, anaemia, steroid treatment—as these will have a negative impact on the healing process.
- Lifestyle and anticipated length of recovery to 'normal' functions: e.g. patient expectation of full recovery will differ depending on their diet and exercise, age, previous abilities.
- Weight: patients who are clinically obese will put more strain on wound closure material and have reduced healing abilities. There may also be impaired healing due to a reduced blood supply caused by the increased amount of adipose tissue.
- Reduced nutritional status will impact on collagen synthesis, which is part of the basis for wound healing.
- Cosmetic expectations: body image and self-esteem post-surgery is very important to patients, especially those who have undergone 'enhancement' surgery, and placement of surgical incisions can determine how well a scar heals.

Classification of surgical wounds

Clean
Elective, not emergency, non-traumatic, primarily closed, no acute inflammation, no break in technique, respiratory, GI, biliary, and genitourinary tracts not entered.

Clean-contaminated
Urgent or emergency that would otherwise be clean, elective opening of respiratory GI, biliary, and genitourinary tract with minor spillage. Not encountering infected urine or bile. Minor break in technique.

Contaminated
Non-purulent inflammation, gross spillage from GI, entry into biliary and genitourinary tract in the presence of infected bile or urine; major break in technique; penetrating trauma <4 hours old.

Dirty
Purulent inflammation, preoperative perforation of GI, biliary, and genitourinary tracts; penetrating trauma >4 hours old.

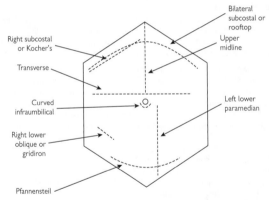

Fig. 18.1 Names of several common abdominal incisions. Reproduced with permission from Tulloh B and Lee D (2007). *Foundations of Operative Surgery: An Introduction to Surgical Techniques*, ISBN 9780199228669, with permission from Oxford University Press, Oxford.

Haemostasis

Haemostasis can be described as the arrest of bleeding by either using the physiological process or by surgical means. If haemostasis is not controlled excessive bleeding can lead to decreasing blood volume and BP, which can eventually result in death.

Physiological process

Vasoconstriction

- Vascular constriction: an immediate response resulting from the contraction of smooth muscle within the vessel wall. Sufficient to close small vessels but only a temporary measure in larger vessels.
- Platelet plug formation: occurs when platelets bind with collagen and then bind with fibrinogen to form a plug. Sufficient to close small tears or cuts.

Coagulation

- Required to close large tears or cuts.
- Requires the formation of a blood clot which is a mesh of protein fibres which bind blood cells, platelets, and fluid.

Surgical methods

During surgery, providing haemostasis will aid the surgeon maintain visualisation of the wound site. It will also assist in the wound healing process as fluid and blood left in the wound site may encourage microbial development leading to infection or prevent direct contact of the wound sides

Haemostasis during surgery is maintained in a variety of ways

- *Sutures and ligatures (ties):* material used to either knot/tie/ligate around medium-to-large bleeding vessels or to bring together sides of a wound. Designed as either absorbable or non-absorbable depending on the requirement. Length of time the material takes to be absorbed is dependent on type of material, patient's health, and speed of wound healing.
- *Metal surgical clips (staples):* used when a vessel has been identified, clips are placed prior to excision. Though it should not be used as the main haemostatic as they can impede further ligation. Non-absorbable.
- Bone wax: a semi-synthetic material used on bone surfaces to halt localised bleeding; absorbable.
- Electrosurgery (*diathermy*): electrical current which heats the bleeding vessel cauterising it (◻ see Electro-surgical equipment, p.358)
- *Ultrasonic:* coagulates blood vessels by vibrating at a frequency 55 500 cycles per sec (55.5KHz). The human ear may hear sounds from longitudinal waves at frequency range between 20 and 20 000 cycles per sec. Heat is generated due to the high frequency vibration of the tissue.
- *Absorbable haemostats:* various types which are presented in a mesh format to provide a matrix for clot formation used on small blood vessels. Absorbed within 7–10 days.

- *Haemostatic forceps (artery clips):* presented in various sizes, dependent on potential use, though generally the smaller ones are used to clamp small blood vessels, prior to being ligated or left until blood clot is formed (2–5 minutes).
- *Tissue adhesives:* similar function as glue, used predominantly in head wounds and as a final skin closure material.
- *Chemical:* silver nitrate in an aqueous environment acts as a strong oxidising agent cauterising small blood vessels. Predominantly used for epistaxis (nose bleeds).

Further reading

Erian M and McLaren G (2004). Ultrasonically activated technology in gynaecologic operative laparoscopy. *Reviews in Gynaecological Practice* **4**(3), 194–8.

Lloyd S, Almeyda, J, Di Cuffa R et al. (2005) The effect of silver nitrate on nasal septal cartilage. *Ear, Nose and Throat Journal* **84**, 41–4.

Inc. Ethicon (1994). *Ethicon Wound Closure Manual. Johnson & Johnson.* Available at: http://www.mitekproducts.com/public/USENG/Ethicon_WCM_042007.pdf

Singh S and Maxwell D (2006). Tools of the trade. *Best Practice & Research Clinical Obstetrics & Gynaecology* **20**(1), 41–59.

Wound closure

Sutures (stitches) are lengths of material used to either knot/tie/ligate around bleeding vessels or to allow for healing through primary intention, i.e. tissues are held in proximity until enough healing occurs to withstand stress without mechanical support. There is no ideal suture—all types have their merits and disadvantages.

Sutures can be divided into 2 main categories

- *Absorbable:* loses most of its tensile strength within 60 days of insertion. Ideally loses its strength at the same rate that the tissue regains its strength, being then absorbed into the body leaving no foreign material. Use on stomach, colon, bladder. Absorbable sutures are now used on the skin as a subcuticular closure. They have the advantage of producing better alignment of the wound edges, leave less of a scar, and do not require removal, making them ideal for use in children.
- *Non-absorbable:* retains strength for a long time, sometimes indefinitely. When used as a skin closure they must be removed once healing has taken place to prevent chronic sepsis. Use on skin, fascia, tendons.

Sutures can be further divided into:

- *Monfilament sutures* have one strand and are considered to be less of an infection risk because the lack of interstices prevents the harbouring of infective organisms. However frequent handling or tying can create weaker areas causing breakage of the suture.
- *Multifilament sutures* are made up of a number of strands which are twisted or braided which improve the tensile strength, pliability, handling, and knot-tying properties. However, they are associated with higher tissue drag and are therefore coated to ensure relatively smoother passage through the tissues. Avoid in areas of high contamination e.g. anus.

Further considerations

- Knot tensile strength: its strength is defined by the force necessary to cause the knot to undo.
- Plasticity, elasticity, and memory are all intertwined, as a suture must be able to allow for wound swelling (plasticity). Though as swelling subsides, the suture should regain its original form and length (elasticity). Memory is related to plasticity and elasticity and enables sutures to return to their original shape after deformation by tying.
- Tissue biocompatibility: suture materials produce varying degrees of tissue reaction, specifically inflammation. Significant inflammation increases the risk of infection and can delay wound healing. Synthetic materials, which are mostly used today, produce a minimal reaction.
- Diameter: sizes of sutures are standardised and relate to a specific diameter range (in mm) of the suture strand that is necessary to produce a certain tensile strength. Sizes are expressed with zeroes, such as 3-0, 4-0, 5-0, and 6-0; more zeroes indicate a smaller size.

Other types of wound closure

Steri-Strips™

These are adhesive skin closures that are sometimes used to close small wounds or in areas where there are cosmetic considerations such as on the face. They might also be used in conjunction with sutures to bring the wound closer together.

Staples

These are the fastest method of closing the skin and they have a low level of tissue reactivity. Skin staples come in pre-loaded different sized dispensers. The edges of the wound should be everted while the stapler is positioned over the line of the incision and a staple placed evenly at each side. Skin staples are removed after 5–7 days using a staple remover and produce an excellent cosmetic result if applied correctly.

Further reading

Inc. Ethicon (1994). *Ethicon Wound Closure Manual. Johnson & Johnson.* Available at:
http://www.mitekproducts.com/public/USENG/Ethicon_WCM_042007.pdf

Singh S and Maxwell D (2006). Tools of the trade. *Best Practice & Research Clinical Obstetrics & Gynaecology* **20**(1), 41–59.

Needles

The needles attached to sutures are divided into three main sections:
- Eye: the majority of sutures are now swagged, i.e. the suture is attached to the needle. Other eyes are closed and spring.
- Body: part of needle grasped by the needle holder:
  - Straight—generally used by hand.
  - Half curved—allows easy access down trocar ports.
  - Curved needle—most commonly used shape.
  - Compound curve (J-shaped)—used in confined spaces.
- Point: designed to penetrate tissues with minimum damage:
  - Cutting—cutting edge uppermost on the needle.
  - Reverse cutting—cutting edge on the underside of the needle.
  - Taper point.
  - Spatula.
  - Taper cut—round.
  - Blunt.

See Fig. 18.2 for shapes of needles and Fig. 18.3 for examples of types of needles.

There are 3 main types of cutting needle:
- Taper cut: used for tough fibrous tissue.
- Conventional cutting: two opposing cutting edges with a third on the edge on the inside curve of the needle.
- Reverse cutting: two opposing cutting edges with a third edge on the outside curve of the needle. It is a triangular-shaped needle. Only the edges near the tip are sharp.

Taper-cut points are used on delicate tissues that are easily penetrated, such as peritoneum, heart, and intestines. The point is designed so that the shaft gradually tapers to a point which results in a very small hole in the tissue.

Blunt-point needles have a rounded end for use with friable tissue such as the kidney or the liver, when neither piercing nor cutting is suitable.

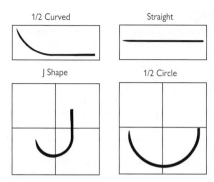

Fig. 18.2 Shapes of needles. Reproduced with permission of Ethicon.

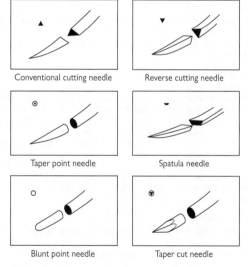

Fig. 18.3 Types of needles. Reproduced with permission of Ethicon.

Dressings

The final stage in the operation is the application of the dressing which is a role usually left to the scrub practitioner to perform. A dressing can be said to perform five basic, but important functions:

- To protect the incision from contamination and trauma.
- To absorb exudates.
- To facilitate haemostasis and minimise swelling.
- Provide support, or to splint or immobilise a body part.
- To enhance the patient's physical and psychological comfort.

Dressings should be appropriately selected for the type of wound. For a straightforward skin-wound dressing there are many proprietary makes of occlusive dressing available, the choice of which will often be down to personal preference. Before the surgical procedure is commenced any allergies that the patient has will have been checked, so care is taken to avoid using an adhesive to which the patient is sensitive.

Application

- The wound and surrounding area is cleaned by the scrub practitioner with a moistened (if necessary) swab and dried using a swab or sterile dressing towel.
- The dressing is prepared as appropriate for the type of wound using a sterile technique and the dressing applied to the wound.
- The drapes can then be removed from the patient while the dressing is held in place.

Specialist dressings

These include:

- Hydrocolloids which contain a matrix and other gel-forming agents such as gelatin and pectin. It promotes autolysis and aids granulation.
- Alginates contain calcium and sodium salts obtained from seaweed. They are useful for heavily exudating wounds.
- Foam dressings can be used for moderately exudating wounds. They deslough by maintaining a moist environment.
- Hydrogels have a high content of water to create a moist wound surface and debrides by hydration and autolysis.
- Debriding agents are useful for difficult to heal surgical wounds. They work by removing necrotic tissue and eschar.

Further reading

Bale S and Jones V (1996). *Wound Care Nursing: A patient-centred approach*. Bailliere Tindall: London.

Grey JE and Harding KG (eds) (2006). *ABC of Wound Healing*. Blackwell Publishing: Oxford.

Wound drains

A drain is a means of providing a conduit for internal fluids (or gas) to be removed from the body.

Main types

- Open usually corrugated, allows the fluid to drain into a receptacle—either a bag or pads.
- Closed: perforated drainage tube is inserted in area of the drainage site and connected to a bag or bottle.
- Free drainage (passive): relies on differences in pressure between cavities and external environment and the build up of fluid
- Low vacuum/suction (active): suction is induced either low or high depending on cavity and drainage site.
- Autologous: patient's own blood is filtered as it drains as can be transfused back into the patient before a nominated time period.

A drain could be a low vacuum closed drain e.g. redivac, chest drain; a open passive drain e.g. Yeates; a closed passive drain e.g. urinary catheter.

There is debate surrounding their effectiveness as drains:

For their use

- Removes fluid from the wound site which if left could provide a source for bacterial growth.
- Facilitates wound healing by preventing the formation of a haematoma or seroma.
- Provides a means of observing blood loss and early detection of haemorrhage.

Against their use

- A conduit for bacteria to enter the cavity, increasing the risk of infection.
- Trauma induced on insertion and removal of the drain.
- Trauma to tissues due to the presence of suction within a cavity.

Some surgeons will use a suture to secure the drain to the skin to prevent accidental displacement of the drain. Through confusion or agitation, patients may inadvertently remove the drain causing further trauma to the wound.

Urinary catheters

Drains urine from the bladder either transurethrally (via the urethra) or suprapubically (via the abdomen).

Rationale for use

- Monitor urine output.
- Allow irrigation of the bladder.
- Bypass an obstruction.
- Obtain a sterile specimen.

Insertion of a catheter is an aseptic technique, despite this urinary tract infections are the most common infections acquired in hospital. Various sizes and lengths and materials used depending on the requirements.

Nasogastric tubes (also known as Ryles tubes)
• Inserted via the nasal passages and passed into the stomach.
• Remove fluid and gas from GI tract.

Rationale for use
• Preparing the patient for emergency surgery such as ectopic pregnancy, ruptured aortic aneurysm; to assist in gastric surgery such as bariatric surgery, keeping the stomach empty to allow the surgeon adequate access to the operative site.
• To drain the gut after surgery during the period of ileus preventing the accumulation of fluid and gas.
• Administer medication and feeding directly into GI tract.
• Obtain specimens of gastric contents.

Further reading

Kumar B (2006). *Working in the Operating Department* (2nd edn). Churchill Livingstone: Edinburgh.

Parker MJ and Roberts C (2007). Closed suction surgical wound drainage after orthopaedic surgery (review). *The Cochrane Collaboration of Systematic Reviews*: Issue 4.

Wilson J (2003). *Infection Control in Clinical Practice*. Bailliere Tindall: Edinburgh.

Surgical equipment

Minimal access surgery

- May also be described as minimally invasive surgery or keyhole surgery.
- Allows access to parts of the body through very small incisions for
  - Diagnosis.
  - Treatment.
- Procedures performed through small natural or surgical holes.

Advantages over open surgery

- Less postoperative pain as the incisions are small.
- Faster recovery and earlier discharge.
- Patient can return to normal activities more quickly.
- Better cosmetic result as the incisions are small.
- Potentially less blood lost during surgery so reduced need for blood transfusion.
- Potential reduction in risk of postoperative wound infection as the incisions are small.
- Opportunities for theatre staff to observe the surgery.
- Useful for teaching. Interesting for theatre staff.
- Photographs or recordings may easily be made for the patient or for future teaching/presentations (with the patient's consent).

Disadvantages

- Equipment is expensive—may have an implication when setting up the service.
- Instruments are more difficult to clean and decontaminate.
- Difficult technique to learn.
- Can be technically challenging for surgical and scrub staff.
- For these reasons, can be a longer procedure than open surgery.

Technique

- A telescope attached to a camera is introduced into the area for surgery.
- At least two incisions are made—one for the telescope and one or more for instruments.
- The area is visualised on a monitor.

Arthroscopy

- Means looking into a joint.
- May be a diagnostic or an operative procedure.
- MRI scanning has largely replaced diagnostic arthroscopy as the quality of the imaging is so good.

Equipment

A camera stack comprising:

- High intensity light source.
- High resolution camera system.
- Monitor screen.
- Recording equipment.

Commonly used for surgery on these joints

- Knee.
- Shoulder.

May also be used for:

- Elbow.
- Wrist.
- Big toe.
- Ankle.
- Hip.

Technique

- Two incisions <1cm long are made in the skin over the joint.
- A port is introduced for the telescope and fluid inflow.
- A telescope attached to a camera is inserted through the port and an instrument through the other incision.
- The instrument may be a probe to assist with visualising the joint or a punch to remove tissue e.g. torn cartilage (meniscectomy).
- Anterior cruciate ligament (ACL) reconstruction may be performed arthroscopically.

Laparoscopy

- Means looking into the abdominal cavity.
- May be a diagnostic or an operative procedure.
- Major surgery may be performed this way e.g. bowel resection.
- May be used alongside other surgical techniques e.g. laparoscopically assisted vaginal hysterectomy (LAVH).
- A small incision may be required to remove tissue or an organ surgically incised e.g. bowel resected laparoscopically.

Equipment and instruments

A camera stack comprising:
- High intensity light source.
- High resolution camera system.
- Monitor screen.
- Recording equipment.
- CO_2 insufflator.

Commonly performed laparoscopic procedures

- Cholecystectomy—removal of gall bladder.
- Inguinal hernia repair.
- Appendicectomy.
- Bowel resection.
- Operations on the kidney—pyeloplasty, nephrectomy.

Technique

- A pneumoperitoneum is achieved using CO_2 gas to create space and allow the organs to be visualised.
- Telescope and instruments are used through the ports to perform surgery.

Risks associated with laparoscopic surgery

Insufflation
- The gas may be introduced using a *Verres needle*. The needle is inserted blind through the abdominal wall and gas introduced.
- The first port may be introduced using a *cut down*. A small para-umbilical incision is made into the peritoneal cavity. A blunt trocar is introduced allowing the peritoneal cavity to be visualised during gas insufflation to minimise the risks of perforation.

Risks
- Perforation of blood vessels or organs caused by the needle being wrongly positioned e.g. into the bowel or into the aorta or vena cava.
- Gas insufflated to the incorrect area potentially causing surgical emphysema if the needle is in the subcutaneous tissue or pneumothorax if in the thoracic cavity.
- Cardiac arrhythmias caused by stimulation of the vagus nerve by the pressure of the gas.
- CO_2 embolism caused by insufflation of gas into a blood vessel.
- Respiratory depression caused by upward displacement of the diaphragm by the pressure from the gas leading to reduction in lung capacity.

- Inadvertent hypothermia caused by insufflation of cold gas over a period of time.

Electrosurgery (diathermy)
- Breaks in insulation on instruments used for diathermy during surgery may result in damage to tissues or organs out of the visual field e.g. the bowel. This may not be noticed at the time of surgery and may not become apparent until a postoperative peritonitis occurs.
- Coupling: the live electrode accidentally touches a non-insulated instrument and causes a burn out of the field of vision.

Endoscopy

- Means looking into the body.
- Uses the body's natural openings without need for incisions.

Commonly performed endoscopic procedures

- *Gastroduodenoscopy*: to examine the inside of the oesophagus, stomach, and duodenum and take biopsies
- *Hysteroscopy*: to examine the cervix and endometrium of the uterus through the vagina, take biopsies and resect fibroids or the endometrium (TCRE = transcervical resection of endometrium).
- *Colonoscopy*: to examine inside the colon, take biopsies, and remove polyps.
- *Cystoscopy*: to examine inside the bladder through the urethra, take biopsies, destroy lesions e.g. cancer, and to resect the prostate gland (TURP = transurethral resection of prostate).
- *Ureteroscopy*: to examine the ureters; accessed through the bladder.

Technique

- For gastroduodenoscopy and hysteroscopy the picture is viewed on a monitor via a camera.
- Air (gastroscopy and colonoscopy) or fluid (hysteroscopy = warm saline or glycine if operative, and cystoscopy = warm water or glycine if operative) are used to dilate the organ to allow visualisation.
- Flexible scopes are widely used for gastroscopy, colonoscopy, and diagnostic cystoscopy and hysteroscopy.
- Rigid scopes are commonly used for resection—TURP, TCRE.

Prosthesis

- The definition for prosthesis is 'the artificial substitute for a missing part of the body for either functional or cosmetic reasons'.
- Most commonly thought of prosthesis are those that replace limbs such as legs and arms.
- Other types of prosthesis are (but not limited to):
  - Joint replacements.
  - Arterial grafts.
  - Ophthalmic lenses.
  - False teeth.
  - Heart valves.
  - Reconstructive appliances—breast, chin, penile implants.
  - Pacemakers.
  - Intervertebral discs.
  - Mesh to support muscles walls.

The manufacture and use of prosthesis is regulated by the MHRA, who are responsible for ensuring that medical devices, such as prosthesis, are fit for use, i.e. are safe and perform to the standard expected. They monitor all medical devices and communicate across healthcare settings any raised concerns regarding devices and suggest action.

The MHRA work closely with the NICE to ensure that best practice, clinical effectiveness and is incorporated into the clinical area when deciding appropriate selection of prosthesis.

Prosthesis can be made of a variety of materials depending on:
- Anticipated usage after implantation: e.g. a young patient receiving a joint replacement would be expected to live longer than the average lifespan of the conventional primary joint prosthesis.
- Site of placement: e.g. replicate action of natural tissue such as a breast implant. Actions of surrounding tissues or chemical e.g. dental implants need to withstand chemical reactions within the mouth.
- Majority of prosthesis are now made of man-made materials such as metallic alloys, ultra-high molecular weight polyethylene (UHMWPE) and ceramics for joint replacements; expanded polytetrafluoroethylene (ePTFE), Dacron®, and polyurethane (PU) for arterial grafts. Although pig valves and human donor grafts have been used for heart valve replacements.

Patients undergoing prosthetic surgery are considered to be at high risk of infection. Therefore certain precautions have been advocated:
- Prophylactic antibiotics.
- Laminar (ultra clean) theatre with high efficiency particulate air (HEPA) filters.
- Instrumentation and 'scrubbed staff' within the laminar flow.
- Minimal movement of staff during surgery.
- Minimal unnecessary conversation during surgery.

Further reading

British Orthopaedic Association (2006). *Primary total hip replacement; A guide to good practice.* British Orthopedic Association: London.

Hampson FG and Ridgway EJ (2005). Prophylactic antibiotics in surgery. *Surgery (Oxford)* **23**(8), 290–3.

Knobben BAS, van Horn JR, van de Mei, HC, et al. (2006). Evaluation of measures to decrease intra-operative bacterial contamination in orthopaedic implant surgery. *Journal of Hospital Infection* **62**, 174–80.

NHS Estates (1994). *Health Technical Memorandum 2025. Ventilation in healthcare premises. Validation and verification.* NHS Estates: London.

Electro-surgical equipment

Diathermy is the use of high frequency electrical current (300kHz to 3MHz) to produce heat. This heat is used in the surgical field to cut or destroy tissues. It can also be used to coagulate bleeding vessels. Due to its high frequency diathermy does not activate nerves and muscles.

Diathermy can be defined as either *bi-polar* or *mono-polar*. Because the diathermy is an electrical system, it needs to complete a circuit to be effective.

Bi-polar diathermy

This is when the two electrodes within the surgical instrument (e.g. forceps) combine. The current passes between the tips of the instrument coagulating the vessels in between and not through the patient; this then completes the circuit. Bipolar diathermy is often used when coagulation only is required as cutting can not take place. It is also used when very precise or "micro-coagulation" is required. It is suggested to be safer for the patient as the electrical pathway is much shorter.

Mono-polar diathermy

This uses a 'grounding plate' to complete the circuit. This plate or pad is applied to the patient and is known as the return or indifferent electrode. Temperature rises at the active electrode (surgical instrument) whenever there is resistance to the flow of currant. This rise in temperature is used to produce the cutting and coagulation effects. Because the indifferent electrode has a significantly larger surface area with much less resistance, the heat is localised at the instrument tip and not at the plate.

Diathermy plate (grounding plate)
- Ensure plate is placed away from:
  - Implants.
  - Scars.
  - Bony prominences.
- Ensure good contact with skin:
  - Remove hair.
  - Avoid spirit based prep near application site.
  - Avoid creases—skin and plate.

Diathermy effects
The effects of the diathermy depend on the current intensity and wave form supplied by the diathermy machine (generator).

Coagulation

The COAG waveform is produced using short blasts (between 50–100 a second) of low frequency waveforms this enables slow drying and coagulation of vessels.

Cutting

Cutting is achieved though the application of the CUT waveform which generates a continuous current with a sinus waveform at a lower voltage but higher current than COAG. Cell explosion occurs due to the intense heat within the localised area, producing a cutting effect.

Complications
- Can interfere with pacemaker function.
- Electrical burns or tissue damage from arcing with surgical instruments and implants.
- Burns under grounding plate if not applied correctly.
- Insulation failure surrounding instrument can cause damage user or surrounding tissues.

Harmonic scalpel

Used for cutting soft tissue and coagulating blood vessels through ultrasound vibration, therefore keeping thermal injury to a minimum. The harmonic scalpel can be used in addition to, or as a direct replacement for, electrosurgery, standard scalpel, and lasers. Electrical energy produced by the harmonic scalpel generator is converted to a mechanical motion in a dedicated handpiece. The hand piece has a blade tip which moves longitudinally at >55 000 cycles a second. This movement produces enough heat to cause the tissue proteins to change in molecular structure producing a coagulum. Coagulation occurs when pressure is exerted upon the tissues between the two tips of the handpiece allowing the coagulum to produce haemostasis. The surgeon can also cut tissues by using different levels of tip pressure, tissue traction, and power levels.

Advantages
- No electrical stimulus to patient.
- Minimal smoke produced, better surgical view.
- Reduces need for ties due to cutting and coagulation effect.
- Lower temperature coagulation: no charring of tissues.

Operating microscopes

Microscopes are used in several surgical specialties including:

- Ophthalmology.
- ENT.
- Neurosurgery.
- Microvascular surgery.

They may be either fixed to the wall or ceiling of an operating theatre, or freestanding so that they can be moved into the theatre when required. Theatre staff need to have an understanding of the use and care of these expensive and complex pieces of theatre equipment and the accessories that accompany them.

It is useful if practitioners who work in specialties that use microscopes understand some of the basic principles of the optics. Microscopes used in surgery are stereoscopic, which facilitates adjustment of the level of magnification. The objective lens is fitted to the bottom of the microscope and the focal length will be determined by the objective length of the lens. Typically a 400mm lens will common in neurosurgery while ophthalmology may require a 175 or 200mm lens. The microscope should be wiped over with a mild detergent solution before and after use and then the optics polished with a soft lens cloth prior to storage. The lens and eyepieces should be inspected for any damaged at this juncture while the light should also be tested prior to use. A spare bulb should be kept and practitioners should be aware how to replace a bulb that has blown. The protective cover is then put over the microscope and it is stored away from traffic and free from dust.

Some centres utilise a sterile polythene drape to cover the microscope for specialities such as ENT and neurosurgery while ophthalmology may use sterilised covers which go over the control knobs. It is important that practitioners are conversant with how to prepare the microscope in the manner appropriate for the type of surgery to be undertaken.

Further reading

Phillips N (2007). *Berry and Kohn's Operating Room Technique* (11th edn). Mosby: St Louis, MO.

Tourniquets

Indications

Tourniquets are used in surgical contexts for 2 reasons:

- Optimising the surgeon's view of the site through the provision of a bloodless operating field achieved by the temporary arrest of circulation of blood distal to the point of application.
- To administer regional anaesthesia to a limb while preventing the local anaesthetic agent entering the general circulation—Bier's block.

Equipment

- Modern tourniquets consist of an inflatable cuff, a source of compressed air or O_2, and a device to select, control, and maintain the pressure to which the cuff is inflated.
- Other types apply the principle of securing a piece of fabric around the limb and have the disadvantage that there is no way of knowing the pressure to which the soft tissues are subjected.
- Tourniquets are manufactured in a range of shapes and sizes to meet a range of applications. It is becoming more commonplace to use disposable cuffs in more recent times.

Preparation and application

Protection of the patient's soft tissue requires application of both skill and knowledge; practitioners who lack the appropriate level of proficiency should not use tourniquets:

- The skin under the tourniquet should be clean and dry.
- The entire circumference of the limb should be covered with lint-free padding to prevent damage from pinching and shearing forces.
- The ends of the tourniquet bladder should overlap by >7cm and <15cm.
- If the limb is tapered due to musculature or obesity a contoured cuff should be used, ensuring adequate skin contact and preventing slippage and shearing forces.
- To prevent maceration and/or chemical burns, accumulation of fluids between skin and tourniquet should be prevented using an occlusive drape.
- The occlusion pressure is usually estimated to be between 30–70mmHg above systolic BP and varies with patient's age and the depth of soft tissue covering the humerus/femur.
- Irreversible damage to nerve and muscle tissue can occur after as little as 60 minutes of ischaemia; 90 minutes is considered the upper limit for tourniquet inflation time.

Exsanguination

Preoperative exsanguination is required to prevent venous thrombosis; there are three recognised methods of exsanguination:

- The optimal method is the application of a Rhys-Davis exsanguinator.
- A secondary option is the tubular application of an Eschmarsh's bandage or other elastic bandage to the level of the tourniquet with 2.5cm overlap on each turn.
- The least satisfactory method is elevation.

Contra-indications

Tourniquets should not be applied to a limb if:
- The patient has a history of peripheral vascular disease.
- The limb is the site of an arteriovenous fistula for dialysis.
- There is an infected lesion of the soft tissue or bone of the limb.

Aftercare

Before deflating the tourniquet consider:
- The anaesthetist should be aware that circulation is about to be restored to the limb.
- The stage of wound closure.
- Regular and frequent documentation of the limb's neurovascular status.

Documentation

The following items should be documented in the patient's record when a tourniquet has been used:
- Site of application.
- Duration of inflation.
- Inflation pressure.
- Condition of the skin before and after inflation.

Maintenance

- Tourniquets should be clean, dry, and checked regularly for cracks or breaks in the outer fabric, and to ensure that the pneumatic bladder, hoses, and joints/connectors do not leak.
- Pneumatic regulators should be calibrated according to the manufacturer's instructions.
- Disposable cuffs must not be re-used.

Further reading

Association for Perioperative Practice (2007). *Standards and Recommendations for Safe Perioperative Practice* (2nd edn). AfPP: Harrogate.

Fortunato N (2003). *Operating Room Technique* (10th edn). Mosby: St Louis, MO.

Groah LK (1996). *Perioperative Nursing*. Appleton & Lange: London.

Use of lasers in surgery

The word 'laser' is an acronym for light amplification by stimulated emission of radiation.

Laser light is an intense narrow beam of light and can be used to vaporise tissue while at the same time sealing small blood vessels and causing minimal damage to surrounding tissues.

Properties of laser light

- Single colour (monochromatic) in a single wavelength. *Ordinary, or white light, is a mixture of all colours.*
- Laser light is very straight in a parallel beam. *Ordinary light spreads out in all directions.*
- Laser light is coherent—the waves all run together in phase. *Ordinary light is incoherent—the waves are all mixed up.*
- Laser light can be concentrated with a lens into a tiny intense spot to cut, coagulate or vaporise tissue. *Ordinary light cannot be concentrated in this way.*

Types of laser

The colour/wavelength of the light is chosen for absorption of the laser by different tissues in the body.

The colour of the laser is determined by the medium used to generate the radiation. Common types include:

- CO_2: infrared light.
- Argon: blue or green light.
- Nd YAG: infrared.
- Others—excimer lasers may be argon, krypton, or xenon fluoride and produce ultraviolet pulses used for correcting eye sight.

Classification of lasers

Ranges from class 1 to class 4. The classification is determined by the potential of damage to the eye caused by the laser, class 1 being the least and class 4 the most hazardous. Class 4 lasers are the ones most usually used in surgery.

Hazards

Effects on the eye

Depend on the wavelength of the light:

- Corneal burns leading to clouding of the cornea.
- Keratitis on the surface of the cornea.
- Retinal damage leading to blind spots.

Effects on the skin

A burn is the main hazard:

- Scarring and possible loss of sensation to touch may occur after healing.
- The reflex action of withdrawing from the pain may limit the damage. Anaesthetised patients will not have this reflex.
- Long-term exposure to ultraviolet lasers may result in pigmentation changes and skin cancer.

Incidental hazards

- Fire: the beam of a surgical laser is a fire risk if it comes into direct contact with surgical drapes and gowns or flammable skin preparations.
- Reflection of the laser beam from shiny surfaces: e.g. stainless steel trolleys
- Laser plume: the smoke generated during vaporisation of tissue may contain potentially hazardous substances including toxic chemicals, carbonised tissue, and viral DNA.

Safety considerations

- Legislation, standards, and guidance govern the safe use of lasers.
- Laser equipment has to have a number of inbuilt safety features including:
  - An audible or visible alarm when the device is being fired.
  - Covered foot pedals to prevent accidental firing.
  - A removable key to prevent inappropriate use.
- *Local rules* must be in place wherever lasers are used and include:
  - A safe system of work for operating the laser.
  - A list of trained, authorised users.
  - The procedure to follow in case of an emergency.
- A *Laser Protection Supervisor* ensures that the laser is used according to the local rules and usually holds the laser key.
- The *laser controlled area* is the room or area where safety precautions specific to that laser apply and may include:
  - Restricted access which may involve the locking of theatre doors.
  - Use of appropriate warning signs.
  - Window blinds or shields.
  - Protective eyewear for staff.

Preparation of the recovery room

Preparing the recovery room

Even in major hospitals the majority of recovery's workload will come from routine elective lists during normal operating hours. Adequate preparation for this work is essential to ensure the unit is prepared to deal with the patients through the day and to have equipment and supplies on hand to cope with any unforeseen incidents. The type of equipment and supplies required will depend on the size of the unit, the type of surgery (elective or elective and trauma/emergency), and the type of patient cared for in recovery e.g., if ventilated high dependency patients are nursed in recovery or admitted directly to an ITU or HDU.

Daily

In each recovery room there will be emergency equipment which will only be used infrequently during critical incidents and emergency situations. This equipment must be checked on a daily basis to ensure it is fully operational, that all required supplies are present and that expiry dates have not passed. All checks must be documented and there should be a system of audit to ensure that regular checks are carried out to the required standard.

- Check resuscitation trolley (adults and children) and defibrillator.
- Restock drug cupboard and check for expired drugs.
- Check emergency drugs are correct and in date.
- Check anaesthetic machine.
- Check all monitoring equipment.

The Resuscitation Council (UK)[1,2] guidelines specify the minimum requirements for equipment, the drugs required, and recommendations for determining specific requirements based on the dynamics of the unit.

The anaesthetic machine and all monitoring should be checked according to the manufacturers' specifications and according to AAGBI guidelines.[3] Alarms should be audible and parameters set according to unit policy.

Between patients

Checking and cleaning each individual bay prior to the day's lists commencing and between each patient is essential to maintaining safety prior to accepting the next patient. Throughout the day the bays should be restocked to replenish anything used for the previous patient.

- O_2 and tubing.
- Suction and tubing.
- Oral and nasal airways.
- 'T' pieces or 'T' bags.
- Ambu bag or water circuit available with facemask and tubing.
- Check emergency bell at each bay.
- Empty sharps and rubbish containers.

Ongoing

Other equipment will be used on a daily basis but not necessarily for every patient. It should be checked and stocked at the beginning of each day and checked and replenished throughout the day following each use.

- Ensure adequate stock of gloves, fluids, giving sets, syringes, needles, dressing supplies etc.

- Ensure adequate supply of blankets and gowns.
- Ensure patient warming system available.
- Ensure adequate supply of drip stands.

References

1. Resuscitation Council (UK) (2004). *Recommended minimum equipment for in hospital adult resuscitation.* UK Resuscitation Council: London.

2. Resuscitation Council (UK) (2003). *Suggested equipment for the management of paediatric cardiopulmonary arrest.* UK Resuscitation Council: London.

3. Association of Anaesthetists of Great Britain and Ireland (2004). *Checking anaesthetic equipment.* AAGBI: London.

Further reading

American Society of PeriAnesthesia Nurses (2006). *Standards of perianesthesia nursing practice.* ASPAN: Cherry Hill, NJ.

Association of Anaesthetists of Great Britain and Ireland (2002). *Immediate post anaesthetic recovery.* AAGBI: London.

Association of Anaesthetists of Great Britain and Ireland (2007). *Recommendations for standards of monitoring during anaesthesia and recovery* (4th edn). AAGBI: London.

Royal College of Anaesthetists (2004). Guidelines for the provision of anaesthetic services for post operative care. RCoA: London.

Royal College of Anaesthetists (2006). *Raising the standard.* RCoA: London.

Recovery personnel

- The provision of care by nurses/ODPs with expertise and experience in the recovery environment is essential.
- Staffing levels should reflect the number of patients on theatre lists.
- An unconscious patient should receive 1:1 nursing care until consciousness is regained and the patient is able to maintain their own airway.

Role of the recovery nurse

The role of the nurse in recovery is to:
- Provide care to the patient in the immediate post-anaesthesia period.
- To assist the patient through emergence from anaesthesia and the postoperative effects of surgery by assessment of their condition.
- Implement nursing interventions to promote recovery and prevent complications of anaesthesia and surgery.

Nurses should have a good understanding of anatomy, physiology, and pharmacology related to anaesthesia and surgery.

Specific skills are required in caring for the unconscious and intubated patient with particular emphasis on airway management and, in some cases, extubation.

Recovery nursing staff should be certified to immediate life support standards as set by the Resuscitation Council (UK).[1]

Priorities for the recovery room nurse include:
- Airway management and difficult airway management.
- Pain management.
- Thermoregulation.
- Control of nausea and vomiting.
- Haemodynamic management.

Care of patients during the post-operative phase also involves caring for medical patients and caring for children and their family. Box 20.1 identifies additional knowledge and skills required of recovery personnel.

Box 20.1 Knowledge and skills required of recovery personnel

Skills
- Excellent interpersonal skills including verbal and non-verbal communication skills.
- Inter-disciplinary teamwork.
- Care of catheters, drains, CVP lines, epidural catheters, arterial lines, and peripheral lines.
- Post-anaesthesia care in a range of surgical specialties.
- Caring for ventilated patient.
- Perioperative teaching and information giving.

Knowledge
- Principles and practices of anaesthesia.
- Pharmacodynamics.
- Pharmacokinetics.
- Principles and practice of cross-infection.
- Evidence-based practice.

Reference

1. Resuscitation Council (UK). Immediate Life Support-General Information. ⌨ www.resus.org. uk/pages/i/sger.htm

Layout of recovery

The recovery period is a critical and potentially vulnerable time for patients.

Location

The recovery room should be situated in close proximity to theatre to enable fast contact with medical personnel when needed.

Observation

- Due to the rapid patient turnover the recovery room should provide an open area to enable constant observation of all patients.
- Ideally the layout should be such that all bays are visible from all points within the room, unhindered by equipment, cupboards, etc.

Size of unit

- There should be two bays for every functioning operating theatre.
- Consideration should be given to the number of theatres and the type of cases/specialties undertaken when deciding on number of bays, e.g. major cases will have a different impact on the recovery room from minor and/or quick turnover lists and will impact on the space required to service these lists.
- The room should provide sufficient space per patient bay for all necessary equipment.
- Space between bays should provide for patient privacy.
- Adequate space between patient bays is also essential in preventing infection between patients.
- The space between bays should also allow for other equipment as necessary such as ventilators, x-ray machines resuscitation equipment, etc.

Equipment

- All bays should have facilities to provide immediate access to all necessary equipment e.g. airways, suction catheters, syringes, dressings, etc.
- All bays must have piped O_2 and suction available.
- Adequate hand-washing facilities must be available and within easy reach of recovery bays.
- An emergency call system must be in place and available from all recovery bays.
- Emergency equipment should be centrally located and easily accessible when required.

Storage

- Adequate, clean storage space should be available for supplies that will be used frequently and need stocking up at individual bays.
- Storage areas for less frequently used equipment/supplies should be close by or readily available when necessary.
- Dirty utility areas should be available within the recovery room for the disposal of soiled and/or contaminated linen and waste.

Purpose

- Preoperative patients should be separated from and cared for in a different area from post operative patients at all times.
- If children are cared for there should be an area designated for this purpose, where practicable, preferably away from adult patients.

References

American Society of Perianesthesia Nurses (2006). *Standards of perianesthesia nursing practice*, ASPAN: Cherry Hill, NJ.

Association of Anaesthetists of Great Britain and Ireland (2002). *Immediate post anaesthetic recovery*. AAGBI: London.

Monitoring equipment in recovery

The AAGBI[1] state the minimum monitoring requirements for patients in recovery are:
• Pulse oximeter.
• Non-invasive BP.

They further state that the following must be immediately available:[2]
• Electrocardiograph.
• Nerve stimulator.
• A means of measuring temperature.
• Capnograph.

In addition to this minimum monitoring equipment the following equipment will also be utilised and should be available as and when required.
• **Suction:** suction could be seen as the most essential equipment in the recovery room. Airway maintenance is the main priority for recovery staff and the ability to clear an airway to maintain its patency is vital.
• **Resuscitation equipment:** the Resuscitation Council (UK) guidelines[3,4] minimum requirements are for airway management equipment, defibrillation equipment, and emergency drugs. Recovery staff should ensure they are familiar with the operation of this equipment and the action of drugs on an ongoing basis as they will be used infrequently but when required must be used correctly and with confidence.
• **Glucose meters:** due to the nature of preoperative preparation (e.g. fasting) and the effects of anaesthesia and surgical procedures, hypoglycaemic episodes may be seen frequently in recovery in all patients, not just diabetics. Recovery staff should be vigilant to monitor for the signs and symptoms of low blood sugar and ensure proficiency in using glucose monitoring equipment.
• **Infusion pumps and syringe drivers:** many postoperative patients will require IV fluids to replace fluid lost during surgery, or have drug infusions commenced for medical conditions pre-existing or intraoperative, or patients may have local analgesia infiltration. Patients should be monitored for the underlying condition in addition to the pumps/drivers to ensure correct infusion rate.
• **PCA pumps:** PCA may be initiated based on preoperative assessment/ surgical procedure or in response to postoperative pain. Adequate pain assessment to identify required analgesia measures and knowledge of the function and effects of PCA pumps is required. Prompt assessment and monitoring following initiation of PCA to ensure efficacy and prevent side effects should be maintained.
• **Epidural pumps:** epidural infusions are frequently used for postoperative analgesia via continuous infusion. The patient should be continually monitored for adequate analgesia and for the development of side effects, e.g. hypotension, bladder distention, ascending block, etc. The pump also needs frequent monitoring to ensure correct infusion rate, and that volume infused equals that expected.
• **Warming blankets:** the perioperative experience (surgical preparation/ procedure, anaesthesia, environmental factors) all contribute to hypothermia in postoperative patients. Adequate monitoring and

prompt intervention to address lowered temperature is essential. Continual monitoring particularly with forced air rewarming blankets is vital to prevent over-warming and burns.
- *X-rays:* many surgical and anaesthetic procedures require check x-rays postoperatively e.g. orthopaedic surgery or following CVP insertion. Staff in the recovery room must be aware of procedures which require this and signs of complications e.g. pneumothorax.

References

1. Association of Anaesthetists of Great Britain and Ireland (2007). *Recommendations for standards of monitoring during anaesthesia and recovery.* AAGBI: London.

2. Association of Anaesthetists of Great Britain and Ireland (2004). *Checking anaesthetic equipment.* AAGBI: London.

3. Resuscitation Council (UK) (2003). *Suggested equipment for the management of paediatric cardiopulmonary arrest.* Resuscitation Council: London.

4. Resuscitation Council (UK) (2004). *Recommended minimum equipment for in hospital adult resuscitation.* Resuscitation Council: London.

Postoperative care

Caring for the post-anaesthesia patient

Transport to recovery

Before transferring the patient to recovery, it should be confirmed that staff are available to receive the patient.

- Consider that the patient may be starting to regain consciousness and therefore orientation will be required.
- Explain briefly that surgery is complete and that he/she is about to be transferred to the recovery room.
- It is essential that the anaesthetist accompanies the patient to the recovery room, assisted by another member of the theatre team.
- The anaesthetist must remain at the head end of the bed or theatre trolley so that he/she can observe the patient during transfer.
- O_2 will be administered to all patients who have had a general anaesthetic.
- The bed/theatre trolley should therefore be equipped with portable O_2 and a mask and breathing circuit.

Patient safety is of paramount importance during transfer.

- Trolley sides should be in the upright position to prevent falls.
- For paediatric or restless patients, it is advisable to cover the trolley sides with protective padding to prevent injury.
- Particular care must also be taken to ensure support equipment e.g. infusions, drains, catheters, etc. remain in situ.

The anaesthetist should decide upon the need for monitoring during transfer.

- Consideration will be given to stability of the patient and proximity of the recovery room to theatre.
- AAGBI guidelines[1] advise that a short interruption of monitoring is only acceptable if the recovery room is adjacent to the theatre.

On arrival in the recovery room, the anaesthetist must provide a comprehensive handover to a qualified theatre practitioner.

Reference

1. Association of Anaesthetists of Great Britain and Ireland (2007). *Standards of Monitoring During Anaesthetics and Recovery.* AAGBI: London.

Further reading

Association of Anaesthetists of Great Britain and Ireland (2002). *Immediate Post Anaesthetic Care.* AAGBI: London.

Patient handover in recovery

The transfer of the patient from theatre to recovery is a crucial event requiring effective communication, both written and verbally.

It is essential that a formal handover of patient care, both from the anaesthetist and theatre nurse, is routinely given for every patient. This will aid continuity of care and minimise the risk of omissions.

All relevant details must be verbally communicated and the following points are indicative of the minimum information required. The anaesthetist should always accompany the patient to recovery and provide handover to a trained member of staff.[1]

Handover from anaesthetist should include:

- Patient's names and age.
- Pre-existing medical conditions.
- Allergies.
- Procedure performed.
- Type of anaesthetic.
- Perioperative vital signs/events/incidents.
- Fluid balance—urine output/blood loss/IV fluids administered and prescribed.
- Drugs and analgesia—administered and prescribed.
- Postoperative instructions.
- Confirmation that a throat pack has been removed, if applicable.
- Patient monitoring required.
- Patient positioning.
- Investigations required e.g. blood tests, chest x-ray.
- Specific patient information e.g. communication needs.
- Where he/she will be if needed.
- Physiological parameters required prior to discharge.
- Anaesthetist to review patient prior to discharge to ward.
- In some units practitioners discharge patients to the wards.

In addition to providing this information, all documentation, including the anaesthetic, prescription, and IV fluid prescription charts must be handed to the recovery nurse/ODP.

Handover from theatre nurse/ODP should include:

- Patient details should be confirmed.
- Procedure performed.
- Confirmation that a throat pack has been removed if applicable.
- Sutures/clips.
- Infiltration of local anaesthetic.
- Dressings—location, type, amount.
- Drains.
- Presence of stoma/catheter.
- Intraoperative events/incidents.

- Amount of blood loss.
- Specific postoperative instructions.
- Patient positioning.
- Skin condition.

The theatre nurse/practitioner should ensure all documentation has been completed and is handed to the Recovery practitioner, along with medical notes, charts, and x-rays.

Reference

1. National Association of Theatre Nurses (2005). *Standards and Recommendations of Safe Perioperative Practice*. NATN: Harrogate.

Further reading

Hatfield A and Tronson M (2008). *The Complete Recovery Room Book* (4th edn). Oxford University Press: Oxford.

Patient assessment in recovery

When there is a patient in recovery who does not meet the discharge criteria, there must be at least two members of staff present.[1]

Remember to follow and correct A B C before proceeding to D E F!

Airway

- Is it clear? Obstruction may be partial or total.
- Noisy breathing indicates obstruction but remember total obstruction may be silent—rapid assessment is essential.
- Head tilt, chin lift to clear airway.
- Gentle suction may be required to remove secretions.
- Consider use of oral/nasal pharyngeal airway.
- Administer O_2 to all patients in recovery.
- Assess patient's level of consciousness.

Breathing

- *Look*: Is the O_2 mask misting? Is the patient's chest rising and falling?
- Observe depth and record rate of respirations—slow/shallow respirations may not provide sufficient oxygenation.
- Observe skin colour for pallor/cyanosis.
- Monitor and record O_2 saturation rate.
- *Listen*: gurgling? Wheezing? Stridor? *Reassess airway*.
- *Feel*: place hand near patient's mouth to feel breath.

Circulation

- Palpate pulse, noting volume and regularity.
- Record BP. Report hypo/hypertension to anaesthetist.
- ECG monitor—record HR and rhythm.
- Maintain circulating volume—administer IV fluids as prescribed.
- Check wound dressing and drainage.

It is essential that any problems identified are rectified immediately. Always ask for help if required.

Drugs

- Note drugs given in theatre and observe for side effects.
- Discuss analgesia prescribed with anaesthetist—what can be given and when?
- Assess site and severity of pain—administer analgesia and observe patient for side effects e.g. respiratory depression.
- Consider patients pre-existing conditions—may need medication or additional monitoring e.g. blood glucose recording.

Elimination

- Urine output—should exceed 1ml/kg/hour.[2]
- Record type and amount of vomit—administer anti-emetics as prescribed.
- Record type and amount of NG tube drainage/aspirate.
- Record type and amount of wound drainage.

Further care

- Reassure and orientate patient.
- Observations specific to surgical procedure.
- Record patient's temperature—consider use of warming interventions.
- Ensure patient's skin is clean and dry, document condition of pressure areas.
- Offer patient oral hygiene.
- Replace personal items e.g. dentures, hearing aid, spectacles, if appropriate to do so.
- Ensure all patient's property is returned.

It is crucial that the written documentation provides a concise, accurate account of the patient's postoperative period.

References

1. Association of Anaesthetists of Great Britain and Ireland (2002). *Immediate Post Anaesthetic Care*. AAGBI: London.

2. Hatfield A and Tronson M (2008). *The Complete Recovery Room Book* (4th edn). Oxford University Press: Oxford.

Neuromuscular junction blockade

Definition

A muscle relaxant (or neuromuscular junction blocker) is a drug that acts at the neuromuscular junction and causes paralysis of skeletal muscle through blocking the effects of acetylcholine by binding to its receptor sites.

Uses

Muscle relaxants are used to:[1]
- Facilitate intubation.
- Relax the diaphragm and skeletal muscle in the abdomen, to negate the need to use deep anaesthesia for muscle relaxation.
- Facilitate ventilation of patients in intensive care.
- Prevent injury to the patient during electroconvulsive therapy.

Classes of muscle relaxant

There are two main classes of muscle relaxants:
- Depolarising.
- Non-depolarising—also known as competitive.

Depolarising muscle relaxants

Suxamethonium (succinylcholine):
- Is the only depolarising muscle relaxant in current use.
- Acts like acetylcholine but is broken down much more slowly.
- Binds to the acetylcholine receptor sites and causes an action potential (seen as muscle twitches) followed by extended depolarisation and flaccid paralysis.
- Is broken down by plasma cholinesterases.
- Has a rapid onset of action and a short duration of action (approximately 2–6 minutes).[2]
- Allows rapid tracheal intubation—useful to prevent aspiration of stomach contents.
- Cannot be reversed.
- Normal dose is 1mg/kg (adult) by IV injection.[2]
- Can be administered by IV infusion for a prolonged effect.

Suxamethonium can be responsible for the development of malignant hyperpyrexia

Should be used with caution in patients who are deficient of plasma cholinesterase as this can lead to prolonged apnoea—check family history.[1]

Non-depolarising muscle relaxants

Two main classes: *benzylisoquoliniums*, includes atracurium, cis-atracurium, gallamine, and mivacurium (can promote histamine release- except cis-atracurium); and *aminosteroids*, includes vecuronium, rocuronium, and pancuronium.[2]

Non-depolarising muscle relaxants:
- Work by competing with acetylcholine at the neuromuscular junction preventing depolarisation.
- Are administered by IV injection/IV infusion.

- Many are excreted unchanged (atracurium and cisatracturium break down spontaneously—useful in renal failure) in urine.
- Are further classified by duration of action:
  - Short-acting 15–30 minutes—mivacurium.
  - Intermediate-acting 30–40 minutes—atracurium, rocuronium, vecuronium, cisatracurium.
  - Long-acting 60–120 minutes—pancuronium.
- Can be reversed by anticholinesterases e.g. neostigmine (dose 50–70 mcg/kg with 0.6–1.2 mg atropine sulphate).[2]

Cautions and care of patients receiving muscle relaxants

- Trained staff must be available to care for patients who have received a muscle relaxant at all times.
- Following administration of muscle relaxants, patients must be intubated with an ET tube and supported with mechanical ventilation; alternatively, some anaesthetists may ventilate patients with an LMA
- Disconnection alarms must be active.
- The patient must be closely monitored—haemodynamically and with pulse oximetry.
- The patient must not be consciously aware, therefore adequate sedation and analgesia must be administered.
- Protective reflexes are absent—beware corneal abrasions, no gag reflex, brachial plexus injuries.

References

1. Howland RD and Mycek MJ (2006). *Lippincott's Illustrated Reviews: Pharmacology* (3rd edn). Lippincott, Williams and Wilkins: Philadelphia, PA.

2. British Medical Association and The Royal Pharmaceutical Society (2007). *British National Formulary 52 September 2007*. BMJ Publishing and RPS Publishing: London.

Intubated/ventilated patients in recovery

Unwanted demands are sometimes placed on a general recovery unit to provide postoperative ventilation. Aps has often emphasised the concern of recovery practitioners who feel they must care for ventilated patients or to deal with overflows of patients from the ITU into their general recovery wards, without them having the skills to achieve this. He has also argued that such practice within a recovery unit that is not adequately and properly developed, staffed, and supported does not allow for the safe conduct of postoperative critical care.[1]

The following assessment should be made before accepting a ventilated patient to the recovery room:
- Assess the skill mix.
- Assess the workload.
- Assess progress of operating theatre lists, if appropriate.

The recovery room should be equipped with the necessary skills and equipment.
- Appropriate equipment necessary for emergency resuscitation and intubation should already be in place within recovery units.
- Additional equipment for artificial ventilation should be easily available.
- Artificial ventilators, CPAP circuits, invasive monitoring, syringe drivers.
- Recovery practitioners should be appropriately qualified (some with a critical care qualification), experienced, and competent to care for ventilated patients in recovery.
- The standard of nursing and medical care should be equal to that within the ITU.[2]
- Consideration should be given to a temporary swap in working environments where an ITU nurse will care for the patient and a recovery practitioner will work in ITU so their staff numbers are not depleted.
- Consideration should also be given to recovery practitioners undertaking an anaesthetic qualification and gaining experience in caring for the perianaesthesia patient.
- A 1:1 patient: practitioner ratio, as for any ventilated patient, is required with the possible attendance of an anaesthetist and/or anaesthetic practitioner at all times.
- Ventilated patients admitted to the recovery room should remain there for a short period only.
- Patients who are expected to require complex or prolonged critical care should be admitted directly to ITU.
- A good working relationship with the ITU is essential.

Possible reasons for admitting intubated patients to recovery might include:
- Prolonged surgical procedure.
- Hypothermia.
- Respiratory compromise.
- Older patients.
- Poor response to reversal agents of muscle relaxant drugs.

On some occasions it might be necessary to extubate patients in recovery. The patient criteria for extubation in recovery should conform to local policy and may include the following:[3]

- The patient should be able to breathe spontaneously and adequately and able to protect own airway against aspiration.
- There should be minimal signs of respiratory depression.

Extubation in recovery

- Extubating patients in the recovery room is the responsibility of the anaesthetist.[2]
- This should be performed by an anaesthetist or suitably trained perioperative practitioner and assisted by an anaesthetic practitioner and/or experienced recovery practitioner.
- Adhere to recommended guidelines and local policy.
- Ensure relevant equipment is available, to re-intubate if necessary.
- Monitor vital signs and pre-oxygenate patient for 3 minutes.
- Ensure working suction is available to remove excess secretions and/or blood.
- Place patient in left lateral position.
- Deflate cuff slowly—in some instances it may be necessary to pass a suction catheter down the ET tube.
- The patient should be encouraged to take a deep breath and whilst applying suction, the anaesthetist can then remove the catheter and ET tube together.
- Give O_2 therapy via mask and encourage patient to continue to take deep breaths and cough.
- Closely monitor vital signs, especially respiratory rate and O_2 saturation levels; patient's colour and observe for signs of hypoxia or hypercarbia.[3]

References

1. Aps C (2004). [Editorial III] Surgical critical care: the Overnight Intensive Recovery (OIR) concept. *British Journal of Anaesthesia* **92**(2), 164–6.

2. Association of Anaesthetists of Great Britain and Ireland (2002). *Immediate post-anaesthetic recovery.* AAGBI: London.

3. Hatfield A and Tronson M (2008). *The Complete Recovery Room Book* (4th edn). Oxford University Press: Oxford.

Caring for patients following spinal and epidural anaesthesia

Patients in the post-anaesthetic care unit may have had their surgery under spinal or epidural anaesthesia, or they may have had an epidural inserted for postoperative pain relief alongside a general anaesthetic or sedation. A combination of local anaesthetics and opioids are used.

Patient assessment and monitoring

Initial assessment of all patients should be the same as for those having general anaesthesia. Monitoring should be include heart rate, respiratory rate, O_2 saturation, and BP.

Specific considerations:
- Ensure the patient remains flat with only one pillow until sensation returns.
- Take care of anaesthetised limbs, ensure they are in alignment and perform passive limb exercises to help prevent DVT.
- Check the injection site for signs of haematoma and leakage.
- Ensure adequate analgesia given at the first complaint of pain as the effects of the spinal block wears off.
- Make sure the patient is warm and comfortable.
- Observe pressure areas and relieve pressure at vulnerable points, e.g., heels and sacrum.
- Reassure the patient that sensation will return.
- Advise the patient not to try and get out of bed without assistance.

If an epidural infusion is in place or is to be commenced:
- Ensure a test dose has been given.
- Check the dressing site for leaks and ensure the catheter is not kinked.
- Check the level of the block by asking the patient to move each of their limbs to demonstrate motor function.
- Check effectiveness of epidural analgesia and if necessary request top up bolus doses. If the epidural is not effective consider other forms of analgesia.
- If PCEA in place:
  - Explain to patient.
  - Observe and check the pump.
  - Record amounts used.

Potential problems

Hypotension
- Close observation of BP.
- Ensure IV fluids are administered

High level of block
- Assess for any weakness in arms.
- Assess for difficulty in breathing.

Respiratory depression
- Observe the respiratory rate carefully.
- Turn off epidural infusion.

- Give O_2 therapy.
- Consider administering naloxone.
- Call anaesthetist for advice.

Local anaesthetic toxicity

Toxic reactions occur when the concentration of the drug present in the circulation exceeds certain limits either due to incorrect dosage or too rapid uptake into the circulation. In a mild toxic reaction, the patient becomes pale and restless and may feel dizzy and have a tingling sensation of the mouth. In a severe reaction, convulsions followed by cardiorespiratory arrest can occur.

If there is any suspicion of a reaction then:
- Stop any local anaesthetic infusion.
- Call the anaesthetist.

Urinary retention

This may be painless due to the effects of the spinal/epidural.
- Monitor urine output.
- Observe abdomen for signs of distension.
- If there is retention a catheter may be required.

Post-spinal headache:

This may be caused following post-dural puncture. If this occurs:
- Lie the patient flat.
- Maintain IV fluids.
- Give paracetamol.
- Seek advice from the pain team.

Discharge from recovery with epidural infusion in progress

Ideally the patient with an epidural should be nursed in HDU/ITU. If the patient is to return to the ward they should only be discharged from recovery if there are appropriately trained practitioners available to care for them and also when:
- Analgesia is adequate.
- There are no serious side effects noted.
- Cardiovascular system is stable.
- Prescriptions are written for an opioid antagonist e.g. naloxone, antiemetic, O_2, and IV fluids.

References and further reading

Association of Anaesthetists of Great Britain and Ireland (2002). *Immediate post-anaesthetic recovery*. AAGBI: London.

Hatfield A and Tronson M (2008). *The Complete Recovery Room Book* (4th edn). Oxford University Press: Oxford.

Caring for children and parents in the recovery room

Children have special needs reflecting fundamental psychological, anatomical, and physiological differences to adults. There should be a designated recovery area that is segregated from tthe adult areas. It should be child orientated and appropriately decorated. This creates a sense of safety and security. Children should be cared for by appropriately trained and competent staff who have undertaken regular paediatric life support training.

Parents

The presence of a parent or guardian in the recovery room should be encouraged. Where possible the parent should be given a bleep so they can be paged to return to the recovery room at an appropriate time. The parent/guardian should be involved in all aspects of the care of their child. However it is important to make sure that the parent/guardian is cared for as well by providing them with information about what happens in recovery beforehand and providing them with a chair where they can sit with their child to comfort them.

Care of the child in recovery

- Provide one-to-one patient care, with another member of staff present.
- Paediatric equipment should be available:
  - Face masks.
  - Breathing systems.
  - Airways.
  - ET tubes.
  - Emergency drugs and equipment.
- Monitoring equipment—O_2 saturation, heart rate, BP.

Use your eyes to observe colour and breathing and feel for a manual pulse! Do not just rely on the monitors as there may be difficulty getting accurate recordings on a child who is agitated and trying to pull the monitoring off.

- O_2 administration should be guided by the O2 saturation.
- Be aware of any loose teeth that may become dislodged.
- Ensure any IV cannulas are secured with a dressing and a bandage if necessary, to avoid being pulled out by the child or accidental displacement.
- Observe wound site, dressings, and drains.
- Be aware of any specific observations required depending on surgery e.g.:
  - Colour, sensation, and movement of limbs in orthopaedics.
  - Bleeding in the airway following dental or ENT surgery.
- Keep the child warm. If they have come to theatre in their own clothes and they had to be taken off, try to put them back on before they wake up so they are not upset at having their clothes removed.
- Ensure that there is padding on the trolley rails to avoid the disorientated child causing themselves injury.

Potential postoperative problems

Airway obstruction

Airway obstruction in children rapidly leads to hypoxia due to higher O_2 consumption than in adults. Factors that contribute are large floppy tongues, epiglottis, tonsils, and adenoids.
- Recover children in the recovery position.
- If required, gently extend the head by either lifting the mandible by placing fingers under the jaw or through chin lift ensuring that soft tissues are not compressed.
- If necessary use gentle suction taking care not to stimulate the back of the throat.

Nausea and vomiting

Frequently affects older children. Increased risk from:
- Inhalational anaesthesia.
- Opioid analgesia, especially morphine.
- Certain types of surgery, e.g., adenotonsillectomy, appendicectomy, middle ear surgery.

Reassure the child, provide with a vomit bowl and give antiemetic if indicated. If prolonged consider IV fluids.

Pain

It is sometimes difficult to assess if the child is distressed due to anxiety or distressed due to pain.
- Reassure the child through touch and 'cuddles' (if appropriate) involving the parent/guardian if present.
- Ask the child about their comfort using pain assessment scales such as visual analogue scale.
- Observe the child for non-verbal signs of pain, e.g., guarding.
- Avoid IM injections.
- Use PCA for children who are able to understand.

Discharge from recovery

The child should be discharged from the recovery when they meet the following criteria:
- Awake with no signs of airway obstruction.
- Clinically stable.
- Little or no pain.
- No nausea or vomiting.
- Warm and comfortable.
- No evidence of bleeding from wound sites.
- Ongoing care prescribed, e.g. pain relief, IV fluids.

References

Association of Anaesthetists of Great Britain and Ireland (2002). *Immediate post-anaesthetic recovery*. AAGBI: London.

Hatfield A and Tronson M (2008). *The Complete Recovery Room Book* (4th edn). Oxford University Press: Oxford.

Documentation

The documentation of care in the post-anaesthetic care unit is the final chapter of the patient's operating theatre journey. Many documents are in use and include:

- Observation charts.
- Fluid balance charts.
- Prescription charts.
- Pain relief charts.
- Care plans.
- Care pathways.
- Electronic records.

What should be documented?

Different units will have their own policies and procedures in place which must be adhered to but consideration should be given to the following.

- Written entries should always be in black ink and signed, name printed, timed, and dated.
- Any errors should be crossed through with a single line and signed with the date and time.
- All care given to the patient in the post-anaesthetic care unit should be documented:
  - Recording of vital signs, fluid input/output.
  - Assessment of wounds, dressings, and drains.
  - Any medication given, including pain relief.
  - Any nausea/vomiting and whether anti-emetics administered.
  - Assessment of pressure areas.
  - Mouth care given.
  - Specific assessments made, e.g., colour, sensation and movement of limbs, vaginal loss, pedal pulses.
- If regional anaesthesia record level of sensation return and mobility of limbs.

Any clinical incident should be recorded in the care plan along with any other departmental reporting mechanisms.

Integrated care pathways

Integrated care pathways may also be used in the perioperative area. In this instance the routine postoperative care of patients is prewritten and only if an action is not met would further documentation be required. This is identified as a variance and the reasons the action had not been met explained. This facilitates a consistent approach to the care given and provides a guideline to evidence-based best practice. Variances can then be audited to establish recurring themes in the perioperative patient's pathway and identify where improvements or changes should be made.

On discharge to the ward

Ensure

- Discharge criteria are met and documented. If there is an exception then this must be reported.
- O_2 therapy, pain relief, and IV fluids/blood are prescribed.

- Any invasive lines not required on the ward are documented as removed.
- The patient has an identification band still in situ.
- All items returned to patient following surgery, e.g., glasses, dentures, are documented as returned.
- All documentation is returned to the ward with the patient.
- Postoperative instructions are clear and documented.

Postoperative problems

The recovery room or the post-anaesthetic care unit (PACU) is where patients are cared for and managed after anaesthesia and following a surgical procedure.

The PACU provides a place where patients are able to be observed and monitored on a one-to-one basis focusing on restoring the patient back to their preoperative physiological state.

It is during this early recovery that adverse postoperative events and/or complications are likely to occur, and detection and treatment of these is imperative. Patients with little or no pre-existing disease may also suffer complications following anaesthesia and in turn this may lead to serious and catastrophic events.[1]

Incidence

The reported incidence of immediate postoperative adverse events in patients admitted to PACU range from 1.3% up to 30%.[2] Minor adverse events are much more likely to occur than major events.

Common postoperative complications

Respiratory complications
- Stridor.
- Laryngospasm.
- Hypoventilation.
- Swelling/oedema.
- Hypoxaemia.
- Low muscle tone of the oropharyngeal muscles—mouth and pharynx.
- Bronchospasm.
- Foreign bodies.
- Blood.
- Pneumothorax.

Cardiovascular complications
- Hypotension.
- Hypertension.
- Bradycardia.
- Tachycardia.
- Dysryhthmias.
- Vasodilatation—dilation of blood vessels.
- MI.
- Cardiac arrest.

CNS complications
- Nausea and vomiting.
- Pain.

Other complications
- Hypothermia.
- Hyperthermia.
- Shivering.

- Delayed emergence.
- Prolonged sedation.
- Hypoglycaemia.

References

1. Kluger MT and Bullock MFM (2002). A review of the Anaesthetic Monitoring Study. *Anaesthesia* **57**, 1060–6.

2. Sewell A and Young P (2003). Recovery and post-anaesthetic care. *Anaesthesia and Intensive Care Medicine* **4**(10), 329–32.

Respiratory distress

Respiratory or airway complications are common in the PACU. These complications are the most likely to be serious and are of immediate threat to the patient. The nature of surgery influences the likelihood of respiratory complications; it is especially common in patients who have undergone abdominal surgery.[1]

Upper airway obstruction is one of the most common respiratory complications and frequently presents itself in the PACU. Other common respiratory complications are hypoventilation, hypoxaemia, and bronchospasm.[2]

Causes of upper airway obstruction

Accounts for approximately 30% of adverse events, the most common cause are the tongue falling back causing obstruction of the pharynx in the unconscious patient.

- Laryngospasm.
- Low muscle tone from residual anaesthetic.
- Soft tissue swelling and/or oedema—more common in children.
- Blood, secretions, or vomit—especially after oral and airway surgery.
- Foreign bodies—throat pack, swabs, teeth.

Causes of hypoventilation

- Defined as respiratory rate of <8 breaths per minute.
- Can be caused by depression of the respiratory centre or impaired respiratory muscles making breathed laboured.

Depression of the respiratory centre

- Drugs.
- Opioid-induced respiratory depression of both respiratory rate and/or depth.
- Benzodiazepines.
- Volatile or inhalational anaesthetic agents.
- High epidural or total spinal.
- Hypothermia.

Impaired respiratory muscles

- Airway obstruction.
- Residual or inadequate reversal of muscle relaxant drugs.
- Pre-existing respiratory disease—COPD, asthma.
- Muscle weakness—muscular dystrophies, Guillain–Barré syndrome.
- Splinting of diaphragm due to the nature of surgery, obesity, or pain.

Causes of hypoxaemia

Low O_2 in arterial blood or haemoglobin, demonstrated as O_2 saturation of 90% or less.

- Increased O_2 consumption—commonly caused by shivering postoperatively.
- Airway obstruction or closure.
- Bronchospasm—more common in patients with an irritable airway (smokers) or pre existing lung disease—asthma, COPD.
- Laryngospasm.

- Pulmonary oedema—may be due to fluid overload.
- Hypoventilation.
- Diffusion hypoxia—reduction of O_2 concentration in the lungs at the end of anaesthesia; the displacement of O_2 by N_2O being the major cause of diffusion hypoxia.
- Pneumothorax.
- Atelectasis—collapse of part or all of the lung; anaesthesia increases the risk, secretions can obstruct the airway and may be caused by insufficient analgesia.

Causes of bronchospasm

Characterised by coughing and wheezing on expiration due to narrowing and obstruction of the airway:

- Most common cause is asthma.
- Anaphylaxis—allergic reaction to drugs or other substances.
- Irritants—irritable airway from smoking or other substances.
- Respiratory infections.

Treatment of airway obstruction

Manual opening of the airway using head tilt, chin lift procedure:

- Administer high flow O_2—100% O_2.
- Using suction or other mechanism clear secretions or remove foreign bodies from the airway.
- Insert an oral/nasal airway.
- If the patient is semi-conscious place in the recovery position.
- If still unresolved positive airway pressure must be applied via facemask.
- If necessary intubation must take place—this occurs in only a very small minority of patients.
- Cricothyroidotomy must be performed if all other attempts at relieving the obstruction have failed and the trachea cannot be intubated.

Treatment of hypoventilation[1]

- Appropriate antagonist or reversal must be used:
- Opioids—naloxone.
- Benzodiazepines—flumazenil.
- Residual neuromuscular block—neostigmine and glycopyrronium bromide.

References

1. Al-Rawi S and Nolan K (2003). Respiratory Complications in the postoperative period. *Anaesthesia and Intensive Care Medicine* **4**(10), 332–4.

2. Peskett MJ (1999). Clinical indicators and other complications in the recovery room or postan-aesthetic care unit. *Anaesthesia* **54**, 1143–9.

Postoperative nausea and vomiting

PONV is one of the most frequently seen side effects following surgery and anaesthesia. It can be very distressing and debilitating for the patient due to its unpleasantness and can cause more concern than pain relief and management of such postoperatively for the patient.

Incidence

PONV has a reported occurrence of approximately 25–30% although in patients considered high risk, a prevalence as high as 70% has been reported.[1]

Implications

The detrimental effect on patients can be both physical and psychological and begins immediately postoperatively.

- **Delayed discharge from PACU:** PONV in the recovery room necessitates immediate treatment with anti-emetic drugs and discharge will be delayed until the PONV is under control and management is shown to be effective for the patient
- **Delayed recovery from surgery:** PONV can cause the patient to suffer with dehydration, electrolyte imbalance, wound dehiscence, and can interfere with nutritional needs and other oral treatments which have a vital and essential part in recovering from surgery.
- **Delayed discharge from hospital and impact on hospital costs:** PONV requires an increased amount and level of care and thus carries an economic burden for the patient and the hospital caring for the patient. Further surgery may be required due to complications suffered.

Risk factors

Predisposing factors for PONV can be identified.

The patient

- Affects females (post puberty) more than males—ratio 3:1.
- Affects children more than adults—peaks at approximately 11–14 years of age.
- Obesity.
- Previous history of PONV or motion sickness.
- Non smoker.[2]

Procedure

The nature of the procedure has more impact on PONV than the type of anaesthetic administered:[3]

- Abdominal.
- Gynaecological.
- ENT.
- Laparoscopic and
- Ophthalmic surgery all increase the incidence of PONV.

The length of surgery also has an influence with the longer the surgery and the longer the anaesthetic, the more likely the patient is to suffer with PONV.

Anaesthetic
Some anaesthetic agents influence the likelihood of PONV.
- The use of N_2O.
- Use of some inhalational anaesthetic agents—sevoflurane and desflurane less likely to cause PONV than enflurane and halothane.
- Administration of opioids.
- Use of induction agents—propofol less likely to cause PONV than etomidate.
- General anaesthesia versus regional anaesthesia—general anaesthetic more likely to cause PONV.

Postoperative[2]
- Pain postoperatively is associated with nausea.
- Opioid analgesics—have known emetic properties.
- Hypotension.
- Dehydration.
- Early resumption of oral intake.
- Movement and mobilisation.

Treatment
PONV is multifactorial and management of such is complex, no single treatment is wholly effective at managing PONV. There are four main classes of drugs:

Anticholinergics
Atropine/hyoscine—act on the vomiting centre, reduce gastric motility.

Antihistamines
Cyclizine/promethazine—useful in middle ear surgery and motion sickness although less effective on agents that stimulate the chemoreceptor trigger zone (CTZ).

D_2 antagonists
Metoclopramide, droperidol, prochlorperazine—act against agents that stimulate the CTZ, such as opioids, anaesthetic drugs and agents, and chemotherapy.

$5HT_3$ antagonists
- Ondansetron, granisetron, dolasetron—effective and successful drug in the prevention of PONV due to blocking of the receptors in the gut, however, it is an expensive treatment.
- Combination therapy is more effective than single therapy and treatment must be prompt.[1]

References
1. Rahman MH and Beattie J (2004). Post-operative nausea and vomiting. *The Pharmaceutical Journal* **273**, 786–8.

2. Taylor R and Pickford A (2003). Postoperative Nausea and Vomiting. *Anaesthesia and Intensive Care Medicine* **4**(10), 335–6.

3. Hines, R, Barash, PG, Watrous G, et al. (1992). Complications occuring in the postanaesthesia care unit. *Anaesthesia and Analgesia* **74**, 503–9.

Sore throat

- General anaesthesia involves using a variety of techniques and adjuncts to ensure breathing is maintained and compromised.
- The nature of surgery and individual presentation will determine which adjuncts are utilised during anaesthesia and each of these may be part of the cause or contribute to sore throat postoperatively.
- Sore throat may only be a minor side effect following surgery and anaesthesia but is still a common complication and can have a detrimental effect on the patient.[1]

Method of airway management

The incidence of sore throat varies depending on the method used.

ET tube

Tracheal intubation is associated with the highest incidence of sore throat—approximately 14–46%.[1,2]

LMA

LMA is less invasive than tracheal intubation and the incidence of sore throat is consistently lower—approximately 4–19%.[3]

Face mask

Face mask is usually used to deliver O_2 and/or inhalational agents. The incidence of sore throat is minimal—approximately 3%.[1]

Other factors

- Females are more likely to suffer with sore throat than males.[1,2]
- Patients undergoing gynaecological surgery are more at risk of experiencing sore throat.[1]

Consideration of the factors that increase the likelihood of sore throat postoperatively can aid in early detection and treatment which in turn may improve the patient experience.

References

1. Higgins PP, Chung F, and Mezei G (2002). Postoperative sore throat after ambulatory surgery. *British Journal of Anaesthesia* **88**(4), 582–4.

2. Christensen AM, Willemoes-Larsen H, Lundby, L *et al.* (1994). Postoperative throat complaints after tracheal intubation. *British Journal of Anaesthesia* **73**, 786–7.

3. Brimacombe J (1995). The advantages of the LMA over the tracheal tube or face mask: a meta-analysis. *Canadian Journal of Anaesthesia* **42**, 1017–23.

Delayed emergence

Patients who undergo surgery and anaesthesia should awaken gradually at the end of the procedure, slowly regaining consciousness. However, some patients will experience delayed emergence from anaesthesia and there are a variety of reasons for this.

Causes

The most common cause for delayed emergence is the continual effect of anaesthesia and the agents used throughout.[1,2] The residual effect of drugs may be from anaesthetic drugs and agents, and excessive sedative drugs or analgesics.

Muscle relaxants

Continued muscle relaxation may be due to incomplete reversal or administration of too much drug.

Benzodiazepines

Midazolam, diazepam, temazepam, and other drugs in this group can be given as pre-medication, all of which enhance the effect of other drugs administered for anaesthesia and may contribute to delayed emergence.

Analgesics

Opioid drugs, also referred to as narcotic drugs that can be given pre-, peri-, and postoperatively may cause hypoventilation. The consequence of hypoventilation during or after anaesthesia is there may be a rise in CO_2 which if high enough can have a sedative effect or render the patient unconscious.

Metabolic disorders

- Hypo- or hyperglycaemia.
- Electrolyte imbalance: may be an associated comorbidity in the patient or due to the surgical procedure—TURP syndrome resulting in hyponatraemia.
- Hypothermia: severe hypothermia alters conscious level.

Neurological complications

Cerebrovascular events or stroke and raised ICP are rare causes of delayed emergence but need to be considered, especially in patients who have undergone carotid or neurosurgery.

Treatment of residual drugs

Reversal of the effect of the specific drug or likely drug can aid wakening.

- Neuromuscular blockers: reverse using neostigmine and glycopyrronium bromide.
- Benzodiazepines: reverse using flumazenil.
- Opioids: reverse using antagonist naloxone; caution needed as reversal of analgesic effect of opioids may occur.

Treatment of metabolic disorders

- Hypoglycaemia: once blood sugar level has been ascertained correct using IV dextrose.

- Hyperglycaemia: once blood sugar level has been ascertained correct using sodium chloride and insulin and supplement with potassium chloride as required.
- Electrolyte imbalance: if TURP syndrome is suspected, surgery must cease immediately with monitoring and correction of electrolytes. Hyponatraemia following TURP: fluid restrict and replace sodium slowly with close monitoring.
- Hypothermia: 📖 see Hypothermia, p.420.

References and further reading

1. Morgan GE, Mikhail MS, and Murray MJ (2005). Care of the patient. *Clinical Anesthesiology* (4th edn). McGraw-Hill Medical, New York.

2. Pescod D (2005) *Postanaesthetic Care Unit Complications*. Available at: 🖥 www.developinganaesthesia.org/index.php?option=com_content&task=view&id=63&Itemid=45

Radhakrishnan J, Jesudasan S, Jacob R (2001). Delayed awakening or emergence from anaesthesia. Physiology. *Update in Anaesthesia* **13**, 1–2. Available at: 🖥 www.nda.ox.ac.uk/wfsa/html/u13/u1303_01.htm

Post-anaesthetic shivering

Post-anaesthetic shivering is a common side effect after general anaesthesia with a reported incidence ranging from 5–65%.[1]

Causes

- Normal mechanisms for temperature control and regulation are dulled with general and regional anaesthesia, therefore it is the anaesthetist's responsibility to manage the patient's temperature.
- Perioperative hypothermia is the main cause of post-anaesthetic shivering followed by the impairment of the body's normal mechanism for temperature control.[2]
- Not all post-anaesthetic shivering is due to hypothermia.
- Post-anaesthetic shivering causes distress for the patient but also has potential serious consequences for the patient.

Risk factors[2]

- Surgery lasting >1 hour.
- Males.
- Children have an increased risk.
- Elderly have an increased risk.
- Patients undergoing combined general/epidural anaesthesia.

Key issues to consider

- Shivering causes an increase in O_2 demand /consumption.
- Exacerbates postoperative pain.
- Increases heart rate.
- Increases BP.
- Interferes with routine monitoring.

Treatment

- Active warming methods such as forced-air warming systems.
- Conventional blankets.
- Increasing ambient temperature.
- Warming IV fluids.
- Drug treatment: pethidine, clonidine, or tramadol can be effective in treating post anaesthetic shivering.

References

1. Crossley AWA (1992). Peri-operative shivering. *Anaesthesia* **47**(3), 193–5.

2. Buggy DJ and Crossley AWA (2000). Thermoregulation, mild perioperative hypothermia and post-anaesthetic shivering. *British Journal of Anaesthesia* **84**(5), 615–28.

Sweating

Sweating (diaphoresis) can be a symptom of over-vigorous warming peri-operatively but is also a physical consequence of some postoperative complications or side effects that must be addressed and treated promptly.

Causes

- High temperature.
- PONV.
- Hypotension.
- Hypoglycaemia.
- Opioids.
- Hypoxia.
- High CO_2—hypercarbia.
- Malignant hyperpyrexia.
- Transfusion reaction.
- Drug reaction.

Transfusion reaction

- A transfusion reaction occurs when sensitivity during a blood transfusion is identified.
- The blood transfusion should be stopped if side effects show an elevated temperature and any other associated effects.

Patient management

- Reassure the patient.
- Inform the anaesthetist.
- Assess pain.
- Monitor vital signs including ECG, SpO_2, and BP.
- Monitor blood glucose.
- Administer O_2 as prescribed.

References

Association of Anaesthetists of Great Britain and Ireland (2002). *Immediate Post Anaesthetic Care*. AAGBI. London.

Hatfield A and Tronson M (2008). *The Complete Recovery Room Book* (4th edn). Oxford University Press, Oxford.

Hypotension

Postoperative hypotension is a common complication in the PACU which must be addressed and treated. There is no absolute figure that is able to define hypotension as the preoperative reading plus individual patient characteristics and preoperative condition will define the figure.[1]

A baseline BP reading is therefore imperative for all patients[2] as deviation from this reading facilitates a diagnosis of hypotension. Subsequent treatment is indicated if a decrease of 20% or more from the systolic preoperative reading or a mean arterial pressure (MAP) of <60mmHg lasts for 15 minutes or longer.

Postoperative hypotension is a cardiovascular complication that is frequently seen in PACU and has a wide range of causes.[3,4]

Key issues to consider

The accuracy of the BP reading **must** be checked as too large or too small a cuff will give a false reading. Monitors are only present to complement visual observation and assessment of the patient.

Causes

- *Hypovolaemia* is one of the most common causes of hypotension.[5,6]
- *Dehydration*: can occur because of inadequate fluid intake or replacement and prolonged NBM status and patients who are generally unwell prior to surgery are more likely to be dehydrated.
  - Certain surgical procedures require patients to undergo bowel preparation prior to surgery which can cause dehydration.
  - Bowel preparation causes huge losses of fluid which if not replaced adequately results in the patient arriving at theatre in a less than optimum state and potentially compromising the patient.
- Anaesthetic drugs/agents.
  - Residual effects of drugs and agents can cause hypotension.
  - Regional anaesthesia causes vasodilatation reducing cardiac output.
  - Induction agents—especially propofol cause a decrease in BP proportional to the amount administered.
  - Volatile agents—cause a decrease in BP proportional to the amount administered.
  - Opioids.
  - Non-depolarising muscle relaxants.

Cardiovascular disease and medication

Pre-existing cardiovascular disease and associated medication can contribute to hypotension postoperatively. Examples are:
- Ischaemic heart disease (IHD), heart failure, dysrhythmias, atrial fibrillation (AF), and complete heart block (CHB) and patients with valve disease.
- Beta-blockers: reduce cardiac output, ACE inhibitors and nitrates.

Other causes

Anaphylaxis causes cardiovascular collapse and therefore hypotension. PE from DVT and air embolus will cause hypotension.

Treatment[1]

- Cause of the hypotension must be identified and managed
  - Surgical cause—bleeding.
  - Anaesthetic cause—regional block.
- Oxygenation must be optimised—increase to 100% O_2.
- Lay patient down—supine position.
- Fluid challenge with IV fluids—individual patient characteristics and associated co-morbidities must be taken into consideration.
- Response to the fluid must be assessed—if hypotension not corrected other causes must be investigated.
- Residual anaesthetic agents and drugs may require vasopressors if fluid bolus is not effective:
  - Ephedrine: 3mg IV boluses.
  - Metaraminol: 0.5–1.0mg IV boluses.
  - Phenylephrine: 0.5 IV boluses.
- Inotropes may need to be considered if management necessitates.

References

1. Beamer JER and Warwick J (2004). Critical incidents: the cardiovascular system. *Anaesthesia and Intensive Care Medicine* **5**(12) 426–9.

2. Osborne A (2006). Hypertension/Hypotension in Postoperative Care. In Colvin JR (ed.), *Raising the Standard: A compendium of audit recipes for continuous quality improvement in anaesthesia* (2nd edn). Royal College of Anaesthetists: London.

3. Kluger MT and Bullock MFM (2002). A review of the anaesthetic monitoring study. *Anaesthesia* **57**, 1060–6.

4. Peskett MJ (1999). Clinical indicators and other complications in the recovery room or post-anaesthetic care unit. *Anaesthesia* **54**, 1143–9.

5. Pescod D (2005) *Postanaesthetic Care Unit Complications*. Available at: 🖳 www.developing anaesthesia.org/index.php?option=com_content&task=view&id=63&Itemid=45

6. Sewell A and Young P (2003). Recovery and post-anaesthetic care. *Anaesthesia and Intensive Care Medicine* **4**(10), 329–32.

Confusion and the violent patient

Anaesthesia affects different people in different ways and is an unknown entity until experienced by individuals.

When patients emerge from anaesthesia they can become very agitated and may need restraining. Occasionally an individual may be aware of previous incidents where they have become violent and this must be taken into account as the individual may become a danger not only to themselves but to staff in PACU.

Patients often become very disorientated, unable to make sense of the place and environment, the situation, and time on emerging from anaesthesia. Whilst they may be able to respond and answer, the responses can be incoherent and muddled, making no sense.

Predisposing factors to confusion
- Elderly.
- Infants and children.
- History of dementia.
- History of drug or alcohol abuse.
- Open heart surgery.
- Intraoperative hypoxia/hypotension.

Pre-existing diseases such as renal and liver problems, electrolyte imbalance, and infection may also contribute to confusion postoperatively.[1,2]

Causes
- Hypoxia: **must** be excluded first and foremost as inadequate O_2 to supply vital organs and tissues can have a damaging and severe effect on an individual.
- Severe pain.
- Infection/sepsis.
- Hypoglycaemia.
- Some drugs: e.g., ketamine, midazolam.

Management
If a patient is *confused:*
- Administer high-flow 100% O_2 and monitor O_2 saturations with pulse oximeter.
- Sedation should be avoided if possible as this may aggravate the situation on the long term.

If a patient is *violent*
- Sedation may be the only option in order to protect the patient from the surrounding environment and staff as much as possible

It is imperative that the patient's airway, breathing, and circulation are supported and managed throughout and on emergence from sedation.[1]

References

1. Hatfield A and Tronson M (2008). *The Complete Recovery Room Book* (4th edn). Oxford University Press: Oxford.

2. Pescod D (2005) *Postanaesthetic Care Unit Complications*. Available at: 🖵 www.developing anaesthesia.org/index.php?option=com_content&task=view&id=63&Itemid=45

Hypoglycaemia

Normal range for blood glucose is 3.3–5.6mmol/L of glucose;[1] however, hypoglycaemia or low blood sugar levels can be considered at a level of <4mmol/L[2] and are associated with fasting prior to anaesthesia which has implications for the surgical patient.[3]

Anaesthesia may inhibit the patient demonstrating the clinical signs of hypoglycaemia which can present as:
• Tachycardia.
• Sweating.
• Confusion.
• Pallor.

Diabetes mellitus is the most common metabolic disorder[2] and causes other diseases within the body systems that have implications for surgery.

During surgery many body systems are potentially compromised and the patient presenting with diabetes will need to be managed appropriately in order to optimise their treatment and not further compromise.

Infection

Diabetic patients are more likely to suffer with infection which in turn affects the control of blood sugar; therefore postoperative wound infections are more common which has numerous implications.[2] Delayed wound healing, less than optimum control of blood sugar, prolonged stay in hospital, and associated costs are all factors.

Respiratory

Diabetic patients are prone to suffer with chest infections, especially so if obese and a smoker, therefore postoperative vigilance and prompt treatment is necessary.

PONV

Prevention of PONV is imperative as nausea and vomiting will have an impact on the patient recommencing oral fluids and diet and therefore returning to their normal preoperative state.

Anaesthesia

Regional anaesthesia has advantages over general anaesthesia:[2]
• Hypoglycaemia is far easier to diagnose in the patient who undergoes regional anaesthesia.
• Oral intake can recommence much sooner in the patient who undergoes regional anaesthesia.
• PONV is much less in the patient who undergoes regional anaesthesia although hypotension following regional anaesthesia is common and can cause PONV.

Critically ill patients often have metabolic disturbances and patients who are septic can often be hypoglycaemic.

Hypoglycaemia must be corrected but the underlying cause must be treated.

References

1. Pleuvry BJ (2005). Pharmacological control of blood sugar. *Anaesthesia and Intensive Care Medicine* **6**(10), 344–6.

2. Webster S and Lewis N (2005). Anaesthetic management of the diabetic patient. *Anaesthesia and Intensive Care Medicine* **6**(10), 3414.

3. Leaper DJ and Peel ALG (2003). *Handbook of Postoperative Complications.* Oxford University Press: Oxford.

Wound dehiscence

What is it?

Wound dehiscence can be either partial or complete and describes a breakdown of a surgically-closed wound. The word dehiscence literally means to split. Be aware that internal wound dehiscence may lead to an incisional hernia forming.

More commonly a late complication of surgery, occurring several days postoperatively; however, complete separation (often known as burst abdomen) can occur at any point postoperatively.

When wound dehiscence is suspected/identified, it should be assumed that the whole wound may be affected until proven otherwise.

Signs

Partial: one part of a surgically closed wound will open up creating a small hole, the remainder of the wound will stay intact. A common pre-cursor to wound dehiscence is a discharge of a 'pinkish' serosanguinous fluid, often seen on the wound dressing. There will be little evidence of systemic disturbance, however signs of infection may be present.

Complete: often called 'burst abdomen' due to the fact that larger wounds (laparotomy) are under greater pressure and therefore have an increased risk of splitting. Obvious signs are a sudden breakdown of the wound, sometimes leading to abdominal contents protruding through. Excessive bleeding can be expected from a complete separation. Patients may experience the feeling of something 'giving way', however if they are unable to communicate this, signs of shock/collapse should be looked for.

Risk factors

Wound dehiscence carries a mortality rate of 15–30% and is classed as a serious complication of surgery.

Pre-disposing factors include:
- Infection.
- Abdominal distension.
- Postoperative coughing.
- Poor surgical technique.
- Inappropriate closure materials.
- Malnourishment.
- Malignancy—underlying causes.
- Smoking.

Treatment

Depending on the severity of the wound breakdown treatment will range from observation-only in simple partial dehiscence, as these type of wound complications will heal themselves over time; to emergency return to theatre.

If active treatment is needed consider the following points:

- *Opiate analgesia:* the patient may experience varying degrees of pain dependent upon the severity of the dehiscence.
- *Sterile dressing to wound:*
  - Pressure may also be needed if bleeding occurs.
  - For complete separation or where abdominal content is visible, a saline soaked sterile dressing should be applied.
- *Fluid resuscitation:*
  - Pressure may also be needed if bleeding occurs.
  - For complete separation or where abdominal content is visible, a saline soaked sterile dressing should be applied.
- *Rapid return to theatre:*
  - Complete dehiscence will need re-closing.
  - This often involves muscle layers so will require the patient to have a general anaesthetic.
- *Antibiotic administration:* in late dehiscence this may not have an effect but should be considered as prevention of increased chance of infection for ongoing management.

Reference

Hatfield A and Tronson M (2008). *The Complete Recovery Room Book* (4th edn). Oxford University Press: Oxford.

Wound dehiscence: images

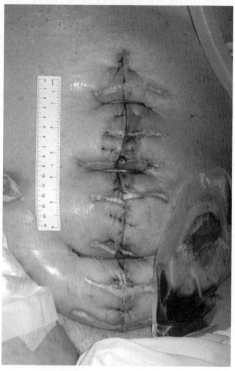

Fig. 21.1 The warning signs: note pressure around sutures and bruising. Courtesy of: Cardiff & Vale NHS Trust (2006).

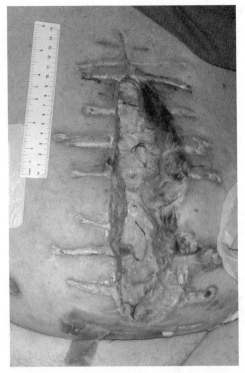

Fig. 21.2 The burst abdomen. Courtesy of: Cardiff & Vale NHS Trust (2006).

Pain in recovery

The majority of patients admitted to the recovery room will experience some level of pain, mainly as a result of their operative procedure. It is important to establish whether the pain is of an acute nature (in response to the surgery) or due to a chronic condition. Acute pain is easier to treat in the recovery room, but often presents more of a problem for patients than chronic pain, due in most part to the sensation of the pain being new.

Appropriate assessment is paramount and the patient's perception of the amount of pain they are in must be believed. Treatment will depend upon the severity of the pain experienced by the patient.

Signs of pain

Other than verbalising their level of pain, patients often exhibit non-verbal cues which should alert the practitioner to the fact that the patient may be in pain. They include:

- Hypertension in severe acute pain, but hypotension in chronic pain.
- Tachycardia in severe acute pain, but bradycardia in chronic pain.
- Increased respiratory rate.
- Nausea and vomiting.
- Grimacing.
- Holding the body rigid.
- Sweating.
- Pallor.
- Reluctance to converse/participate in surroundings.

Common causes

Aside from the procedure itself, several things can contribute to a patient experiencing pain in the recovery room. Obviously the type of operation the patient undergoes will have an effect as the larger the surgery the more chance there is of pain as a result.

- Having an anaesthetic can also cause patients to experience pain postoperatively, e.g., patients may complain of a sore throat from intubation, or be agitated by a venous cannula.
- It is important to address any aspect of the patient's procedure that may be causing them distress.
- Talking to the patient and keeping them informed will help them to rationalise their pain and hopefully result in a reduction of their perception of the pain.

Non-surgical related causes and treatment

Often the pain from the actual wound/procedure is relieved pre-emptively by analgesia given during anaesthesia. However, there are causes of pain which cannot be so easily anticipated, they include angina, positioning, headache, a full bladder, and nerve damage.

- *Angina:* give high-flow O_2, reassure the patient, and give glyceryl trinitrate (GTN) sublingually to dilate coronary arteries thus improving O_2 supply. Pain relief such as opiates may also be required.
- *Positioning:* assess skin integrity to eliminate open skin sores, ensure the patient is repositioned more comfortably (if appropriate), and

offer padding in the form of more pillows. Warm compresses and/or massaging the affected area can also relieve pain.

- *Headache:* if possible move the patient to a quieter area, dim the lights and provide a cool compress. Paracetamol should be given unless contra-indicated.
- *Full bladder:* encourage the patient to pass urine! If this is not possible catheterisation will be required. If the patient experiences bladder spasm an antispasmodic such as hyoscine hydrobromide 20mg given intravenously is an effective remedy.
- *Nerve damage:* the most effective way to treat pain from nerve damage is to inform the patient of the reason for the pain, reassure them, and provide analgesia, the strength of which will depend upon the severity of the pain experienced; however, in most cases this will be a mild-to-moderate level of discomfort alleviated by a weak pain killer.

Reference

Hatfield A and Tronson M (2008). *The Complete Recovery Room Book* (4th edn). Oxford University Press: Oxford.

Hypothermia

Hypothermia occurs when a patient's core body temperature falls below 36°C, and if left untreated can become a life-threatening complication.

The perioperative aspect of a patient's stay in hospital is one of the most crucial in the possibility of a patient becoming hypothermic, and for this reason it is imperative that measures are taken to prevent its likelihood.

Causes
- Cold environment.
- Shivering (a way the body warms itself) abolished by general anaesthesia.
- Vasodilation.
- Scant clothing.
- Evaporative heat loss, particularly of core temperature during intra-abdominal surgery.
- Infusion of cold fluids.
- Cold/dry anaesthetic gases.

Age may be a pre-disposing factor as older adults and children are more susceptible to hypothermia

Effects
Milder consequences include:
- Patient discomfort.
- Impaired wound healing.
- Increased risk of infection.

Serious effects include:
- Reduction in cough reflex, increasing the risk of aspiration.
- Tachycardia.
- Reduced tissue perfusion.
- Atrial fibrillation/ventricular fibrillation.
- Delay in metabolism/excretion of drugs.
- Increased blood viscosity, impeding flow.
- Shivering is significant cause of increased O_2 consumption and leads to hypoxia.

If a patient's temperature falls below 33°C they will stop shivering and loss of consciousness is not far away!

Treatment
- Patients should not be rapidly warmed, and it can take >12 hours to safely re-warm a severely hypothermic patient.
- Monitoring is important to ensure a steady increase in temperature and to identify any cardiovascular changes.

Monitor:
- Core temperature.
- BP.
- HR/ECG.
- Glucose level.
- Urine output, this will increase as hypothermic kidneys fail to concentrate urine.

Actively warming with the use of a forced air heater. Use fluid warmers for any infusions, the hypothermic patient may also become hypotensive so fluid should be used to maintain circulating volume.

It is important to administer high concentrations of O_2 to prevent hypoxia, especially when the patient is shivering, as O_2 consumption is increased during the shivering process. Re-warm at a rate no faster than 0.8°C per hour.

Although hypothermia can lead to death, there is a positive chance of successful resuscitation after warming as when a patient is severely hypothermic (temperature below 32°C) some cellular damage is prevented.

Treatment for hypothermia
Patient temperature between 35–35.9°C
- Do not re-expose to cold conditions.
- Keep warm for several hours.
- Watch for a drop in temperature.
- Do not massage cold limbs—this can cause cellular damage.

Patient temperature between 33–34°C
- Assess for cardiac arrhythmias.
- Warm only the trunk of the body.
- Give humidified, warmed O_2.
- Warm any IV fluids—but do not overload.
- Monitor HR, ECG, BP, respiration rate.

Patient temperature between 30–32°C
- Any sudden movements of the patient at this stage could induce cardiac arrest.
- NBM.
- Check airway.
- May need to artificially ventilate using bag and mask.
- Intubate if unable to maintain airway.
- Cardio pulmonary resuscitation.
- Defibrillation may be required—but only if core temp above 30°.

Continue to treat—don't give up until the patient is sufficiently warmed.

References
Davey A and Ince CS (2000). *Fundamentals of Operating Department Practice*. Oxford University Press: Oxford.

Hatfield A and Tronson M (2008). *The Complete Recovery Room Book* (4th edn). Oxford University Press: Oxford.

Post-dural headache

A post-dural headache occurs following spinal or epidural block and is defined as a dural puncture with a 16-gauge needle causing severe headache.[1] Excessive CSF in the epidural space causes traction on the meninges in the brain.[2] The evidence identifying the incidence of this postoperative complication is conflicting but it can occur in up to 2% of patients and sometimes occurs in the recovery room.

Treatment

- Maintain hydration with fluid therapy.
- Fluid therapy should be continued for 24 hours even if the patient is eating and drinking.
- Simple analgesia.
- If the headache fails to subside, a blood patch is recommended to arrest the CSF leak.

Postoperative care

- Psychological support should be provided until symptoms subside.
- Maintain fluid therapy.
- Administer analgesia as prescribed.

Blood patch

- A blood patch should only be undertaken in the absence of sepsis or pyrexia.
- It is effective in the majority of patients.
- Approximately 20mL of the patient's own blood is injected into the epidural space under sterile precautions.
- This blood should clot and block the CSF leak.
- It is necessary to lay patients flat following this procedure for 2 hours.
- Complications of blood patch can occur if the clot becomes infected within the epidural space.
- Although it is rare, if an abscess develops then paraplegia may occur.

References

1. Carpenter M (2003). Postoperative complications related to anaesthesia and intensive care. In: Leaper DJ and Peel ALG (eds) *Handbook of Postoperative Complications*. Oxford University Press: Oxford.

2. Hatfield A and Tronson M (2008). *The Complete Recovery Room Book* (4th edn). Oxford University Press: Oxford.

Extravasation

Extravasation occurs when an IV cannula becomes displaced. Occurrence can be reduced by careful siting away from joints.

Risk factors

Those at increased risk of extravasation include:
- Older people.
- Children.
- Infants.
- Patients with fragile veins.
- Confused patients.
- Unconscious patients.

Symptoms

Symptoms of extravasation can include:
- Pain.
- Delay in onset of action of the drug administered.
- Swelling.
- Leakage at the site of injection.
- Erythema of the skin around injection site.

Treatment

If extravasation is suspected:
- Stop infusion or administration of IV drug.
- Inspect the site for leakage.
- Inform anaesthetist/medical team.
- Remove cannula and dress accordingly.
- Problems associated with extravasation must be addressed at the earliest opportunity to prevent tissue damage and preserve future venous access.
- Symptoms can be relieved by applying warm or cold compresses.
- Re-site cannula: a different site should be used to administer the remainder of the drug.
- Treatment should be in line with local policy.

Postoperative care

- Psychological support to the patient should be provided.
- Inform patient that the site may be sore for a few days.
- Observe site regularly.
- Ensure patient's comfort.
- Provide analgesia as prescribed.
- Elevate the limb to reduce swelling.
- Documentation.
- Depending on the severity of the extravasated site and the toxicity of drug injected, plastic surgery may be necessary to remove damaged tissue although this is a very rare occurrence.

References and further reading

Hatfield A and Tronson M (2008). *The Complete Recovery Room Book* (4th edn). Oxford University Press: Oxford.

Lister S (2004). Drug administration: general principles. In Dougherty L and Lister S (eds) *The Royal Marsden Hospital Manual of Clinical Nursing Procedures* (6th edn). WileyBlackwell: Oxford.

Inadvertent intra-arterial injection

Drugs that are inadvertently administered intra-arterially are irritant and are likely to cause a reaction in the artery and surrounding vessels. It usually occurs when IV injections are attempted in the ante-cubital fossa region.[1]

Symptoms can include:
- Severe pain.
- Delay in onset of action of the drug administered.
- Blanching of the area affected.

Treatment
- Treatment should be in line with local policy.
- The drug administered should be diluted.
- Flush the artery with saline.
- If there is marked arterial spasm then a sympathetic block may be helpful as this will produce vasodilation.

Later care
- The patient should be fully informed and provided with appropriate support.
- Elevation of the arm to reduce oedema.
- Analgesia.
- Detailed documentation listing the chain of events in nursing and medical notes is vital.
- Review by a vascular surgeon may be necessary.

Reference
Hatfield A and Tronson M (2008). *The Complete Recovery Room Book* (4th edn). Oxford University Press: Oxford.

Discharge from the recovery room

Clear discharge criteria are essential in the recovery room to enable the safe and timely discharge of patients. A detailed policy outlining such criteria should be in place so that the recovery room nurse can discharge patients that achieve discharge criteria. Policy should also be in place to provide guidance to deal with those patients who do not achieve discharge criteria; this would usually require confirmation from an anaesthetist for discharge

Discharge criteria

Neurological

Anaesthetic agents will impact on the patient's neurological functioning and the recovery nurse must be confident that the patient has returned to previous neurological status and is not suffering any after effects of anaesthesia or has experienced any untoward events while in theatre e.g. CVA. The following criteria should be assessed prior to discharge:

- Eye opening to name.
- Orientated to person and place.
- Obeys commands.
- Muscle strength to sustain head lift for 5 seconds and strong hand grips.
- Neurological assessment consistent with the patient's preoperative status is acceptable if these criteria are not met.

Respiratory

Anaesthesia, with its sedative drugs and muscle relaxants, impair breathing. Full recovery of respiratory function is essential prior to discharge, especially as observation on the ward will not be as constant and direct as in recovery. The following criteria should be present prior to discharge:

- Spontaneous breathing at rate between 10 and 24 breaths per minute.
- Able to maintains patent's airway without artificial airway, clears oral secretions, and able to cough.
- Room air O_2 saturation >93%.
- O_2 removed **or** no O_2 treatment adjustments for 15 minutes prior to discharge.

Cardiovascular

Anaesthetic agents can affect cardiovascular function in some way. In addition, most surgical procedures will involve some degree of blood loss and/or potential for blood loss postoperatively. The recovery room nurse must ensure that cardiovascular stability is present prior to discharge:

- Pulse >45 and <120 beats per minute.
- Mean arterial pressure >60 and <120 mmHg.
- Systolic BP >95 and <185mmHg; diastolic BP <110mmHg.

Genitourinary

Particular attention should be given to genitourinary function postoperatively due to the effects of muscle relaxants if undergoing general anaesthetic, and the loss of sensation and function if given regional technique. The patient will also have received IV fluids intraoperatively. The bladder should be palpated and not be distended

Surgical sites

Assessment of the patient's surgical site should be carried out prior to discharge to ensure there are no complications. Surgery-specific assessments should be within normal parameters, e.g., drain output, wound drainage, perfusion, or swelling. Movement, sensation, and perfusion to extremities should be consistent with surgery, anaesthesia, and patient's preoperative neurovascular status.

Pain control

Pain level should be assessed and be at a level acceptable to the patient. Local policy should determine the minimum stay following analgesia administration, in particular after IM opioid, IV opioid, and bolus epidural medication. Minimum stay following initiation or change in epidural infusion rate should also be identified.

Thermoregulation

An adequate temperature is vital for postoperative recovery. Surgical procedures which open the body cavities to the environment, anaesthetic agents which cause vasodilation, cool theatre temperatures and prep solutions which cool the skin all contribute to a lowered body temperature post operatively. It can affect pain management as well as impair wound healing and reduce the body's ability to fight infection. Core temperature should be 35.4–38.6 °C.

Discharge procedure

Once discharge criteria have been met, the patient should be prepared for transfer, e.g., positioned safely, drains and catheters emptied and secured, O_2 for transfer if required, and any special equipment obtained as required (e.g. monitors, suction).

References

Aldrete JA (1998). Modifications to the post-anesthesia score for use in ambulatory surgery. *Journal of PeriAnesthesia Nursing* **13**(3), 148–55.

American Society of Perianesthesia Nurses (1998). *Standards of Perianaesthesia Nursing Practice*. ASPN: Thorofare, NJ.

Drain CB and Cristoph SS (1994). *The Post Anaesthesia Care Unit*. WB Saunders Co.: Toronto, ON.

Litwack K (ed) (1993). *Core curriculum for post anaesthesia nursing practice* (3rd edn). WB Saunders Co.: Toronto, ON.

Royal College of Anaesthetists (2000). *Raising the standard*. RCoA: London, UK.

Patient discharge to intensive treatment unit

Why and when?

- Sometimes patients will need to be transferred to the intensive care unit (ITU).
- A number of patients will be taken to ITU straight from theatre, sedated and ventilated; whilst some patients may need to be admitted following deterioration in the recovery room.
- The position of the ITU should be relatively close to the theatre department, ideally on the same floor, to allow for a swift transfer.

Preparation

- …is the key to a successful transfer to ITU.
- The period of transfer is a critical one for a patient; they are often very unwell and therefore need careful management and attention.
- Detailed planning before transfer will ensure as smooth a transition as possible. It is imperative that all healthcare professionals involved in the transfer are informed and ready throughout the process.

Responsibilities

- The overall responsibility for the transfer lies with the anaesthetist/intensivist in charge of the patient's care.
- The qualified practitioner caring for the patient has a responsibility to ensure a safe and timely discharge and that all equipment is available and ready for use.
- Communication is vital between perioperative and critical care staff; local policies should be in place regarding transfers and admissions from theatre to ITU and from recovery to ITU.
- The receiving ITU staff have a responsibility to ensure the area is prepared and adequately staffed to safely receive the patient.

Equipment needed

Equipment must be checked on a daily basis and sufficient stock levels maintained. The basic equipment needed for most patients includes:

- Portable ventilator (with adequate O_2 for the whole journey).
- Secondary O_2 supply.
- Equipment for manual ventilation:
  - Oropharyngeal airways.
  - Ambu-bag/waters circuit.
  - Face masks.
- ECG monitor.
- Pulse oximeter.
- Portable suction.
- Emergency drugs and items required for venous access.
- Infusion pumps.

Depending upon the patient's condition and aspects of care, other equipment may be needed during the transfer. It is important that any equipment needed is gathered before moving the patient, preventing any delays/disruption in the care of the patient.

Handover

Just the same as discharging a patient to a ward, when discharging to ITU a comprehensive handover of care must be provided to enable continuity of care for the individual patient.

Medical handover
- Details of cardiovascular status, including relevant history.
- Outline of treatment and reason for the need for ITU care.
- Pharmacological interventions (received and needed).
- Investigations and results.
- Immediate plan of care.

Nursing handover
- Details of patient, including admitting ward.
- Description of interventions during theatre/PACU phase.
- Re-affirm details given during medical handover regarding cardiovascular status, drugs given, fluid balance, and patient history.
- Give details of infusion pumps, drips, drains, and catheters.

Always remember to contact the admitting ward to notify them that the patient has gone to ITU. This will allow the ward staff to inform any relatives or carers of the location of the patient, but may also enable the ward bed to be utilised.

References and further reading

Association of Anaesthetists of Great Britain and Ireland (2007). *Recommendations for standards of monitoring during anaesthesia and recovery* (4th edn). Association of Anaesthetists of Great Britain and Ireland: London.

Hadfield A and Tronson M (2008). *The complete recovery room book* (4th edn). Oxford University Press: Oxford.

Overnight intensive recovery

What is it?

- Overnight intensive recovery (OIR) or surgical intensive care (SIC) is, in essence, a recovery space that is set up and staffed to provide intensive care for postoperative surgical patients over a short period of time.
- The development of an OIR service can provide a safe period of recovery time for patients who are not well enough to be returned to a ward immediately postoperatively, but may not require an extended period of time in a critical care unit.
- The utilisation of such a service can protect critical care beds for elective patients, thus reducing cancellations and preserving ITU beds for acutely ill patients.
- Most recovery units could be adapted to encompass such a service, and the set-up costs would be far less than in the development of a separate stand-alone facility.
- Each OIR bed would need 24-hour staffing and it is imperative that the OIR and ITU collaborate in care provision.
- Recovery nurses should be appropriately qualified (some with a critical care qualification), experienced, and competent to care for those patients requiring OIR, and that the service is not utilised in an inappropriate way.

Benefits

There are benefits for patients, staff, and the organisation in the utilisation of an OIR as outlined next:

The patient:

- A reduced chance of elective surgery cancellations.
- An appropriate level of care postoperatively (1:1 nurse care opposed to ward-based patient groups).
- A reduction in possible episodes of premature extubation due to lack of critical care beds.
- Appropriately trained staff to care for the patient.

Staff:

- A clear delineation of role between recovery and intensive recovery staff.
- A reduced likelihood of an over-busy unit which could have resulted in staff needing to stay on past end of shift.
- Development opportunities.
- Broader scope of practice.
- Constant nearby availability of an anaesthetist and surgeon.

Organisation:

- Reduced chance of recovery spaces being 'blocked' by ITU patients.
- Extra critical care beds for the acutely sick.
- Reduced chance of cancelled operations, resulting in lowered waiting times.
- A workforce with the appropriate skills to deliver a higher level of postoperative care.

Considerations

- Although benefits to patients, staff, and the organisation have been outlined it is important to consider the feasibility of creating and running such a service, and the possible drawbacks associated with an OIR unit.
- A major consideration is staffing and skill mix.
- An OIR unit can only be successful if it is properly resourced and the staff working there are competent and confident to care for the type of patient admitted.
- It must be viewed by the organisation and its staff as an extra facility and not simply more critical care bed space to fill.
- The criteria of patients only staying overnight (as the name suggests) or 24 hours must be rigidly adhered to.

References

Aps C (2002). Critical care for the surgical patient. *British Journal of Perioperative Nursing* **12**(7), 258–65.

Aps C (2004). Surgical critical care: the overnight intensive recovery (OIR) concept. *British Journal of Anaesthesia* **92**(2) 164–6.

Postoperative ward assessment

Postoperative patients should remain in the recovery room until conscious with stable vital signs.

On return to the ward area a *full comprehensive handover* must be received by the nurse caring for the patient from the recovery staff. This should include:
- Anaesthetic notes.
- Operation notes.
- Recovery notes.
- Full postoperative instructions.

Monitor immediately: A B C
- Airway.
- Breathing.
- Circulation.

Assess:
- The patient's colour.
- Vital signs.
- O_2 saturation levels.
- Level of consciousness.
- CVP/ECG if patient's condition requires.

The frequency of the routine observations will be determined by the nature of the surgery, the pre-disposing medical condition of the patient, and their recovery.

Observe and record:
- Drains: nature and volume of drainage.
- Wound dressings: for strike through or haemorrhage.
- NG tube: note aspirate, drainage, content, colour.
- Urinary output: >30mL/hour.
- Fluid balance: fluid replacement/blood transfusion.
- Pain management.
- O_2 therapy via nasal cannula or face mask: encourage deep breathing.

NB observe for complications:
- Nausea and vomiting.
- Pulmonary complications.
- Cardiac complications.
- Urinary complications.

The first 24 hours:
- Continue to assess, monitor, observe, and record.
- Good communication will help reduce anxiety.
- Regular pain assessment: administration of appropriate prescribed pain relief.

References
Hatfield A and Tronson M (2008). *The Complete Recovery Room Book* (4th edn). Oxford University Press: Oxford.

Perioperative pharmacology

Principles of drug action

Wide ranges of drugs are required throughout the perioperative phase, particularly within the anaesthetic and recovery room, and in some circumstances they are needed urgently. With the growth of interest in the fields of drug interaction, drug surveillance, and clinical pharmacology, knowledge of drug interactions in anaesthesia and post anaesthesia care should be a mandatory tool ensuring a high quality delivery of care to perioperative patients.[1]

The aim of drug therapy is to prevent, cure, or control various disease processes. To achieve this goal, adequate drug doses must be delivered to the target tissues so that therapeutic, yet non-toxic levels are obtained. It is essential that clinicians working in anaesthetics and recovery recognise that the speed of onset of drug action, the intensity of the drug's effect, and the duration of drug action are controlled by four fundamental pathways of drug movement and modification in the body.[1]

Pharmacology can be divided into two disciplines:
- *Pharmacokinetics*, which considers medicine disposition and the way the body affects the medicine with time, i.e. the factors that determine its absorption, distribution, metabolism, and excretion.
- *Pharmacodynamics*, which deals with the effects of the medicine on the body.

Pharmacokinetics

The pharmacokinetic phase comprises the medicine absorption, its distribution to the tissues, its biotransformation or metabolism, and its excretion from the body. Individual variations occur because of:
- Difference in body weight.
- Age.
- Diet and nutrition.
- Pathologic disease state.
- Immunopharmacology.
- Psychologic and environmental factors.
- Genetics

Plasma concentration and half-life
- For many medicines, disappearance from the plasma follows an exponential time course characterised by the plasma half-life.
- Plasma half-life, in the simple case, is directly proportional to the volume of distribution, and inversely proportional to the overall rate of clearance.
- With repeated dosages or sustained delivery of a medicine, the plasma concentration approaches a steady value within 3–5 plasma half-lives.

Reference
1. Howland RD, Mycek MJ, Harvey RA, et al. (2005). *Pharmacology* (3rd edn). Lippincott, Williams & Wilkins: London.

Further reading
Rang HP, Dale MM, Ritter JM, et al. (2007). *Rang and Dale's Pharmacology* (6th edn). Churchill Livingstone: London.

Absorption and distribution

There are four fundamental pathways of drug movement and modification in the body: absorption, distribution, metabolism, and elimination.[1]

Medicine absorption

Bioavailability takes into account both absorption and metabolism and describes the proportion of the medicine that passes into the systemic circulation. This will be 100% after IV injection, but following oral administration the following factors affect drug absorption:

- Formulation.
- Stability to acid and enzymes.
- Motility of gut.
- Food in stomach.
- Degree of first-pass metabolism.
- Lipid solubility.

Since medicines must cross membranes in order to enter cells or to transfer between body compartments, medicine absorption will be affected by both chemical and physiological factors, i.e., cell membranes, molecular size, and pH.

Distribution

Following absorption or administration into the systemic blood, a medicine distributes into interstitial and intracellular fluids.

- Cardiac output, regional blood flow, and tissue volume determine the rate of delivery and potential amount of medicine distributed into tissues.
- Initially, liver, kidneys, brain, and other well-perfused organs receive most of the drug, whereas delivery to muscle, most viscera, skin, and fat is slower.
- The second distribution phase may require several hours before the concentration of medicine in the tissues is in distribution equilibrium with that in blood. The second phase accounts for most of the extravascularly distributed medicine.

Tissue distribution is determined by partitioning of medicine between blood and the particular tissue. Lipid solubility and pH are important determinants of such uptake.

Reference

1. Howland RD, Mycek MJ, Harvey RA, et al. (2005) *Pharmacology* (3rd edn). Lippincott, Williams & Wilkins: London.

Further reading

Rang HP, Dale MM, Ritter JM, et al. (2007). *Rang and Dale's Pharmacology* (6th edn). Churchill Livingstone: London.

Metabolism and elimination

Medicine metabolism

Metabolism

Medicines are metabolised in:
- Liver (major site).
- Tissues.
- Kidney.
- Lung.
- GI tract.

The sequential metabolic reactions that occur have been categorised as:
- Phase 1 metabolic reactions including:
  - Oxidation.
  - Reduction.
  - Hydrolysis.
- Phase 2 metabolic reactions:
  - Occur in the liver.
  - Involve conjugation of the medicine.
  - Conjugates are less active and polar molecules which are readily excreted by kidney.

Factors affecting metabolism

- *Enzyme induction*: some medicines and pollutants (e.g. polycyclic aromatic hydrocarbons in tobacco smoke) increase activity of drug-metabolising enzymes (Table 22.1).
- *Enzyme inhibition:* may cause adverse drug interactions. Medicines may inhibit different forms of cytochrome P_{450} and so affect the metabolism only of medicines metabolised by that particular isoenzyme (Table 22.1). *Genetic polymorphisms:* the study of determinants that affect medicine action is called pharmacogenetics, e.g. 8% of the population have faulty expression of CYP2D6, leading to prolonged responses to medicines such as propranolol and metoprolol.
- *Age:* hepatic microsomal enzymes and renal mechanisms are reduced at birth. In the elderly, hepatic metabolism of medicines may be reduced but declining renal function important for medicine dosages.

Table 22.1 Examples of medicines that induce or inhibit medicine metabolism

Enzyme inducers	Enzyme inhibitors
Phenobarbital	Allopurinol
Rifampicin	Chloramphenicol
Phenytoin	Corticosteroids
Ethanol	Cimetidine
Carbamazepine	MAO inhibitors
	Erythromycin
	Ciprofloxacin

Elimination

Medicines are eliminated from the body either unchanged by the process of excretion (elimination) or converted to metabolites.

Excretory organs eliminate polar compounds more efficiently than substances with lipid solubility. Lipid-soluble medicines thus are not readily eliminated until they are metabolised to more polar compounds.

Excretion of medicines can occur in various ways:
- *Renal excretion:*
  - Glomerular filtration, tubular reabsorption (passive and active) and tubular secretion all determine the extent to which medicine will be excreted by the kidneys.
  - Renal disease will affect excretion of certain medicines.
- *GI excretion:*
  - Medicine conjugates excreted into bile.
  - These released into intestines.
  - Hydrolysed back to parent compound and reabsorbed.
  - This 'enterohepatic circulation' prolongs effect of the medicine.
- *Lungs* into exhaled air.
- *Medicines* may also leave body through *breast milk* and *sweat*.

Further reading

Rang HP, Dale MM, Ritter JM, *et al.* (2007). *Rang and Dale's Pharmacology* (6th edn). Churchill Livingstone: London.

Pharmacodynamics

Pharmacodynamics is the study of the biochemical and physiological effects of medicines and their mechanisms of action.

Two types of effects are delivered by medicines:
- *Primary effect*: reason for which medicine is administered.
- *Secondary effect*: side effect of the medicine that may or may not be desirable.

Time responses

A period of time after a medicine is administered until the pharmaceutical response is realised is referred to as the medicine's time response. There are three types of time responses:
- Onset: time for the minimum concentration of medicine to cause the initial pharmaceutical response.
- Peak: when the medicine reaches its highest blood or plasma concentration.
- Duration: length of time that the medicine maintains the pharmaceutical response.

All three parameters are used when administering medicines in order to determine the therapeutic range, i.e.:
- When medicine will become effective.
- When it will be most effective.
- When the medicine is no longer effective.

It also determines when a medicine is expected to reach toxic levels.

Therapeutic index and therapeutic range

The medicine's therapeutic index identifies the margin of safety of the medicine. Drugs that have a low therapeutic index have a narrow margin of safety e.g. aminoglycosides (gentamicin), anticonvulsants (carbamazepine), immunosuppresants (ciclosporin); digoxin; lithium; theophylline.

Peak and trough levels

Plasma concentrations of a medicine must be monitored for medicines that have a narrow/low therapeutic index. Therapeutic index is referred to as the ratio between the toxic dose and the therapeutic dose of a drug, used as a measure of the relative safety of the drug for a particular treatment.
- *Peak level*: highest plasma concentration at a specific time. This indicates the rate the medicine is absorbed in the body and is affected by the route of administration. Blood samples are drawn at the time of estimated peak plasma concentration based on the route of administration. Samples are usually taken 30–60 minutes after medicine administration.
- *Trough level*: lowest plasma concentration of the medicine and measures the rate at which the drug is eliminated. Blood is drawn immediately before the next dose is given.

Further reading

Rang HP, Dale MM, Ritter JM, et al. (2007). *Rang and Dale's Pharmacology* (6th edn). Churchill Livingstone: London.

Medicine response relationships

Drugs are administered by a certain route of administration, at a certain dosage, with the expectation of achieving a desired response. There are many factors that affect the time of onset, the intensity, and the duration of action of a particular drug:[1]

- The concentration of a medicine at the site of action controls the effect of the medicine although this may be non-linear.
- Whether the drug works by binding to a receptor or a chemical interaction, the dose (regardless of route) and the concentration at a cellular level will make the relationship more complex.
- The dose of any medicine should produce a sufficient response but not cause excessive adverse effects.

Dose response

Pharmacodynamics

- There is a hypothetical dose-response curve (Fig. 22.1) where the X-axis plots concentration (dose) and the Y-axis plots the response.
- This is related to potency, maximal efficacy (ceiling), and degree of response per unit dose.
- The higher the affinity for the receptor, the lower the concentration at which it produces a given level of occupancy.
- Biologic variation (age, weight, general health) will influence response.

Medicine actions

- An *agonist* is a medicine that causes a response. If various concentrations of an agonist are administered, the dose-response curve will rise as the concentration increases from low (the left) to high (the right).
- A *full agonist* (A) is a medicine that produces a full response in the tissues. A *partial agonist* provokes a less than maximum response (i.e. less than the *full agonist*).
- An *antagonist* is a medicine that does not cause a response itself but by binding to a receptor will prevent access by the natural *agonist*.

Drug response definitions[1]

- *Efficacy* refers to the maximum effect that can be produced by a drug.
- *Hyporeactivity* indicates that a person requires excessively large doses of a drug to obtain a therapeutic or desired effect.
- *Potency* refers to the dose required of a particular drug to produce an effect similar to another drug.
- *Tolerance* is a type of hyporeactivity that is acquired during chronic exposure to a drug in which unusually large doses are required to reach a desired effect.
- *Cross-tolerance* occurs when two drugs with similar actions are given to a patient who has developed tolerance to that category of drugs e.g. opiates—the amount of each drug must be increased to achieve the desired effect. An example of this is a heroin addict receiving high doses of opiates to maintain minimal analgesia.

- *Hypersensitivity* refers to a drug-induced antigen–antibody reaction. The particular hypersensitivity reaction can be either a type 1 or anaphylactic reaction or a type 4 delayed reaction.
- *Meta reactivity* is when a drug produces unusual side effects unrelated to the dosage strength. It is also referred to as an idiosyncratic reaction e.g. the occurrence of muscular-skeletal pain and increased intra-ocular pressure following the administration of suxamethonium.

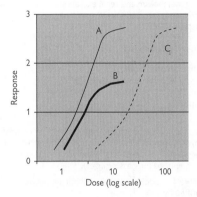

Fig. 22.1 Dose response curve: The full agonist (A) is more potent than medicine B. Medicine B is more potent than medicine C, but its maximum efficacy is lower.

Reference

1. Howland RD, Mycek MJ, Harvey RA, *et al.* (2005). *Pharmacology* (3rd edn). Lippincott, Williams & Wilkins: London.

Further reading

Rang HP, Dale MM, Ritter JM, *et al.* (2007). *Rang and Dale's Pharmacology* (6th edn). Churchill Livingstone: London.

Medicine compatibility

Refers to the possibility of interactions between active medicines and their excipients and includes:
- Chemical and alcohol interactions.
- Pharmacokinetic interactions:
  - Affecting absorption.
  - Changes in protein binding.
  - Affecting metabolism and renal excretion.
- Pharmacodynamic interactions:
  - At receptor sites.
  - Between medicines affecting the same system.
- Due to altered physiology.

IV medicine compatibility

Types of medicines administration includes:
- Continuous IV.
- Intermittent IV.
- Bolus IV.

Ideally medicines should be infused separately. Most compatibility data is based on physical compatibility. Information on reconstitution and dilution identifies the suitable diluents (e.g. water for injection etc.) and delivery systems (e.g., the need for glass syringes).

Incompatibility of a medicine and its diluent or between two medicines may be identified by:
- Change in colour of the medicine.
- Clouding of the medicine.
- Development of a haze.
- Precipitation.

pH values

- pH values help predict possible physical incompatibility among medicines where no compatibility data exists.
- It is not advisable to co-administer medicines with divergent pH values as this can lead to precipitation or inactivation of either or both medicines.

References

Rang HP, Dale MM, Ritter JM, et al. (2007). *Rang and Dale's Pharmacology* (6th edn). Churchill Livingstone: London.

Common medicine problems

Medication related adverse events can be minimised by adhering to the five 'Rs' of safe medicine administration:
• *Right* patient.
• *Right* medicine.
• *Right* dose/amount.
• *Right* route—epidural, IT, IV.
• *Right* frequency.

Adverse reactions

Sensitivity

Previous exposure to a medicine or a similar medicine may result in the formation of antibodies. On subsequent administration these antibodies react with the medicine (the allergen) and initiate an allergic reaction by the release of chemicals such as histamine. Sensitivity may manifest as:
• Urticaria.
• Pruritus.

Allergic emergency (anaphylactic shock)

A severe reaction to an allergen that may manifest itself as a rash, swollen tongue or throat, respiratory distress, shock, pallor, or cyanosis and may lead to a cardiac arrest. Treatment for anaphylaxis includes:
• Airway management.
• Adrenaline (epinephrine) IM stat which may need to be repeated

📖 See Types of shock, p.558 for practical guidance.

Idiosyncrasy

• An abnormal reaction owing to a genetic abnormality, e.g. the lack of the enzyme cholinesterase prolongs the action of the muscle relaxant suxamethonium.

Adverse events related to injected medicines

Inappropriate site selection and poor technique may result in:
• Pain.
• Nerve injury.
• Bleeding.
• Abscess formation.

Tolerance, dependence, addiction, and withdrawal

Tolerance

Diminished response to the same dose of the same medicine taken on a regular basis. Often seen with opioids (e.g. morphine and diamorphine) where dose escalation is needed on a regular basis.

Dependence

• Psychological: intense mental cravings occur if the medicine is unavailable or withdrawn.
• Physical: a person is dependent on taking the medicine to achieve everyday functions (activities of daily living) or an endpoint. Abrupt cessation of the medicine would lead to withdrawal within 8 hours that may last for 7 days.

Addiction

Addiction is defined as compulsive drug seeking behaviour that results from recurring drug intoxification.

Withdrawal

- Signs and symptoms include, but are not limited to:
- Restlessness.
- Runny nose and sweating.
- Aggressive behaviour and restless sleep.
- Backache and muscle spasm.
- Hypertension and hypotension.
- Nausea, vomiting, and diarrhoea.

Dose adjustment

It may be necessary to adjust the dose in some populations for some medicines. Therefore it might be necessary to check the following prior to administration:

- Infants and children—age and weight.
- Pregnancy status.
- Breastfeeding status.
- Presence of hepatic or renal disease.

The older person has undergone physical changes, such as an alteration in body fat content, therefore dose adjustment may be necessary. Since the older person usually takes more medicines, this increases the risk of adverse effects and interactions.

Further reading

Rang HP, Dale MM, Ritter JM, et al. (2007). *Rang and Dale's Pharmacology* (6th edn). Churchill Livingstone: London.

Suspected adverse reactions

This is an unwanted effect of the medicine and is also known as an adverse effect or side effect (see Box 22.1). Since medicines are distributed throughout the body their actions are unlikely to be restricted to a single organ or tissue.

Box 22.1 Yellow card system

Suspected adverse reactions to any medicine or therapeutic agent should be reported using the yellow card system to:

Medicines and Healthcare Products Regulatory Agency
CSM
Freepost
London
SW8 5BR

or at 🖵 www.yellowcard.gov.uk

The yellow card system may be used by all health professionals and patients. Yellow cards may be found in the back of each BNF.

Suspected adverse reactions

Adverse event
An adverse event refers to any untoward occurrence in a patient to whom a medicine has been given. This includes occurrences which are not necessarily caused by, or related to, the medicine.

Adverse reaction
An adverse reaction refers to any untoward and unintended response in a patient which is related to any dose of a medicine that has been administered.

Unexpected adverse reaction
This is known to be an adverse reaction that is 'unexpected' if its nature and severity are not consistent with the information about the medicine found in the summary of product characteristics.

Serious adverse reaction/event
An adverse reaction is 'serious' if it:
- Results in death.
- Is life threatening.
- Requires prolongation of existing hospitalisation.
- Results in persistent or significant disability or incapacity.

Suspected serious adverse reaction (SSAR)
Any adverse reaction that is classed as serious and which is consistent with the information listed in the summary of product characteristics (SPC).

Suspected unexpected serious adverse reaction (SUSARs)
Any adverse reaction that is classed as serious and is suspected to be caused by a medicine that is **not** consistent with the information in the SPC.

Risk of adverse reactions

This may be reduced by:
- Checking sensitivities and allergies.
- Checking use of herbal remedies and supplements.
- Do not use the medicine unless there is a good indication.
- Use as few medicines as possible.
- Dose adjustment may be needed in patients with extremes of age or who have hepatic or renal impairment.

Types of adverse reactions

These vary in intensity. Clinically relevant side-effects of all licensed medicines are listed in the BNF.

Examples of side effects and associated medicines include:
- Nausea and vomiting, e.g. opioids especially tramadol.
- Constipation, e.g. $5HT_3$ antagonists, strong opioids.
- Ulceration of the oral mucosa, e.g. NSAIDs, chemotherapy.
- Teeth staining, e.g. chlorhexidine.
- Dry mouth, e.g. opioids.
- Extrapyramidal effects, e.g. metoclopramide.
- Rashes.
- Drowsiness, e.g. opioids.
- GI side effects including discomfort, bleeding and ulceration NSAIDs.
- Hypersensitivity reactions, e.g. aspirin.
- Renal failure, e.g. NSAIDs.

Further reading

Rang HP, Dale MM, Ritter JM, *et al.* (2007). *Rang and Dale's Pharmacology* (6th edn). Churchill Livingstone: London.

Routes of medicine administration

'The route of drug administration is determined primarily by the properties of the drug such as water or lipid solubility and ionisation, and by the therapeutic objectives which is the desirability of a rapid onset of action or the need for long term administration or restriction to a local site.'[1]

See Fig. 22.2 for examples of medicine administration routes.

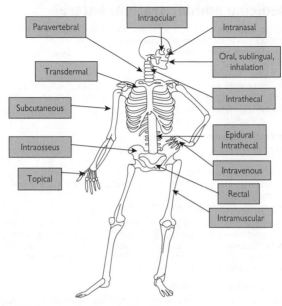

Fig. 22.2 Examples of medicine administration routes.

Reference

1. Howland RD, Mycek MJ, Harvey RA, *et al.* (2005). *Pharmacology* (3rd edn). Lippincott, Williams & Wilkins: London.

Medicine administration: enteral

The administration of medicines can be achieved by a variety of routes but there are two major routes of drug administration:
- Enteral drug administration.
- Parenteral drug administration.

> Enteral pertains to the intestinal tract and is commonly used to mean medicines administered by the oral route (including via NG or nasojejeunal tubes) and rectal routes.

Enteral drug administration

Enteral drug administration includes drugs given by the following routes:
- Oral, e.g. tablets, capsules, linctus.
- Sublingual, e.g. tablets, sprays.
- Buccal, e.g. mucosal linings of the nasal, rectal, vaginal, ocular, and oral cavity.
- Rectal, e.g. enemas, suppositories, creams.

The enteral (oral) route is preferred wherever possible as it is the simplest, most convenient, and usually cheapest route. The choice of route will be dependent upon the patient's tolerability and the pharmacodynamics (what the drug does to the body) and pharmacokinetics (what the body does to the drug) of the medicine.

Oral drug administration

Oral preparations are those which are administered via the mouth and subsequently swallowed. This is the preferred route in patients able to tolerate oral fluids. Absorption of medicines from this route usually occurs in the small intestine and is dependent upon:
- The formulation of the medicine as this will affect the disintegration and dissolution of tablets or capsules—plain versus coated, drug particle size.
- Stomach contents.
- Gastric motility.
- Splanchnic blood flow—gut perfusion.

The absorption process can also be affected by the alteration of the gastric volume and pH caused by preoperative drugs or anaesthesia and surgery.

Regular oral paracetamol reduces opioid requirements thus reducing the incidence of opioid induced side-effects. Other drugs that may be given by the oral route include NSAIDs, immediate release opioids and antiemetics (cyclizine, ondansetron, granisetron). The oral route is contraindicated for patients experiencing nausea and vomiting or who have delayed gastric emptying.

The choice of analgesic agent requires careful thought if there is some evidence of impaired renal function. Dose reduction may be necessary in some patients as drug and active metabolite may accumulate. Codeine, dihydrocodeine, and morphine should be avoided in patients with renal dysfunction. Fentanyl and oxycodone should be used in preference.

Modified release strong opioids are contraindicated in the first postoperative 24 hours because of the risk of dumping secondary to delayed gastric emptying. Oral pethidine should be avoided due to the accumulation of the metabolite *norpethidine* which is toxic.

Oral drugs given in recovery have some distinct disadvantages; nausea and vomiting may occur which reduces the amount of the drug available for absorption by the small intestine.[1] Oral drugs given orally in recovery include paracetamol, tramadol, codeine, and morphine sulfate solution.

Box 22.2 First-pass metabolism

Once a drug has been absorbed from the gut it must pass through the liver (where it may be metabolised) before reaching the systemic circulation. Some drugs are almost completely metabolised during this time. These medicines (such as naloxone) are said to undergo complete first-pass metabolism thus making them unsuitable for oral administration. First-pass metabolism varies between individuals.

Medicine administration: transmucosal (buccal and sublingual)

Sublingual drug administration

- The medicine is placed under the tongue which avoids first-pass metabolism and allows for rapid absorption
- The most commonly used sublingual analgesic is buprenorphine (which should be used with caution as it is a partial opioid agonist and can displace more effective opioids from their receptor sites).
- The sublingual route allows the drug to diffuse into the capillary network and therefore to enter the systemic circulation directly
- Administration of a drug by this route means that the drug bypasses the intestine and liver and is not inactivated by first-pass metabolism.[1]
- Drugs such as nifedipine, glyceryl trinitrate, and buprenorphine are given sublingually.
- Both the sublingual and the rectal routes of administration have the additional advantage that they prevent the destruction of the drug by intestinal enzymes or by low pH in the stomach.[1]

Rectal drug administration

- This route of administration relies on passive diffusion like medicines in the upper GI tract.
- Medicines are usually given in the form of a fatty suppository which facilitates transport of the drug to the rectal fluid.
- The rectum has a good blood supply but venous drainage occurs into both the portal (mostly the upper part of the rectum) and systemic (the lower part of the rectum) circulations.
- Due to individual variations in rectal venous drainage an unpredictable proportion of an absorbed drug will escape first-pass metabolism.
- Therefore a suppository (e.g. diclofenac) placed low in the rectum will have a higher proportion of its drug delivered directly to the systemic circulation.
- Patient consent is required for the administration of rectal medicines.
- Rectal medicines (e.g. paracetamol) are often available in a variety of doses for infant, child, and adult use.
- The rectal route is useful if a drug induces vomiting when given orally or if the patient is already vomiting. Drugs given rectally include diclofenac, paracetamol, metronidazole, and occasionally antiemetics.

Buccal drug administration

The medicine is placed between the upper lip and lining of the upper gum and left in place where it forms a gel. The drug is absorbed transmucosally into the systemic circulation, thus bypassing first-pass metabolism. Rapid absorption can be achieved if medicines are lipophilic (fat soluble) e.g. fentanyl. Prochlorperazine is available in a buccal preparation for the treatment of nausea and vomiting. This is a useful route for patients who are unable to tolerate oral medicines (NBM) but should be used with caution in patients who have oral ulceration (e.g. post-chemotherapy).

Transmucosal

The medicine is absorbed through the oral mucosa rather than swallowed. Fentanyl is available as a lozenge which is 'painted' onto all surfaces of the mouth and tongue over a 10–15-minute period. This route is useful for managing procedural and breakthrough cancer pain but should be avoided in patients with a dry mouth or who have mucosal ulceration. It is anticipated that a buccal fentanyl preparation will be available in the near future.

References and further reading

1. Howland RD, Mycek MJ, Harvey RA, *et al.* (2005). *Pharmacology* (3rd edn). Lippincott, Williams & Wilkins: London.

Dougherty L and Lister S (2008). The Royal Marsden Hospital Manual of Clinical Nursing Procedures (7th edn) Wiley Blackwell: Oxford.

Hatfield A and Tronson M (2008). *The Complete Recovery Room Book* (4th edn). Oxford University Press: Oxford.

Parenteral drug administration: 1

Parenteral refers to the administration of medicines other than via the GI tract.

- Parenteral drug administration is used for drugs that are poorly absorbed from the GI tract and for agents such as insulin that are unstable in the GI tract.[1]
- Parenteral administration is used perioperatively in unconscious patients and under circumstances that require a rapid onset of action.
- It provides the most control over the actual dose of the drug delivered to the body.
- The three major parenteral routes most commonly used within the perioperative environment include:
  - IV.
  - IM.
  - SC.

IV drug administration

The administration of medicines via the IV route allows rapid therapeutic blood levels as the drug is delivered directly into the systemic circulation, bypassing the first-pass metabolism.

The IV route is commonly used for the bolus administration of analgesia in the recovery room and for continuing postoperative opioid PCA. Repeated bolus administration or a continuous infusion results in steady plasma analgesic concentrations within the 'therapeutic window' (see Fig. 22.3).

This route is suitable for most patients (including paediatrics and the elderly) but should be used with expert input in the known or suspected drug user. Examples of drugs given intravenously in the perioperative environment include:
- Anaesthetic induction agents.
- Muscle relaxants.
- Opiates *and* antagonists.
- Antiemetics.
- Antibiotics.
- Resuscitation drugs.
- Reversal agents *and* respiratory stimulants.

Commonly administered IV analgesics include:
- Morphine.
- Fentanyl.
- Remifentanil.
- Oxycodone.
- Paracetamol.
- Parecoxib—a selective COX-2 inhibitor.

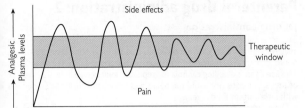

Fig. 22.3 Achievement of analgesic therapeutic window by repeat bolus administration.

Reference

1. Howland RD, Mycek MJ, Harvey RA, *et al.* (2005). *Pharmacology* (3rd edn). Lippincott, Williams & Wilkins: London.

Parenteral drug administration: 2

IM drug administration

The intermittent delivery of drugs into muscular tissues for continuing analgesia after surgery is out of vogue due to local complications—pain, nerve damage, haematoma formation, and scarring (also see Box 22.3). The use of an indwelling cannula for repeated injections can lessen the risk of these, but does not avoid the peaks and troughs of analgesia associated with intermittent IM delivery.

- Drugs administered via the IM route are absorbed relatively slowly into the bloodstream.
- It reaches quite a high peak level and then declines over the next 2–3 hours. This means that pain relief is slow, and lasts a short time.
- The result is a pattern of severe pain, injection, side effects, and short-lived analgesia.
- IM drug administration in the perioperative environment is now uncommon with the exception of anti-D which is given to patients following and evacuation of retained products of conception (ERPC). This is very often administered in theatre when the patient is still un/semi conscious.
- IM drug administration also requires absorption and is slower than the IV route.
- It requires simple diffusion from the site of injection into the systemic circulation.
- It does not provide a reliable rate of systemic absorption.

Box 22.3 Warning!

'A drug administered by IM or SC injection to a patient who is hypothermic will probably not achieve the desired effect as hypothermia causes vasoconstriction. When a patient is re-warmed, the drug can be rapidly liberated from the injection site, causing large concentrations of the drug into the systemic circulation. This can be dangerous especially when opiates are administered.'[1]

SC

A hypodermic needle is used to deliver drugs under the horny keratinous layer of the skin. Administration may be intermittent or continuous. Used commonly in palliative care for symptom control the SC route is sometimes used for acute pain when patients are unable to take oral preparations. An indwelling butterfly cannula may be used. If swelling or a local reaction occurs the cannula site will need rotation. PCA can be administered by this route.

Commonly used SC medicines include:
- Oxycodone.
- Diamorphine.
- Cyclizine.
- Heparin.
- Insulin.

Reference

1. Howland RD, Mycek MJ, Harvey RA, *et al.* (2005). *Pharmacology* (3rd edn). Lippincott, Williams & Wilkins: London.

Further reading

Dougherty L and Lister S (2008). *The Royal Marsden Hospital Manual of Clinical Nursing Procedures* (7th edn) Blackwell Publishing: Oxford.

Hatfield A and Tronson M (2008). *The Complete Recovery Room Book* (4th edn). Oxford University Press: Oxford.

Neuraxial analgesia

Neuraxial analgesia refers to the administration of medicines into the epidural (peridural, extradural) or intrathecal (subarachnoid, spinal) spaces to provide relief from pain.

The vertebral column consists of 7 cervical, 12 thoracic, and 5 lumbar vertebrae together with the sacrum and the coccyx. The spinal cord lies in a protective tunnel within the vertebral column and is surrounded by 3 layers of membrane (also known as meninges): the dura mater (on the outside), the arachnoid mater (middle layer), and the pia mater (inside layer).

Epidural analgesia

Indications:
- Management of postoperative pain.
- Management of the pain of labour.
- Amelioration of the stress response to surgery.

Contraindications to epidural analgesia:
- Central or spinal neurological disease.
- Systemic sepsis or local (in the region of the catheter) sepsis.
- Coagulation disorders, e.g. haemophilia, von Willebrand's disease.
- Severe hypovolaemia.

Precautions with epidural analgesia
- Patients receiving LMWH thromboprophylaxis:
  - The smallest dose should be administered.
  - LMWH therapy should be delayed as long as possible for at least 12–24 hours postoperatively.
- Patients receiving treatment doses of heparin.
- Patients receiving anti-platelet therapy: anti-platelet or oral anticoagulant medications should not be given in combination with LMWH due to increased risk of spinal haematoma.
- Patients receiving oral anticoagulation, e.g. warfarin.
- Presence of a dural puncture.

Identifying the epidural space
The epidural space lies outside the protective dural membrane. It is a potential space composed of fat, nerves, lymph tissue, and blood vessels. The most common way to identify the epidural space is the loss of resistance (LOR) to saline technique. The epidural catheter is advanced through the internal lumen of the Tuohy needle until 3–5cm of catheter is in the epidural space. The needle is then withdrawn leaving the catheter in situ. The catheter is connected to a bacterial and particulate filter and is affixed to the skin using a clear occlusive dressing.

Medicines used in epidural analgesia
Most commonly two types of drugs are used to provide epidural analgesia: local anaesthetics and opioids. A combination of both produces a synergistic effect thus reducing the required dose of each. It is recommended that these infusions are commercially prepared and that a limited number of combinations are provided to reduce confusion. The specific drugs

and concentrations should be clearly stated in local protocols and on the epidural prescription. An example would be levobupivacaine 0.125% + fentanyl 4mcg/mL 0-12mL/hour.

Local anaesthetics
- Reversibly block the sodium channels of nerve cell membranes thus inhibiting nerve conduction.
- Amide local anaesthetics with a long duration of action are used in preference.
- Ropivacaine and levobupivacaine are recommended in preference to bupivacaine as they are considered to be less cardiotoxic.

Local anaesthetic effects include:
- Sympathetic blockade (resulting in vasodilatation) which may unmask hypovolaemia.
- A high, low, or patchy block.
- Urinary retention.
- Reduction in the stress response.
- Local anaesthetic toxicity.

Opioids
- Bind to opioid receptors in the substantia gelatinosa in the dorsal horn of the spinal cord and in the brain.
- Lipophilic (fat soluble) opioids, e.g. fentanyl is most commonly used but has a short duration of action.
- Lipophilicity determines the onset and duration of action but lipophilic drugs need to be delivered close to the incision.

Opioid effects include:
- Pruritus.
- Nausea and vomiting.
- Drowsiness which may lead to over sedation.
- Urinary retention.

Rarely a patient may experience back pain and a change in sensation in limb sensation and motor function. An epidural haematoma or abscess must be ruled out by the use of MRI imaging.

IT analgesia
- The IT space lies beneath the dura and contains the spinal cord and nerve roots which are bathed in CSF.
- The indications and precautions of spinal analgesia are similar to that for epidurals.
- Opioids are most commonly used as a single dose.
- Opioids IV infusions can be used for postoperative analgesia.
- Doses are small and a single dose of preservative-free morphine 0.5mg may provide analgesia for 24 hours.

References and further reading

Howland RD, Mycek MJ, Harvey RA, *et al.* (2005). *Pharmacology* (3rd edn). Lippincott, Williams & Wilkins: London.

Rang HP, Dale MM, Ritter JM, *et al.* (2007). *Rang and Dale's Pharmacology* (6th edn). Churchill Livingstone: London.

Respiratory medicines administration

Refers to the administration of medicines via the respiratory tract and includes:
• Inhalation.
• Intranasal.
• Intratracheal.

> **Box 22.4 Indications for respiratory medicines administration**
>
> These are unclear and under investigation. However, these routes have the advantage of avoiding first-pass metabolism.
>
> The factors that must be considered for these routes include:
> • Medicine absorption and bioavailability.
> • Speed of onset of analgesia, efficacy.
>
> Duration of action and side effects—both systemic and related to the route of administration.

Intranasal

The nasal mucosa is very vascular and permits rapid absorption of drugs into the bloodstream. The maximum volume that can be administered by this route is limited to 150 microlitres. Medicines that are lipophilic are preferred.

Any swallowed component will be absorbed from the stomach or small intestine and be subject to first-pass metabolism. Some medicines have a bitter taste.

Medicines include:
• Sufentanil—pre-medication and PCA for postoperative pain.
• Fentanyl.
• Alfentanil.

Pulmonary

Medicines are delivered as a nebulised aerosol. Absorption is dependant on the size of the molecule which should be <20 micron to be absorbed. New drug delivery systems increase the bioavailability of opioids up to 100%.
Medicines include:
• Morphine.
• Fentanyl.
• Diamorphine.

Intratracheal route

Suitable for the administration of lipid-soluble drugs only, including lidocaine, adrenaline (epinephrine) atropine, and naloxone (which has the mnemonic 'LEAN'). The drug must be diluted up to 5mL to aid absorption.

Indications

Resuscitation in patients with no IV access. Five adequate tidal breaths must be given after medicine administration.

Inhalational drug administration

- Inhalation provides the rapid delivery of a drug across the large surface area of the mucous membranes of the respiratory tract and pulmonary epithelium.[1]
- It produces an effect almost as quickly as IV injection.
- This route is used for drugs that are gases or those that can be expelled in an aerosol.
- It is effective for patients with respiratory complaints such as asthma or COPD.
- Inhalation drugs are delivered directly to the site of action and systemic side effects are minimised. Drugs commonly used in the perioperative environment include:
  - Anaesthetic volatile agents.
  - Bronchodilators.
  - O_2.
  - N_2O.
  - Entonox.

References and further reading

1. Howland RD, Mycek MJ, Harvey RA, et al. (2005). *Pharmacology* (3rd edn). Lippincott, Williams & Wilkins: London.

Dougherty L and Lister S (2008). The Royal Marsden Hospital Manual of Clinical Nursing Procedures (7th edn) Blackwell Publishing: Oxford.

Hatfield A and Tronson M (2008). *The Complete Recovery Room Book* (4th edn). Oxford University Press: Oxford.

Rang HP, Dale MM, Ritter JM, et al. (2007). *Rang and Dale's Pharmacology* (6th edn). Churchill Livingstone: London.

Topical analgesia

Topical refers to the transdermal administration of medicines and includes local anaesthetics and opioids e.g. buprenorphine and fentanyl. Both have a low molecular weight, are lipophilic and avoid first pass metabolism as they are taken up directly into the systemic circulation.

Indications
The management of pain including:
- Pre-emptive e.g. the application of EMLA at least 60 minutes prior to cannulation or 10 minutes prior to ablation of genital warts.
- Treatment e.g. severe opioid responsive pain.

Contraindications/precautions for transdermal opioids
Management of acute postoperative pain in an opioid naïve patient. This is because of:
- The lack of opportunity for dosage titration in the short term.
- Possibility of significant respiratory depression.
- Products are unlicensed for postoperative pain
- The elderly.
- Patients with renal or hepatic dysfunction.

Medicines
Local anaesthetics
- Lidocaine (lignocaine) e.g. Versatis® 5% medicated plaster licensed for post-herpetic neuralgia but may be useful for acute neuropathic pain but must not be applied to wounds.
- EMLA® cream 5% is a mix of lidocaine 2.5% and prilocaine 2.5% and should be applied under an occlusive dressing for most uses. It has been used to provide analgesia for split skin grafting.

Opioids
Buprenophine is available in two transdermal matrix presentations neither of which is licensed for postoperative pain:

BuTrans® (5mcg/hour, 10mcg/hour, 20mcg/hour)
- Treatment for severe opioid responsive pain conditions which are not adequately responding to non-opioid analgesics.
- The patch should be changed every 7 days.

Transtec® (35mcg/hour, 52.5mcg/hour, 70mcg/hour)
- Licensed for moderate to severe cancer pain and severe pain not responding to non-opioid analgesics.
- Not suitable for acute pain.
- The patch should be changed twice weekly.

Fentanyl is available as both a reservoir and matrix patch which should not be interchanged. They are indicated for the treatment of chronic intractable pain only and are contra-indicated in acute pain because of the lack of opportunity for dosage titration in the short term and the resultant possibility of significant respiratory depression.

Iontophoresis

- An iontophoretic fentanyl patch is currently being investigated for PCA use for acute postoperative pain.
- Iontophoresis is the facilitated movement of ions across a membrane under the influence of an externally applied, small electrical potential difference.
- The technology has been successfully applied to the delivery of a number of medicines with poor absorption profiles across the skin (including fentanyl). Absorption into the systemic circulation is achieved without delay.
- The passage of ionised medicines through the epidermis and particularly the stratum corneum of the epidermis is limited and slow. Opioid medicines such as fentanyl are usually highly ionised.
- This system could enable the patient to control the frequency of administration of the programmed dose without the need for a cannula or bulky PCA device (□ see Patient-controlled analgesia, p.466).

References and further reading

Howland RD, Mycek MJ, Harvey RA, et al. (2005). Pharmacology (3rd edn). Lippincott, Williams & Wilkins: London.

Rang HP, Dale MM, Ritter JM, et al. (2007). Rang and Dale's Pharmacology (6th edn). Churchill Livingstone: London.

Patient-controlled analgesia

PCA is defined as the administration of analgesia (usually opioids) by a patient to manage pain. Although PCA delivery may occur by a variety of routes e.g. epidural, it usually refers to the IV route.

IV opioid PCA

Indications
The management of acute pain including:
- Acute, e.g. sickle cell crisis.
- Postoperative.
- Procedural, e.g. dressing changes.

Contraindications/precautions for opioid PCA
- The possibility of significant respiratory depression if additional opioids are administered by a different route.
- Products are unlicensed for postoperative pain.
- The elderly.
- Patients with renal or hepatic dysfunction.

Epidural PCA

Epidural PCA combines the benefits of a continuous epidural with the advantage of the patient being in control.

Indication
The management of acute postoperative pain.

Contraindications/precautions to epidural PCA
- Central or spinal neurological disease.
- Systemic sepsis or local (in the region of the catheter) sepsis.
- Coagulation disorders, e.g. haemophilia, von Willebrand's disease.
- Severe hypovolaemia.

Advantages
- Patient controlled.
- Improved patient satisfaction.
- Synergistic effect of low dose opioid and local anaesthetic.

Box 22.5 PCA terminology

- *Loading dose:* a single dose usually administered intraoperatively or in the recovery room before PCA maintenance therapy is commenced.
- *Bolus dose:* the amount of drug a patient receives when they press the demand button. This is measured in mg or mcg.
- *Background infusion:* a continuous infusion of analgesic that may be administered concurrently through the PCA.
- *Lockout time:* a pre-determined time when the PCA device will not deliver a dose if requested. Range 4–10 minutes
- *4-hour limit:* offers the possibility to pre-set a maximum amount of PCA that a patient may receive in any 4-hour period.

Table 22.2 PCA examples

PCA examples	Bolus dose	Lockout time	Comments
Morphine:	1 mg	5 minutes	Gold standard
100mg in 100mL NaCl 0.9%			Metabolites may accumulate
Fentanyl:	10mcg	3–5 minutes	
1000 mcg in 100mL NaCl 0.9%		No metabolites	
Oxycodone:	2–3 mg	5 minutes	
200mg in 100mL NaCl 0.9%			No metabolites

Further reading

Howland RD, Mycek MJ, Harvey RA, *et al.* (2005). *Pharmacology* (3rd edn). Lippincott, Williams & Wilkins: London.

Rang HP, Dale MM, Ritter JM, *et al.* (2007). *Rang and Dale's Pharmacology* (6th edn). Churchill Livingstone: London.

Pain management

Acute pain

The principles of acute pain management

Pain is a subjective experience and we are reliant upon patients to report their experience. There is no objective measure. Acute pain can be defined as pain that occurs as a result of an injury and lasts for <3 months. The pain is predominantly nociceptive and self-limiting.

Acute pain management should aim to:
- Improve the patient journey and reduce hospital length of stay.
- Provide evidence-based relief from pain.
- Minimise or effectively treat analgesia-related side effects.
- Minimise the risk of complications from immobility.
- Facilitate early discharge.
- Reduce the risk of persistent pain after surgery.

Pain assessment (Box 23.1)

Pain assessment is fundamental to managing pain effectively and the patient's report should be believed. It may be performed using a uni-dimensional (e.g. numerical rating scale or Wong-Baker FACES of pain scale) or multi-dimensional pain assessment tool (e.g. Brief Pain Inventory, McGill Pain Questionnaire).

> **Box 23.1 Use a structured approach to basic pain assessment**
>
> - Location—where is it, does it radiate?
> - Pattern—is it continuous, intermittent or brief?
> - Intensity—how strong is it? See numerical rating scale (Fig. 23.1).
> - Onset—when did it start?
> - Triggers—what makes it worse?
> - Relievers—what makes it better, what has worked in the past?

Pain should be assessed and recorded as the 5th vital sign
- On arrival in recovery and at regular intervals—e.g. every 15 minutes.
- After every pain relieving intervention.
- On the ward—minimum 4-hourly.
- Until discharge from hospital.

Unidimensional pain assessment (pain intensity)
- As a minimum pain intensity may be assessed and recorded. This may take the form of the use of numbers, text or a combination of both (Fig. 23.1). If patients are pre-verbal or are cognitively impaired an alternative would be to use a pain assessment tool with faces that indicate pain intensity.

Multi-dimensional pain assessment tools
- The British Pain Society provides open access to assessment tools in a variety of languages and scripts on its website.[1]

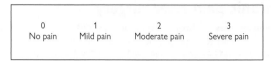

0	1	2	3
No pain	Mild pain	Moderate pain	Severe pain

Fig. 23.1 A numerical rating scale with intensity descriptors.

Pain ladder

The WHO devised the original pain ladder over 30 years ago for cancer pain but this has been adapted for acute pain and is widely used. If an analgesic or analgesic combination results in inadequate analgesia (pain persists or increases) the prescriber should move up the ladder (Fig. 23.2).

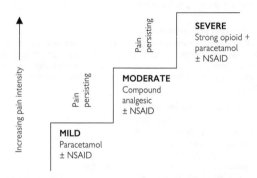

Fig. 23.2 An adaptation of the WHO analgesic ladder. NSAID, non-steroidal anti-inflammatory drug; compound analgesic, mixture of paracetamol + a mild opioid (e.g. codeine or dihydrocodeine).

Reference

British Pain Society. Available at: 🖳 www.britishpainscoiety.org

Chronic pain after surgery

The principles of chronic pain management

These are similar to those for acute pain management. The prevalence of chronic pain after surgery is widely underestimated. Pain that persists for >3 months is described as chronic. Some potential causes of chronicity are listed in Box 23.2. There is scant evidence for the use of pre-emptive analgesia in humans.

> **Box 23.2 Causes of chronic pain after surgery**
> - Unrelieved (poorly managed) acute pain.
> - Certain forms of surgical exposure or surgery e.g. thoracotomy, inguinal hernia repair, amputation, mastectomy.
> - Pre-existing chronic painful conditions.

Multi-dimensional pain assessment

Patients with chronic pain or at risk for chronicity require multi-dimensional pain assessment noting the words used to describe the pain (descriptors) as shown in Table 23.1. This will identify patients experiencing persistent post-acute (nociceptive) rather than neuropathic pain which results from nerve injury.

Diagnosis of neuropathic pain

- Pain history to ascertain underlying cause.
- Examination especially skin changes.
- MRI imaging for central lesions.
- Diagnostic local anaesthetic blocks.
- Electrophysiological studies e.g. nerve conduction.
- Sural nerve biopsy where involved.

Treatment options for neuropathic pain

Pharmacological

- Topical agents e.g. lidocaine plasters, capsaicin cream.
- Opioids e.g. tramadol, oxycodone—neuropathic pain is only partially responsive to opioids.
- Anticonvulsants e.g. pregabalin, carbamazepine.
- Tricyclic antidepressants e.g. amitriptyline, nortriptyline, dosulepin.
- NMDA receptor antagonists e.g. ketamine.
- Membrane stabilisers e.g. lidocaine.

Interventional

- Cognitive behavioural therapy (CBT).
- Transcutaneous electrical nerve stimulation (TENS).
- Acupuncture.
- Massage.
- Exercise.
- Trigger point injections with local anaesthetic.
- Regional blockade e.g. intercostal nerve block with local anaesthetic or neurolysis with alcohol or phenol.
- Radiofrequency ablation of nerve root.

- Neuraxial blockade.
- Spinal cord (dorsal horn) stimulation.

Table 23.1 Characteristics of acute nociceptive and neuropathic pain

Acute nociceptive (<3 months)	Neuropathic (any duration)
• Sharp	• Numb
• Stabbing	• Pins and needles
• Lancinating	• Burning
• Splitting	• Pricking
	• Stinging
	• Shooting

Non-pharmacological pain management

Non-pharmacological approaches to managing pain includes but is not limited to CBT, acupuncture, TENS, aromatherapy, and hypnotism. The combination of pharmacological (medicines) and non-pharmacological strategies is often more successful than a single strategy.

CBT

CBT is a biopsychosocial approach to pain management based on behavioural and cognitive theories which can help patients manage their pain more effectively. Psychologists commonly use this technique for patients with chronic painful conditions (e.g. back pain, sickle cell anaemia).

Cognitive theory

The principle of this theory is that early experiences shape our core beliefs from which we develop rules for life (assumptions).

Behavioural theory

This theory consists of two principles;
- Classical conditioning such as a response initiated by a stimulus—Pavlov's dogs.
- Operant conditioning where a behaviour results in a reward.

Acupuncture

This technique involves piercing the skin with fine metal needles in order to relieve symptoms, cure disease, and promote health. Two main contemporary approaches to acupuncture exist in UK practice.

Traditional Chinese

This complex system results from the influence of a number of philosophies and concepts including *Yin & Yang* and *Qi* (life energy or vital force). Needling points along *Qi* meridians can exert a therapeutic effect.

Western Medical approach

This approach requires an orthodox clinical diagnosis with points chosen on neurophysiological principles. This includes the needling of trigger points and segmental needling.

TENS

TENS is the safe application of electrical current from a hand-held generator via self-adhesive electrodes through intact skin to activate nerve fibres in tissues underneath the electrodes. This current produces physiological actions that lead to relief from pain. TENS can also be used to reduce postoperative nausea and vomiting and post-surgical symptoms.

Aromatherapy

This approach uses plant-derived essential oils to enhance physical and psychological well being.

Lavender oil

Patients in recovery who received lavender oil therapy expressed greater satisfaction with pain management and had a reduced opioid consumption.

Peppermint oil
Patients received peppermint oil had less intense postoperative nausea and vomiting.

Hypnotism

The power of suggestion is one of the oldest therapeutic tools. Hypnosis can be defined as the induction of a subjective state in which perception or memory can be elicited by suggestion.

Breast surgery
The combination of analgesia and preoperative hypnosis has been shown to provide superior analgesia and reduced fatigue, discomfort, and nausea in patients scheduled for breast surgery.

Oral and maxillofacial surgery
Adult patients who received intraoperative hypnosis during oral and maxillofacial surgery under local anaesthesia expressed greater postoperative satisfaction.

Children
Children can be easier to hypnotise than adults. Hypnotism has been successfully used for procedural pain associated with bone marrow aspiration and lumbar puncture.

Role of the pain management service

The development of the majority of Acute Pain Services in the UK was stimulated by the publication of the report by the RCoA and the Faculty of Anaesthetists in 1990.

An effective PMS will:

Be multidisciplinary with input from;
- Nurses.
- ODPs.
- Recovery staff.
- Anaesthetists.
- Surgeons.
- Physiotherapists.
- Pharmacists.
- Psychologists and
- Patients.

Educate:
- Patients and carers with information about the choices, risks, and benefits of different perioperative pain management techniques.
- Provide targeted education to all members of the multidisciplinary team to meet specific needs including:
  - Sessions on the principles of pain assessment, physiology, pharmacology, and the management of analgesia-related side effects.
  - Study days that focus on acute and chronic pain.
  - Epidural study days for staff involved in the care of patients receiving epidural analgesia; attendance is mandatory and competency must be assessed and recorded; an update session is essential at least every 3 years.

Advise:
Provide staff with an expert opinion on the biopsychosocial management of pain in individual patients.

Modernise:
Ensure prompt access to modern, standardised:
- Equipment—including infusion devices and administration sets.
- Infusions—opioid and local anaesthetics.
- Labels.
- Guidelines, protocols, and policies.

Measure quality using audit:
Undertake regular audits of pain standards to demonstrate compliance with local protocols for:
- Staff competency.
- Pain assessment documentation.
- Pain intensity.
- Analgesia consumption.
- Patient satisfaction.

- Adverse event reporting.
- Specific patient groups e.g. children, the elderly, the pregnant patient.

Guide

Ensure that evidence-based policies, procedures and guidelines are in place to support the care delivered to patients in acute and chronic pain.

Perioperative drugs

Overview

There is a wide variety of drugs which may be used in isolation or in conjunction with each other to produce the ideal conditions for the operative procedure. Most perioperative drugs are given intravenously.

Pre-medication

- These are drugs given in advance of any anaesthetic or surgical procedure.
- Examples include:
  - Temazepam to reduce anxiety.
  - Ranitidine to suppress gastric acid secretion.
  - Oral analgesia.
  - Pupil dilators for cataract surgery.

Local anaesthetics

- Local anaesthetic drugs are introduced directly around the site of procedure by various routes (topically, subcutaneously, deep tissue injection) to create localised loss of sensation.
- They are injected around large nerves to give regional anaesthesia.
- They are also injected/infused into the subarachnoid/epidural space to give spinal/epidural anaesthesia.
- Examples include:
  - Lidocaine.
  - Bupivacaine.
  - Levobupivacaine.

Sedatives

- Sedative drugs are intended to produce a state of sedation, where the patient can still be roused by verbal stimulus.
- Most often given to distressed patients having procedures under local, regional, or spinal/epidural anaesthesia.
- May also be given as pre-medication part of general anaesthetic induction, e.g., midazolam

Anaesthetic agents

- Produce complete loss of consciousness for general anaesthesia.

IV anaesthetic agents

- Used for the induction of general anaesthesia, e.g., propofol, thiopental, etomidate, ketamine
- Propofol can be used as a continuous infusion for maintenance.

Inhalational anaesthetic agents

- May be used for induction of general anaesthesia, but are more frequently used for maintenance, e.g., isoflurane, sevoflurane, desflurane.
- May also be for induction if:
  - Veins are poor.
  - There is a potential for airway obstruction, e.g., foreign body.
  - Patient request!

Volatile agents

Volatile agents (isoflurane, sevoflurane, desflurane) are stored in liquid form, but evaporate at room temperature and are introduced into the anaesthetic breathing circuit through a calibrated vaporiser.

Some anaesthetic agents can also be used as sedatives.

Analgesics

- Used for intra- and postoperative pain relief.
- Although unconscious, patients under general anaesthetic can still be affected by painful stimuli during surgery; to reduce the impact of these stimuli and thus reduce the need for anaesthetic agent, analgesics are used.
- Analgesics work on a number of different pathways to reduce the perception of pain, and so different types may be used in to produce a 'balanced analgesia'.
- Examples include morphine, fentanyl, tramadol, paracetamol, diclofenac.
- Local, regional, epidural, or spinal anaesthesia can also be used as a form of analgesia.

Muscle relaxants

- Used to produce muscle relaxation, commonly termed 'paralysis'.
- Given intravenously these drugs block the neuro-muscular junction, causing complete loss of tone and control in all striated muscle (but not smooth muscle).
- This creates conditions suitable for ET intubation and mechanical ventilation, and for certain types of surgery, e.g., laparotomy.
- Muscle relaxants are categorised into two groups, depolarising (suxamethonium) and non-depolarising.
- Suxamethonium causes depolarisation of striated muscle on administration, has rapid onset of action (about 30 seconds IV) and is short acting (about 3–5 minutes duration).
- Non-depolarising (e.g. atracurium, cisatracurium, rocuronium, and vecuronium) do not cause depolarisation, but create a competitive blockade at the neuromuscular junction.
- These drugs have slower onset and are longer acting than suxamethonium.

Reversal agents

- The action of non-depolarising muscle relaxants can be reversed under certain conditions.
- Neostigmine (an anticholinesterase) is the only reversal agent used, and should be given in conjunction with an anticholinergic (e.g. glycopyrronium bromide or atropine) to counteract bradycardia and increased airway secretions which may also be caused by neostigmine.
- Neostigmine is available premixed with glycopyrrolate, or as a single drug.

Anti-emetics

- A number of drugs given in the perioperative phase produce nausea, especially morphine and N_2O, as well as procedures such as middle ear, ophthalmic, and gynaecological surgery.

- Anti-emetics are often given prophylactically for this reason.
- Cause of postoperative nauseas and vomiting can be related to the patient, the anaesthetic, and the surgical procedure.
- Examples include cyclizine, ondansetron, dexamethasone.
- Propofol is sometimes selected as the anaesthetic agent of choice as it not only produces very little nausea, but it is also thought to have anti-emetic properties.

Emergency drugs

- In preparation for giving an anaesthetic emergency drugs are drawn up, but not necessarily given, unless required.
- Most often atropine for bradycardia and ephedrine for hypotension are prepared to correct any cardiovascular complications caused by anaesthetic drugs or surgery.
- Suxamethonium is also drawn up for emergency ET intubation.

Surgery

- There are drugs which are administered solely to aid the practice of surgery, for example adrenaline used to produce vasoconstriction at surgical wound sites—this must be used with caution however.
- Antibiotics are often administered prophylactically in the perioperative phase, especially for orthopaedic or implant surgery.

References and further reading

Allman KG and Wilson IH (eds) (2006). *Oxford Handbook of Anaesthesia* (2nd edn). Oxford University Press: Oxford.

British National Formulary. Available at: http://bnf.org/bnf/

Sasada M and Smith S (2003). *Drugs in anaesthesia and intensive care* (3rd edn). Oxford University Press: Oxford.

Oxygen therapy

Definition
- The administration of O_2 at a concentration greater that that of ambient air.
- Effective delivery of O_2 is predicated on the maintenance of a patent airway.

Indications
- Cardiac or respiratory arrest.
- Acute hypotension.
- Carbon monoxide poisoning.
- Trauma.
- Post-anaesthesia recovery.
- Use of opiates or other respiratory depressant drugs.
- Low cardiac output and metabolic acidosis (bicarbonate <18mmol/L).
- Respiratory distress (respiratory rate >24/minute).

Equipment
Two basic types of device are used for delivery of O_2 (Table 24.1):
- Variable flow devices: deliver a variable concentration of O_2 which is dependent on patient's respiratory rate, e.g., nasal specula, Hudson (MC) mask, simple mask with reservoir bag (non-rebreather).
- Fixed flow devices: deliver a fixed concentration of O_2 independent of the patient's respiratory rate, e.g., Venturi masks.

Table 24.1 O_2 delivery devices

Devices	% oxygen delivered	Uses
Nasal cannulae	Varible – flow rate dependent Maximum 40%	Post operative recovery when maintaining patent airway unassisted Procedures under local anesthesia Endoscopy Long-term home oxygen therapy
Hudson/Mc mask	Variable – flow rate dependent Maximum 50% at 15 L/min	Severe asthma Left acute ventricular failure Trauma
Simple mask with reservoir bag (non-rebreather)	Variable – flow rate dependent Maximum 60–70%	Severe sepsis N.B. min. flow rate 5 L/min
Venturi mask	Fixed variable (see table 2 for details 24–60%)	Controlled treatment of chronic respiratory failure

Risks associated with O_2 therapy

O_2 therapy in COPD

Caution should be exercised as high concentrations of O_2 reduce the hypoxic drive to breathe. This in turn causes CO_2 retention that can result in potentially fatal respiratory acidosis.

Table 24.2 Fixed concentration (Venturi) masks

Colour	Flow rate (L/min)	% O_2 delivered
Blue	2	24
White	4	28
Yellow	6	35
Red	8	40
Orange	12	60

In cardiac or respiratory arrest the absence of O_2 *will* be fatal!

O_2 toxicity

When high concentrations of O_2 (>60%) have been inhaled for >48 hours damage the alveolar membrane can occur resulting in adult respiratory distress syndrome (ARDS).

O_2 therapy in neonates

- Prolonged exposure to high concentrations of oxygen can result in retinopathy of prematurity (ROP)(formerly known as retrolental fibroplasia).
- Supplemental O_2 should only be used when explicitly indicated, e.g., respiratory distress or cyanosis.
- As with COPD, in emergencies O_2 should be used without restriction as *hypoxia will kill.*

Long-term O_2 therapy

When administered for a minimum of 15 hours daily prolongs survival in some patients with chronic obstructive pulmonary disease.

Intermittent O_2 therapy

- Episodes of breathlessness not relieved by other treatment;
- In patients with severe COPD.
- Interstitial lung disease.
- Heart failure.
- Palliative care.

References

British National Formulary (2008). Available at: 🖳 www.bnf.org

Green D, Ervine M, and White S (2003). *Fundamentals of Perioperative Management*. Greenwich Medical Media: London.

Anaesthetic induction agents

Drug	Indications	Contraindications/cautions	Side effects	Drug route	Dose
Propofol (Diprivan) Provides a smooth rapid induction	Induction of anaesthesia Total IV anaesthesia Sedation/hypnotic effect To treat nausea in chemotherapy Treatment of status epilepticus in repeated fits with no return of consciousness	Not to be used for the sedation of ventilated children and adolescents under 17 years old due to risk of potentially fatal effects, e.g., metabolic acidosis, cardiac failure Caesarean section Epilepsy Allergy to eggs, soya, soybean oil and peanuts Reduce dose for elderly or haemodynamically unstable patients A bolus injection can cause significant respiratory depression and bronchodilation IV infusion can cause a reduction in tidal volume	Pain on injection Bradycardia Discoloration of hair and urine may occasionally occur Epileptiform movements Facial parasthesiae Decrease in BP Cardiac output can decrease by 20% and vasodilation can occur as secondary response	IV injection IV infusion	*Adult dose (IV injection 1%):* 1.5–2.5mg/kg (20–40mg every 10 seconds) *Paediatric dose (IV injection 1%):* 2.5mg/kg (over 8 years) 2.5–4mg/kg in younger child
Thiopentone Thiopentaal	Induction of anaesthesia of short duration Anticonvulsant Hypnotic	Hepatic impairment Sedative effects may persist up to 24 hours	Arrhythmias and myocardial depression Injection site reaction Hypotension	IV injection PR	*Adult dose (IV injection):* 100–150mg over 10–15 seconds

				Paediatric dose (IV injection): 2–7 mg/kg
	Avoid intra-arterial injection Extravasation causes severe pain Porphyria	Coughs and sneezing Hypersensitivity reaction (rash) Necrosis if injected intra-arterial Rare—severe anaphylactoid reaction	IV injection	Adult dose: 300mcg/kg slowly Elderly: 150–200 mcg/kg slowly Paediatric dose: 300mcg/kg slowly
Etomidate (hypnomidate) Induction of anaesthesia Treatment of Cushing's syndrome prior to surgery Rapid recovery usually without hangover effect	Patients with porphyria can cause problems with homeo/haemostasis Pregnancy Breast feeding	Pain on induction (can be reduced with Lidocaine) Decreased respiratory rate and tidal volume Hypotension Venous thrombosis Thrombophlebitis if injected into small vein Involuntary muscle movements may occur on induction May suppress adrenocortical function		
Reasonably cardio-vascularly stable				

References

Allman KG and Wilson IH (eds) (2006). *Oxford Handbook of Anaesthesia* (2nd edn). Oxford University Press: Oxford.

British National Formulary. Available at: 🖳 http://bnf.org/bnf/

Sasada M and Smith S (2003). *Drugs in anaesthesia and intensive care* (3rd edn). Oxford University Press: Oxford.

Opiate analgesic drugs

Drug	Indications	Contraindications/cautions	Side effects	Drug route	Dose
Morphine	Moderate to severe pain Used intraoperatively to complement general anaesthesia Postoperative pain relief	Raised ICP Head injury Risk of paralytic ileus Allergy Hypotension Asthma Hepatic impairment Renal impairment Other opiates administered	Respiratory depression Nausea; vomiting Sweating Flushing or itching Drowsiness or confusion Bronchospasm Hypotension Urinary retention Constipation	IV injection Intrathecal Epidural IM SC Oral	*Adult dose (IV):* 2.5mg every 4 hours / more frequently during titration *Paediatric dose (IV):* 100–200mcg/kg every 4 hours *Neonates (IV):* 40–100mcg/kg every 6 hours
Pethidine (Pamergan®)	Often used as an alternative for patients with morphine allergy / sensitivity Moderate-to-severe pain Postoperative analgesia Obstetric analgesia	Severe renal impairment Raised ICP Head injury Risk of paralytic ileus allergy Hypotension Asthma Hepatic impairment Renal impairment Other opiates administered *Less potent than morphine and shorter acting*	Convulsions in overdosage Respiratory depression Nausea; vomiting; sweating Flushing or itching Drowsiness or confusion Bronchospasm; hypotension Urinary retention; constipation	IV injection IM Oral	For postoperative pain: *Adult dose (SC/IM):* 25–100mg every 2–3 hours *Paediatric dose:* 0.5–2mg/kg (IM)

Diamorphine	Severe pain Administered as part of planned pain management strategy	Raised ICP Head injury Risk of paralytic ileus *More potent than morphine and shorter acting*	Respiratory depression Nausea; vomiting; sweating Flushing or itching Drowsiness or confusion Bronchospasm; hypotension Urinary retention; constipation	IT or epidural in the perioperative setting IV as PCA	For acute pain: *Adult dose (IM/SC):* 5mg every 4 hours
Codeine phosphate	Mild to moderate pain Suppression of cough Postoperative analgesia	Raised ICP Head injury Risk of paralytic ileus, allergy Hypotension Asthma Hepatic impairment Renal impairment Other opiates administered	Respiratory depression Nausea; vomiting; sweating Flushing or itching Drowsiness or confusion Bronchospasm; hypotension Urinary retention; constipation	IM injection Oral	*Adult dose (IM):* 30–60mg every 4 hours *Paediatric dose:* Orally 3mg/kg daily
Tramadol	Moderate pain Used postoperatively in recovery *Tramadol acts on opiate and other receptors*	Raised ICP Head injury Risk of paralytic ileus, epilepsy Must be given by slow injection when administered intravenously Less effective than other opiate analgesia	Less respiratory depression than morphine Convulsions Hallucinations in the elderly	IV injection IM Oral	*Adult dose:* 50–100mg every 4–6 hours (IV infusion)

Continued

Opiate analgesic drugs—continued

Drug	Indications	Contraindications/cautions	Side effects	Drug route	Dose
Fentanyl	Intraoperative analgesia	Raised ICP Head injury Risk of paralytic ileus Significantly more potent than morphine Shorter acting	More marked respiratory depression than morphine Bradycardia	IV injection IT Epidural	*Adult dose (IV):* 50–100mcg *Paediatric dose:* 1–3mcg/kg (IV)
Alfentanil	Intraoperative analgesia	Raised ICP Head injury Risk of paralytic ileus Significantly more potent than morphine Shorter acting than fentanyl	More marked respiratory depression than morphine Bradycardia	IV injection	*Adult dose (IV):* 50–500mcg *Paediatric dose:* 10–20mcg/kg (IV) with assisted ventilation
Remifentanil	Intraoperative analgesia *Remifentanil is rapidly metabolised; the effects of the drug wear off soon after IV infusion has stopped*	Raised ICP Head injury Risk of paralytic ileus Significantly more potent than morphine Should be administered as an IV infusion with dose/rate calculated to patients' ideal body weight	More marked respiratory depression than morphine Bradycardia	IV infusion	*Adult dose (IV):* 0.25–1 mcg over 30 seconds *Paediatric dose (IV):* Over 12 years: 0.25–1 mcg over 30 seconds

| Co-codamol 30/500 | Postoperative analgesia | Hepatic impairment Renal impairment | Liver damage with overdose | Oral | *Adult dose:* 1–2 tablets every 4 hours *Paediatric dose:* Not recommended |

References

Allman KG and Wilson IH (eds) (2006). *Oxford Handbook of Anaesthesia* (2nd edn). Oxford University Press: Oxford.

British National Formulary. Available at: 🖥 http://bnf.org/bnf/

Sasada M and Smith S (2003). *Drugs in anaesthesia and intensive care* (3rd edn). Oxford University Press: Oxford

Non-opiate analgesic drugs and NSAIDs

	Drug	Indications	Contraindications/cautions	Side effects	Drug route	Dose
Non-opiate analgesic drugs	Paracetamol	Mild-to-moderate pain Used intra- or postoperatively Pyrexia	Hepatic impairment Renal impairment	Liver damage with overdose Blood disorders Rash Hypotension on infusion	IV infusion PR Oral	*Adult and child > 50kg* (IV infusion): 1g every 4–6 hours over 15 minutes *Adult and child 10–50kg:* (IV infusion) 15mg/kg every 4–6 hours over 15 minutes
Non-steroidal anti-inflammatory drugs	Diclofenac	Mild-to-moderate pain Postoperative analgesia Can be given preoperatively	Gastric ulceration Anti-coagulant therapy ACE inhibitor therapy Aspirin asthmatics High blood loss during surgery; Hypovolaemia Hepatic impairment Renal impairment Care with elderly patients Use of other NSAIDS	Hypersensitivity reactions (rash, bronchospasm, angioedema) GI irritation (ulceration, bleeding) Fluid retention Hypertension	IV infusion IV bolus IM PR Oral	*Adult dose* PR: 75–150mg daily *Paediatric dose* 1–2mg/kg PR

Ketorolac	Moderate-to-severe pain Only to be used postoperatively	Gastric ulceration Anti-coagulant therapy ACE inhibitor therapy Aspirin asthmatics High blood loss during surgery; hypovolaemia Hepatic impairment Renal impairment Care with elderly patients Use of other NSAIDS	Hypersensitivity reactions (rash, bronchospasm, angioedema) GI irritation (ulceration, bleeding) Fluid retention Hypertension	IV IM	*Adult dose* 10mg IV over 15 seconds *Paediatric dose* Not recommended
Parecoxib	Moderate pain Only to be used postoperatively Parecoxib is a COX II specific inhibitor	Gastric ulceration Dehydration Anti-coagulant therapy ACE inhibitor therapy Aspirin asthmatics High blood loss during surgery; hypovolaemia Inflammatory bowel disease	Heart disease Hypersensitivity reactions (rash, bronchospasm, angioedema) GI irritation (ulceration, bleeding) Fluid retention Hypertension	IV IM	*Adult dose* 40mg 20mg for elderly/ patients <50kg *Paediatric dose:* not recommended

References

Allman KG and Wilson IH (eds) (2006). *Oxford Handbook of Anaesthesia* (2nd edn). Oxford University Press: Oxford.

British National Formulary. Available at: http://bnf.org/bnf/

Sasada M and Smith S (2003). *Drugs in anaesthesia and intensive care* (3rd edn). Oxford University Press: Oxford.

Depolarising muscle relaxants and non-depolarising muscle relaxants

Drug		Indications	Contraindications/cautions	Side effects	Drug route	Dose
Depolarising muscle relaxant	**Suxamethonium**	To facilitate endotracheal intubation when rapid neuromuscular block is required	Avoid use if patient has a family history of malignant hyperthermia; hyperkalaemia; major trauma; severe burns; major muscle wasting and immobilisation; congenital myotonic disease and muscular dystrophy. Caution is advised for patients who are known to have an atypical pseudocholinesterase enzyme, which has very little ability to break down the drug, thus prolonging its effect (suxamethonium [Scoline] apnoea)	Skeletal muscle pains Tachycardia and other dysrhythmias Rise in intraocular pressure Rash and flushing is common Bronchospasm and severe anaphylaxis can occur	IV injection IV Infusion IM injection	*Adult dose:* 1mg/kg (IV injection) *Paediatric dose:* Infant over 1 year: 1mg/kg Infant under 1 year: 2mg/kg
	Atracurium	Muscle relaxation for surgery of short to intermediate duration	Pregnancy Breast feeding Avoid excessive dosages in obese patients The activity of the drug is prolonged in patients with myasthenia gravis	Bradycardia Histamine release Possible hypotension and bronchospasm	IV injection	*Adult dose:* 300–600 mcg/kg(initial) 100–200 mcg/kg (maintenance) *Paediatric dose:* For child over 1 month 300–600 mcg/kg (initial) 100–200mcg/kg (maintenance)
	Mivacurium	Muscle relaxation for surgery of short duration	Patients with hepatic impairment, renal impairment and the elderly. The activity of the drug is prolonged in patients with myasthenia gravis	Transient cutaneous flushing is common Hypotension Tachycardia,	IV injection	*Adult dose:* 70–250mcg/kg 100 mcg/kg (maintenance) *Paediatric dose:*

Vecuronium	Muscle relaxation for surgery of intermediate duration	The activity of the drug is prolonged in patients with myasthenia gravis, and in neonates and infants, requiring a longer recovery period.	Anaphylactic reactions are very rare, unexpected sustained neuromuscular blockade can occur in neonates.	IV injection	*Adult dose:* 80/100 mcg/kg *Paediatric dose:* 60/100 mcg/kg BNF advises test dose of 10–20 mcg/kg in children
Pancuronium	Muscle relaxation for surgery of intermediate duration	Patients with hepatic impairment, renal impairment and pregnancy The activity of the drug is prolonged in patients with myasthenia gravis	Vagolytic and sympathomimetic effects can cause mild to moderate tachycardia and occasional increase in BP	IV injection	*Adult dose:* 50–100mcg/kg *Paediatric dose:* 60–100mcg/kg
Rocuronium	Muscle relaxation of moderate duration of action to facilitate surgery	Fatal anaphylactioid reactions to rocuronium have been reported The activity of the drug is prolonged in patients with myasthenia gravis Caution advised for patients with hepatic and renal impairment Pregnancy Breast feeding	Causes pain on injection; its mild vagolytic effects can counteract any bradycardia caused during surgery	IV injection	*Adult dose:* 600mcg/kg *Paediatric dose:* 600mcg/kg

Non-depolarising muscle relaxant drugs

References

Allman KG and Wilson IH (eds) (2006). *Oxford Handbook of Anaesthesia* (2nd edn). Oxford University Press: Oxford.

British National Formulary. Available at: 🖳 http://bnf.org/bnf/

Sasada M and Smith S (2003). *Drugs in anaesthesia and intensive care* (3rd edn). Oxford University Press: Oxford.

Anti-coagulant drugs

Drug	Indications	Contraindications /Cautions	Side effects	Drug route	Drug dose
Heparin	Treatment of DVT, fat embolus, PE, DIC Prophylactic prevention of VTE with LMWH	Spinal and epidural anaesthesia with treatment doses of heparin Thrombocytopenia Haemophilia Acute bacterial endocarditis Hypertension Cerebral haemorrhage Hepatic impairment Renal impairment Pregnancy; elderly	Haemorrhage Thrombocytopenia Injection site reactions Skin necrosis Priapism Hyperkalaemia Osteoporosis Hypersensitivity reactions	IV injection IV infusion SC injection	*For prophylaxis:* 5000 units 2 hours prior to surgery and every 8–12 hours until the patient is ambulant
Tinzaparin	Treatment of DVT, fat embolus, PE, unstable angina and acute peripheral arterial occlusion Prophylactic prevention of VTE with LNWH	Spinal and epidural anaesthesia with treatment doses of heparin Thrombocytopenia Haemophilia Acute bacterial endocarditis Hypertension Cerebral haemorrhage Hepatic impairment Renal impairment Pregnancy; breastfeeding; Elderly	Haemorrhage Thrombocytopenia Injection site reactions Skin necrosis Priapism Hyperkalaemia Osteoporosis Hypersensitivity reactions	SC injection	*For prophylaxis:* 3500 units two hours prior to surgery and every 24 hours until the patient is ambulant

| Danaparoid sodium | Prophylactic prevention of VTE with LMWH | Spinal and epidural anaesthesia with treatment doses of danaparoid
Haemophilia
Hypertension
Thrombocytopenia
Cerebral haemorrhage
Hepatic impairment
Renal impairment
Recent bleeding
Risk of bleeding
Pregnancy; breast feeding | Haemorrhage
Hypersensitivity reactions | IV injection
SC injection | *For prophylaxis:*
750 units 1–4 hours prior to surgery and BD until the patient is ambulant |

References

Allman KG and Wilson IH (eds) (2006). *Oxford Handbook of Anaesthesia* (2nd edn). Oxford University Press: Oxford.

British National Formulary. Available at: http://bnf.org/bnf/

Sasada M and Smith S (2003). *Drugs in anaesthesia and intensive care* (3rd edn). Oxford University Press: Oxford.

Obstetric drugs

Drug	Indications	Contraindications / Cautions	Side effects	Drug route	Drug dose
Nitrous oxide (Entonox®)	Analgesia used in obstetrics (as Entonox® 50% N_2O : 50% O_2)	Susceptibility to malignant hyperthermia. Can significantly increase the size of a pneumothorax Renal impairment	Respiratory depression with a decrease in tidal volume and an increase in respiratory rate; Diffusion hypoxia Loss of consciousness Cerebral blood flow is increased. Nausea and vomiting Can cause neonatal respiratory depression in third trimester of pregnancy	Inhalation (50% N_2O : 50% O_2)	Self-administered using a demand valve
Oxytocin	Induction of labour To reduce postpartum haemorrhage Aid expulsion of the placenta following delivery and evacuation of retained products of conception To promote lactation	Pregnancy induced hypertension or cardiac disease Foetal distress Pre-eclampsia Cardiovascular disease Monitor for DIC Caudal anaesthesia	Increases the force and frequency of contractions Nausea; vomiting Arrhythmia : vasodilation Tachycardia; Uterine spasm; headache Fluid retention Hypersensitivity Uterine hyperstimulation Fetal distress Placental abruption	IV injection IV infusion	*Caesarean section:* 5 units by slow IV injection immediately following delivery *Postpartum haemorrhage:* 5–10 units by slow IV injection followed by 5–30 units in 500mL of fluid IV infusion if severe

Continued

	Missed and incomplete abortion	Amniotic fluid embolus Hyponatraemia and convulsions in prolonged use	
Ergometrine	To control haemorrhage	Vasoconstriction Hypertension Increased CVP Nausea; vomiting headache; dizziness palpitation; chest pain; dyspnoea; bradycardia; bronchospasm	Hypertension Cardiac disease Vascular disease Severe hepatic impairment Severe renal impairment Sepsis Eclampsia Multiple pregnancy	IV injection IM injection	*Postpartum haemorrhage:* 250–500mcg via IV injection
Anti-D immunoglobulin	To prevent Rhesus-negative mother from forming antibodies to foetal Rhesus-positive cells Should be administered following birth, miscarriage and abortion within 72 hours			IM injection	*Antenatal prophylaxis:* 500 units at 28 weeks' gestation and 34 weeks' gestation 500 units immediately following birth 250 units following abortion up until 20 weeks' gestation 500 units after 20 weeks' gestation

Continued

Obstetric drugs—continued

Drug	Indications	Contraindications / Cautions	Side effects	Drug route	Drug dose
Sodium citrate	To reduce gastric acidity To reduce the effect of acid aspiration (Mendelson's syndrome)	Renal impairment Cardiac disease Hypertension	Mild diuretic	Orally *Should be drawn up fresh as shelf-life is short*	*General anaesthesia:* 30mL of 0.3 molar solution before induction
Ranitidine	To reduce gastric acidity To reduce the risk of acid aspiration (Mendelson's syndrome)	Renal impairment Breastfeeding Porphyria	Diarrhoea; dizziness Headache; rash GI disturbances Rarely alopecia, tachycardia, visual disturbance	IV injection IV infusion IM injection Orally	*Onset of labour:* 150mg orally *General anaesthesia:* 50 mg 45–60 minutes before induction via IM injection or slow IV injection diluted to 20mL

References

Allman KG and Wilson IH (eds) (2006). Oxford Handbook of Anaesthesia (2nd edn). Oxford University Press: Oxford.

British National Formulary. Available at: 🖳 http://bnf.org/bnf/

Sasada M and Smith S (2003). Drugs in anaesthesia and intensive care (3rd edn). Oxford University Press: Oxford.

NICE (2002) Routine antenatal anti-D prophylaxis for Rhesus-negative women. London: National Institute for Clinical Excellence.

Yentis S, May A, Malhotra S (eds) (2007). Analgesia, anaesthesia and pregnancy: a practical guide (2nd Edition). Cambridge University

Inhalational drugs

Drug	Indications	Contraindications/cautions	Side effects	Drug route
Isoflurane	Mainly used for the maintenance of anaesthesia during surgery It has been used as sedation during intensive care	Susceptibility to malignant hyperthermia Can cause hepatotoxicity sensitive patients Can cause neonatal respiratory depression in third trimester of pregnancy	Decreases mean arterial pressure while increased doses will lower the BP and increase the depth of anaesthesia simultaneously which tends to prevent reflex tachycardia Heart rhythm is generally stable, although heart rate can rise particularly in younger patients Respiratory depression with decreased tidal volume; the drug is irritant to the respiratory system which can lead to coughing, breath holding, and increased bronchial secretions. The drug has little analgesic effect; cerebral blood flow is increased leading to increased ICP; muscle relaxation occurs and the effects of the muscle relaxant drugs are potentiated.	By inhalation via a calibrated vaporiser
Sevoflurane	Mainly used for the maintenance of anaesthesia during surgery It can be used for the induction of anaesthesia	Susceptibility to malignant hyperthermia Manufacturer recommends caution in cases of renal impairment Can cause neonatal respiratory depression in third trimester of pregnancy	Decreases systolic BP although the heart rate is generally stable Increased respiratory rate with no change to the minute volume; it inhibits hypoxic pulmonary vasoconstriction and appears to relax bronchial smooth muscle constricted by histamine or acetylcholine The drug produces general anaesthesia Agitation often occurs in children	By inhalation via a calibrated vaporiser

| Nitrous oxide | Mainly used for the maintenance of anaesthesia during surgery

It can be used for pain relief during labour | Susceptibility to malignant hyperthermia.

Can significantly increase the size of a pneumothorax

Manufacturer recommends caution in cases of renal impairment.

Can cause neonatal respiratory depression in third trimester of pregnancy.

May increase gas embolus size e.g. with neurosurgery

Patients with intraocular gas should be avoided | Slight respiratory depression with a decrease in tidal volume and an increase in respiratory rate;

May cause diffusion hypoxia at the end of surgery

CNS is depressed by N_2O if administered in high concentration, (over 80%) resulting in loss of consciousness in most subjects.

Cerebral blood flow is increased.

Nausea and vomiting post operatively

Agitation often occurs in children | By inhalation via appropriate patient breathing circuits |

References

Allman KG and Wilson IH (eds) (2006). *Oxford Handbook of Anaesthesia* (2nd edn). Oxford University Press: Oxford.

British National Formulary. Available at: 🖥 http://bnf.org/bnf/

Sasada M and Smith S (2003). *Drugs in anaesthesia and intensive care* (3rd edn). Oxford University Press: Oxford.

Anti-muscarinic drugs

Drug	Indications	Contraindications/ cautions	Side effects	Drug route	Dose
Atropine	Reduces salivary function Reversal of bradycardia With anticholinesterase, reversal of non-polarising neuromuscular block	Myasthenia gravis Paralytic ileus Prostate enlargement Pyloric stenosis Cardiovascular disease Children and elderly Down syndrome	Transient bradycardia, followed by tachycardia, palpitations, arrhythmias, dry mouth Reduced bronchial secretions Urinary urgency and retention, dilated pupils Occasionally nausea, vomiting, confusion, giddiness	IV IM SC Orally	**For intraoperative bradycardia** *Adult dose:* 300–600mcg via IV injection *Paediatric dose:* **Not licensed** 10–20mcg/kg via IV injection (1–12 years)
Glycopyrronium bromide	Reversal of bradycardia Drying secretions Reversal of non-polarising neuromuscular block with neostigmine *Glycopyrronium bromide is incompatible with thiopental, diazepam and methohexitone*	Myasthenia gravis Paralytic ileus Prostate enlargement Pyloric stenosis Cardiovascular disease Children and elderly Down syndrome	Transient bradycardia, followed by tachycardia, palpitations, arrhythmias Dry mouth Reduced bronchial secretions Urinary urgency and retention, dilated pupils Occasionally nausea, vomiting, confusion, giddiness	IV IM	*Adult dose:* 200–400mcg via IV injection *Paediatric dose:* 4–8mcg/kg via slow IV injection (max 200mcg) Repeat dose if required (1 month–18 years)

References

Allman KG and Wilson IH (eds) (2006). *Oxford Handbook of Anaesthesia* (2nd edn). Oxford University Press: Oxford.

British National Formulary. Available at: http://bnf.org/bnf/

Sasada M and Smith S (2003). *Drugs in anaesthesia and intensive care* (3rd edn). Oxford University Press: Oxford.

Anti-cholinesterase drugs

Drug	Indications	Contraindications/cautions	Side effects	Drug route	Dose
Neostigmine	Reversal of non-depolarising blockade Myasthenia gravis *Neostigmine has a longer duration of action than edrophonium*	Intestinal or urinary obstruction Asthma, arrhythmias, recent MI, bradycardia, hypotension, epilepsy, pregnancy, breastfeeding	Nausea, vomiting, diarrhoea, increased salivation, Overdose includes lacrimation, increased bronchial secretions, excessive sweating, heart block, hypotension Rare—cardiac arrest	IV IM SC Orally	50–70mcg/kg usually with glycopyrronium or atropine
Edrophonium chloride	Diagnosis of myasthenia gravis	Intestinal or urinary obstruction Asthma, arrhythmias, recent MI, bradycardia, hypotension, epilepsy, pregnancy, breast feeding Extreme caution in respiratory distress	Nausea, vomiting, diarrhoea, increased salivation, Overdose includes lacrimation, increased bronchial secretions, excessive sweating, heart block, hypotension	IV IM	500–700mcg/kg usually with or before atropine

References

Allman KG and Wilson IH (eds) (2006). *Oxford Handbook of Anaesthesia* (2nd edn). Oxford University Press: Oxford.

British National Formulary. Available at: 🖥 http://bnf.org/bnf/

Sasada M and Smith S (2003). *Drugs in anaesthesia and intensive care* (3rd edn). Oxford University Press: Oxford.

Anxiolytic benzodiazepine drugs

Drug	Indications	Contraindications/cautions	Side effects	Drug route	Dose
Diazepam	Premedication	Respiratory depression	Drowsiness and light-headedness the following day	IV	*Adult dose:*
	Sedation with amnesia and local anaesthetic	Neuro-muscular weakness		IM	10 mg over 3–4 minutes via IV injection prior to surgical procedure repeated if necessary after 10 minutes
	Short-term use in anxiety or insomnia	Sleep apnoea	Amnesia	Orally	
	Status epilepticus	Severe hepatic impairment	Confusion	Rectal	
	Febrile convulsions	Second period of drowsiness can occur several hours after	Muscle weakness		
		Hepatic impairment	Ataxia		
		Renal impairment	Occasionally headache, hypotension, GI disturbances, vertigo		
		Pregnancy			
		Breastfeeding			
Midazolam	Sedation with amnesia	Neuro-muscular respiratory weakness including unstable myasthenia gravis	GI disturbances	IV	*Adult dose:*
	Sedation in intensive care		Increased appetite	IM	For conscious sedation
	Premedication	Severe respiratory depression	Cardiac arrest	Continuous infusion	2mg per minute prior to procedure via slow IV injection
	Induction of anaesthesia	Acute pulmonary insufficiency	Jaundice		
	Status epilepticus	Cardiac disease	Anaphylaxis		*Paediatric dose:*
		Respiratory disease	Thrombosis		For conscious sedation
	The effects of midazolam can be reversed with flumazenil, glycopyrronium and physostigmine	Myasthenia gravis	Laryngospasm		50–100mcg/kg via slow IV injection over 2–3 minutes (6months–5years)
		Neonates and children	Bronchospasm		
		History of drug or alcohol abuse	Confusion		
			Headache, vertigo		

	Midazolam has controlled drug status	Reduce dose in elderly and debilitated		Dizziness Amnesia		
Temazepam	Preoperative medication Anxiety Hypnotic Temazepam has controlled drug status	Respiratory depression Neuro-muscular weakness Sleep apnoea Severe hepatic impairment Second period of drowsiness can occur several hours after	Drowsiness and light-headedness the following day Amnesia, confusion Muscle weakness Ataxia, headache, hypotension, GI disturbances, vertigo	Orally	*Adult dose:* 20–40mg orally prior to surgery *Paediatric dose:* 1mg/kg orally prior to surgery

References

Allman KG and Wilson IH (eds) (2006). *Oxford Handbook of Anaesthesia* (2nd edn). Oxford University Press: Oxford.

British National Formulary. Available at: 🖳 http://bnf.org/bnf/

Sasada M and Smith S (2003). *Drugs in anaesthesia and intensive care* (3rd edn). Oxford University Press: Oxford.

Antagonists for central and respiratory depression and respiratory stimulants

Drug	Indications	Contraindications/cautions	Side effects	Drug route	Dose
Naloxone	Reversal of opiate induced respiratory depression Overdose of opiate drugs Reversal of neonatal respiratory depression following opiate administration to mother during labour	Cardiovascular disease Opiate dependence *Short duration of action so repeated doses may be necessary*	Reverses effects of analgesia Hypotension; hypertension Ventricular tachycardia and fibrillation Cardiac arrest Hyperventilation Dyspnoea Pulmonary oedema	IV IM SC	*Adult dose:* 1.5–3mcg/kg 100mcg every 2 minutes until desired effect *Paediatric dose:* 10mcg/kg initially Followed by 100mcg/kg until desired effect *Neonatal dose:* 10mcg/kg every 3 minutes
Flumazenil	Reversal of sedative effects of benzodiazepines in anaesthesia. To reverse sedative effects in intensive care and endoscopy During 'wake-up' test for scoliosis surgery Reduces postoperative shivering	Raised inter-cranial pressure Status epilepticus Any life threatening condition controlled by benzodiazepine drugs Benzodiazepine dependence Prolonged benzodiazepine therapy for epilepsy History of panic disorders Hepatic impairment Head injury Elderly, children Breast feeding	Nausea, vomiting Anxiety, agitation Hypertension Headache Transient increase in BP and heart rate in intensive care patients	IV injection IV infusion	300–600mcg 200mcg slowly initially then followed by 100mcg every minute if necessary

| Respiratory stimulants | Doxapram | Postoperative respiratory depression
Acute respiratory failure
Postoperative shivering | *Short duration of action so repeated doses may be necessary*
Severe hypertension
Status asthmaticus
Coronary artery disease
Epilepsy
Thyrotoxicosis
Give O_2 in severe irreversible airway obstruction
Hypertension
Hepatic impairment
Pregnancy | Perineal warmth
Dizziness, restlessness
Excessive sweating
Slight increase in BP and heart rate
During postoperative period, muscle fasciculations, confusion, hallucinations, laryngospasm, bronchospasm, sinus tachycardia, bradycardia, nausea, vomiting, salivation | IV injection
IV infusion | *Adult dose:*
1–1.5mg/kg by IV injection
Repeated every hour if required
Paediatric dose:
Not recommended |

References

Allman KG and Wilson IH (eds) (2006). *Oxford Handbook of Anaesthesia* (2nd edn). Oxford University Press: Oxford.

British National Formulary. Available at: 🖳 http://bnf.org/bnf/

Sasada M and Smith S (2003). *Drugs in anaesthesia and intensive care* (3rd edn). Oxford University Press: Oxford.

Anti-emetic drugs

Drug	Indications	Contraindications/ cautions	Side effects	Drug route	Drug dose
Prochlorperazine	Nausea and vomiting Vertigo Labyrinthitis Cytotoxic therapy Radiotherapy Emesis caused by opiates and general anaesthesia Psychosis	Hypotension likely after IM injection Elderly Comatose state Hepatic impairment Renal impairment Epilepsy Parkinson's disease	Extra pyramidal symptoms Jaundice Rashes Respiratory depression	IM injection Orally	*Adult dose:* 12.5mg via IM injection
Metoclopramide	Postoperative nausea and vomiting Cytotoxic therapy Radiotherapy	GI obstruction Haemorrhage Breast feeding Hepatic disease Renal impairment Epilepsy Pregnancy Elderly; children	Dystonic reactions Restlessness Drowsiness Depression Rashes Diarrhoea Pruritus	IV injection IM injection Orally	*Adult dose:* 10mg via IV / IM injection / orally *Paediatric dose:* 1–5mg via IV / IM injection / orally (1–14years titrated according to body weight)
Cyclizine	Nausea; vomiting Labyrinthitis; vertigo	Severe heart failure Prostatic hypertrophy	Drowsiness Tachycardia	IV injection IM injection	*Adult dose:* 50mg via IV or IM injection

Drug	Uses	Cautions	Side effects	Route	Dose
	Motion sickness Radiation sickness	Hepatic disease Renal impairment Urinary retention Susceptibility to angle-closure glaucoma Pyloroduodenal obstruction May counteract haemodynamic benefits of opioids; children; elderly	Dysrhythmias Antimuscarinic effects such as urinary retention, dry mouth, blurred vision, and GI disturbances. Headache, Psychomotor impairment Less sedating effect	Orally	*Paediatric dose:* 25mg orally (6–12 years)
Ondansetron (Zofran®)	Prophylactically for postoperative nausea and vomiting Prophylactically before cytotoxic therapy *Ondansetron has been known to reduce the incidence of postoperative shivering*	Hepatic impairment QT interval prolongation Pregnancy Breastfeeding	Headache Flushing Constipation Reactions at injection site Rarely hiccups, anaphylaxis, chest pain Bradycardia, hypotension, arrhythmias, movement disorders, seizures On IV administration, rarely dizziness, transient visual disturbances (very rarely transient blindness) suppositories may cause rectal irritation	IV injection IM injection Oral Rectal	*Adult dose:* Prophylactically for postoperative nausea and vomiting 4mg via IM or slow IV injection prior to anaesthesia *Paediatric dose:* Treatment of postoperative nausea and vomiting 100mcg/kg via IM or slow IV injection prior, during or following induction of anaesthesia (over 2 years)

Continued

Anti-emetic drugs—continued

Drug	Indications	Contraindications/ cautions	Side effects	Drug route	Drug dose
Dexamethasone	Vomiting associated with chemotherapy *Can be used alone or with metoclopramide, prochlorperazine or a 5HT₃ antagonist*	Systemic infection Caution in children and elderly patients, hypertension, renal impairment, glaucoma, pregnancy, breastfeeding, epilepsy, recent MI	GI disturbances, osteoporosis, Cushing's syndrome, weight gain, impaired healing, bruising, fluid and electrolyte disturbances	IV injection IM injection IV infusion Oral	*Adult dose:* 0.5mg–24mg via IM or slow IV injection or infusion *Paediatric dose:* 200–400mcg/kg daily via IM or slow IV injection or infusion

References

Allman KG and Wilson IH (eds) (2006). *Oxford Handbook of Anaesthesia* (2nd edn). Oxford University Press: Oxford.

British National Formulary. Available at: 🖳 http://bnf.org/bnf/

Sasada M and Smith S (2003). *Drugs in anaesthesia and intensive care* (3rd edn). Oxford University Press: Oxford.

Local anaesthetic drugs

Drug	Indications	Contraindications/cautions	Side effects	Drug route	Dose
Lidocaine	Local anaesthesia Local infiltration Postoperative analgesia Ventricular arrhythmias Dental procedures with adrenaline	Hypovolaemia Complete heart block Respiratory impairment, impaired cardiac conduction, epilepsy, Bradycardia, Porphyria, Severe shock Myasthenia gravis; Elderly or debilitated patients Hepatic impairment; renal impairment; pregnancy	Respiratory depression Confusion Convulsions Hypotension and bradycardia (may lead to cardiac arrest); Rarely—hypersensitivity	IV Local infiltration SC Topical	Plain 3mg/kg With adrenaline 7mg/kg
Bupivacaine	Peripheral nerve block Local infiltration Epidural anaesthesia Sympathetic block IT anaesthesia	Hypovolaemia Complete heart block Respiratory impairment, impaired cardiac conduction, epilepsy, bradycardia, Porphyria, Severe shock Myasthenia gravis; Elderly or debilitated patients Hepatic impairment; renal impairment; pregnancy	Respiratory depression Confusion Convulsions Hypotension and bradycardia (may lead to cardiac arrest); Rarely—hypersensitivity	IV injection IV infusion Epidural injection IT injection	Plain 2mg /kg With adrenaline 3 mg/kg Marcain Heavy® 5mg (2–4mL for IT anaesthesia)
Prilocaine	Nerve block Infiltration anaesthesia	Hypovolaemia Complete heart block	Respiratory depression Confusion	Local infiltration	Plain 6mg/kg

					With adrenaline 8 mg/kg
	Severe or untreated hypertension; Severe heart disease; elderly or debilitated; pregnancy Respiratory impairment, impaired cardiac conduction, epilepsy, Bradycardia, Porphyria, Severe shock; Myasthenia gravis; Elderly or debilitated patients; Hepatic impairment; renal impairment; pregnancy	Convulsions Hypotension and bradycardia (may lead to cardiac arrest); Rarely—hypersensitivity			
Ropivacaine	Surgical anaesthesia Surface anaesthesia	Hypovolaemia Complete heart block Respiratory impairment, impaired cardiac conduction, epilepsy, bradycardia, Porphyria, Severe shock; Myasthenia gravis; Elderly or debilitated patients; Hepatic impairment; renal impairment; pregnancy	Respiratory depression Confusion Convulsions Nausea, vomiting, rigors, Hypotension and bradycardia; hypertension, tachycardia; headache, urinary retention; back pain Rarely—hypersensitivity	Epidural injection Epidural infusion	Plain 4 mg/kg

References

Allman KG and Wilson IH (eds) (2006). *Oxford Handbook of Anaesthesia* (2nd edn). Oxford University Press: Oxford.

British National Formulary. Available at: 🖳 http://bnf.org/bnf/

Sasada M and Smith S (2003). *Drugs in anaesthesia and intensive care* (3rd edn). Oxford University Press: Oxford.

Anti-bacterial drugs

	Drug	Indications	Contraindications/ cautions	Side effects	Drug route	Drug dose
Penicillins	Amoxicillin	Broad-spectrum antibiotic for Gram positive and Gram negative bacteria Respiratory tract infection Endocarditis; otitis media Urinary tract infection	Renal impairment Penicillin hypersensitivity History of allergic reactions	Nausea, vomiting, diarrhoea, Sore throat; rash; joint pains; urticaria;	IV injection IV infusion IM injection Oral	500mg–1g by IV injection or infusion every 6–8 hours
	Ampicillin	Broad-spectrum antibiotic for Gram positive and Gram negative bacteria Respiratory tract infection Endocarditis; ear, nose, and throat infection; septicaemia; meningitis Urinary tract infection	Renal impairment Penicillin hypersensitivity History of allergic reactions	Nausea, vomiting, diarrhoea, Sore throat; rash; joint pains; urticaria;	IV injection IV infusion IM injection Oral	500mg–2g by IV injection or infusion every 4–6 hours
	Co-amoxiclav	Broad-spectrum antibiotic for Gram positive and Gram negative bacteria Respiratory tract infection Urinary tract and abdominal infection; cellulitis	Renal impairment Hepatic impairment Penicillin hypersensitivity History of allergic reactions Pregnancy	Nausea, vomiting, diarrhoea, Sore throat; rash; joint pains; urticaria;	IV injection IV infusion Oral	*Surgical prophylaxis:* 1.2g by IV injection or infusion on induction of anaesthesia

Drug	Uses	Cautions	Side effects	Route	Dose
Flucloxacillin	Surgical prophylaxis; Respiratory tract infection; Otitis externa endocarditis; Skin and soft tissue infection	Hepatic impairment; Renal impairment; Penicillin hypersensitivity	Gastro-intestinal disturbances; Central nervous system disturbances; nausea; Sore throat; rash; joint pains; urticaria; diarrhoea; Rarely hepatitis, jaundice	IV injection; IV infusion; IM injection; Oral	*Surgical prophylaxis:* 1–2g by slow IV injection or infusion on induction of anaesthesia
Piperacillin	Broad-spectrum antibiotic for Gram positive and Gram negative bacteria used for: Surgical prophylaxis; Respiratory and urinary tract infection; Abdominal sepsis; septicaemia; meningitis; Gynaecological and obstetric infections	Renal impairment; Penicillin hypersensitivity; Pregnancy; Breast feeding	Nausea, vomiting, diarrhoea, Sore throat; rash; joint pains; urticaria; Rarely hepatitis, abdominal pain, constipation, jaundice	IV injection; IV infusion; IM injection	4g every 6–8 hours via slow IV infusion
Ceftazidime	Surgical prophylaxis; Infections due to sensitive Gram-positive and Gram-negative bacteria	Cephalosporin hypersensitivity; Renal impairment; Pregnancy; Breast feeding	Nausea and vomiting; abdominal discomfort; diarrhoea; headache; pruritus; rash, urticaria, anaphylaxis; jaundice; thrombocytopenia; Sleep disturbances, confusion, hallucinations, hypertonia, dizziness	IV injection; IV infusion; IM injection	*Surgical prophylaxis:* 1g by IV injection on induction of anaesthesia

Cephalosporins & beta-lactam antibiotics

Continued

Anti-bacterial drugs—continued

Drug	Indications	Contraindications/cautions	Side effects	Drug route	Drug dose
Cefuroxime	Surgical prophylaxis Infections due to sensitive Gram-positive and Gram-negative bacteria	Cephalosporin hypersensitivity Renal impairment Pregnancy Breast feeding	Nausea and vomiting; abdominal discomfort, diarrhoea; headache; pruritus; rash, urticaria, anaphylaxis; jaundice; thrombocytopenia sleep disturbances, confusion, hallucinations, hypertonia, dizziness	IV injection IV infusion IM injection Oral	*Surgical prophylaxis:* 1.5g by IV injection on induction of anaesthesia
Imipenem	Surgical prophylaxis Infections due to sensitive Aerobic and anaerobic Gram-positive and Gram-negative bacteria Hospital acquired septicaemia	Cephalosporin hypersensitivity Renal impairment Pregnancy Breast feeding	Nausea and vomiting; hearing loss; blood disorders; taste disturbances; pruritus; urticaria; convulsions; confusion	IV infusion IM injection	*Surgical prophylaxis:* 1g by IV infusion on induction of anaesthesia
Tetracycline	Broad-spectrum antibiotic used for: Respiratory, urinary GI tract infection Ear, nose, and throat infection *Incompatible with thiopental*	Hepatic impairment Myasthenia gravis History of allergic reactions Breast feeding	Nausea, vomiting, diarrhoea; renal impairment; hepatic impairment; dysphagia; oesophageal irritation; urticaria; rash; headache; tooth staining; increased ICP	IV injection Intrapleural injection IM injection Oral	0.5–1g via IV every 12 hours

Tetracyclines

		Uses	Cautions	Side effects	Route	Dose
Aminoglycosides	Gentamicin	Urinary tract infection Respiratory tract infection Septicaemia Neonatal sepsis Biliary tract infection Renal infection	Renal impairment Pregnancy; elderly; neonates and infants; Myasthenia gravis May prolong the effect of non-depolarising muscle relaxants Should be administered by injection for systemic infection	Nephrotoxicity Vestibular and auditory damage; blood disorders Nausea; vomiting; rash; headache; colitis; Altered liver function	IV injection IV infusion IT injection IM injection	60–80mg by IM or IV injection or slow IV infusion every 8 hours
Macrolides	Erythromycin	Infections associated with the respiratory tract; skin, joint, eye, oral and Campylobacter; Prophylaxis of bacterial endocarditis	Hepatic impairment; renal impairment; Breast feeding; porphyria; neonates May potentiate the action of midazolam, warfarin, digoxin	Nausea, vomiting, diarrhoea, hepatitis; Rarely hearing loss, jaundice, pancreatitis, chest pain, arrhythmias	IV infusion Oral	50mg/kg daily by IV infusion

Continued

Anti-bacterial drugs—continued

Drug	Indications	Contraindications/cautions	Side effects	Drug route	Drug dose
Clarithromycin	Infections associated with the respiratory tract; skin and tissue infections; otitis media *Helicobacter pylori*	Hepatic impairment; renal impairment Breast feeding; porphyria; neonates May potentiate the action of midazolam, warfarin, digoxin	Nausea, vomiting, diarrhoea, hepatitis, dyspepsia, headache, smell and taste disturbances, glossitis Rarely hearing loss, jaundice, pancreatitis, chest pain, arrhythmias	IV infusion Oral	500mg twice daily by IV infusion
Ciprofloxacin	Infections associated with respiratory, urinary and GI tract; skin, joint, eye, nose, throat; septicaemia; pelvic and intra-abdominal infection	Myasthenia gravis; pregnancy; breast feeding; epilepsy; renal impairment; children	Nausea, vomiting, diarrhoea, abdominal pain; rash; headache; Rarely anorexia; confusion; drowsiness; restlessness; anxiety Rarely convulsions when taking NSAIDS	IV infusion Oral	200–400mg daily via IV infusion

Quinolones

Metronidazole	Surgical prophylaxis	Hepatic impairment;	Nausea, vomiting,	IV infusion	Surgical prophylaxis:
	Anaerobic infections	pregnancy;	diarrhoea, anorexia,	Oral	500mg via IV
	Helicobacter infection	Breast feeding;	taste alterations, rash,	PR	infusion at
	Alternative to penicillin	porphyria; alcohol	darkening of urine		induction of
		May prolong	Rarely hepatitis,		anaesthesia
		the effect of	pancreatitis, jaundice,		
		vecuronium	dizziness, headache,		
			drowsiness, ataxia		

References

Allman KG and Wilson IH (eds) (2006). *Oxford Handbook of Anaesthesia* (2nd edn). Oxford University Press: Oxford.

British National Formulary. Available at: 🖳 http://bnf.org/bnf/

Sasada M and Smith S (2003). *Drugs in anaesthesia and intensive care* (3rd edn). Oxford University Press: Oxford.

Bronchodilating drugs

Drug	Indications	Contraindications/cautions	Side effects	Drug route	Dose
Aminophylline	Severe asthma Chronic obstructive pulmonary disease Heart failure *Aminophylline infusion reduces the recovery time from enflurane/N2O anaesthesia*	Cardiac disease Epilepsy Hypertension Peptic ulcer; Hyperthyroidism Elderly; fever Avoid in porphyria Hepatic impairment Pregnancy Breastfeeding	GI disturbances Nausea Headache Insomnia Tachycardia Palpitation, Arrhythmias Convulsions if given rapidly by IV injection;	IV Injection IV infusion Oral	*Adult dose:* 5mg/kg (250–500mg) by slow IV injection *Paediatric dose:* 5mg/kg by slow IV injection
Salbutamol	Asthma COPD Premature labour *There is a possibility that salbutamol potentiates non-depolarising muscle relaxing drugs*	Cardiovascular disease Arrhythmias Hyperthyroidism Diabetes	Myocardial ischaemia Tachycardia Arrhythmias, palpitation headache, anxiety Insomnia Hypokalaemia Muscle cramps Peripheral vasodilation Sleep and behaviour disturbances	SC IM IV injection IV infusion Inhalation	*Adult dose:* 250mcg by slow IV injection *Paediatric dose:* 5mcg/kg by slow IV injection (1 month–2 years) 15mcg/kg by slow IV injection (2–18 years)

| Ipratropium bromide | Asthma
COPD
Rhinitis | Prostatic hyperplasia
Bladder outflow obstruction
Angle-closure glaucoma | Dry mouth, unpleasant taste
Nausea
Headache
Rarely—constipation palpitation, tachycardia urinary retention, blurred vision, angle-closure glaucoma, rash, urticaria, and angioedema | Aerosol inhalation
Nebulised inhalation | *Adult dose:*
250–500mcg via nebulised solution (3–4 times daily)
Paediatric dose:
125–250 mcg via nebulized solution (under 5 years)
250mcg via nebulized solution (6–12 years) |

References

Allman KG and Wilson IH (eds) (2006). *Oxford Handbook of Anaesthesia* (2nd edn). Oxford University Press: Oxford.

British National Formulary. Available at: http://bnf.org/bnf/

Sasada M and Smith S (2003). *Drugs in anaesthesia and intensive care* (3rd edn). Oxford University Press: Oxford.

Nitrates

Drug	Indications	Contraindications/cautions	Side effects	Drug route	Drug dose
Glyceryl trinitrate (nitroglycerin)	Prophylaxis and treatment of stable and unstable angina Perioperative hypertension Left ventricular failure Extravasation *Glyceryl trinitrate might increase the duration of pancuronium-induced neuromuscular blockade*	Hypersensitivity to nitrates Hypotension; hypovolaemia Aortic stenosis Cardiomyopathy Cardiac tamponade Anaemia; hypothyroidism Malnutrition; hypothermia Head trauma Cerebral haemorrhage Recent MI, hypoxaemia Hepatic impairment Pregnancy, breastfeeding Susceptible to angle-closure glaucoma	Postural hypotension Sinus tachycardia Headache Dizziness Rarely—nausea, vomiting, heartburn, flushing, rash	Sublingual tablet Aerosol spray IV infusion Transdermal patch	400mcg via aerosol spray 10–200mcg per minute via IV infusion
Isosorbide dinitrate	Prophylaxis and treatment of angina Left ventricular failure	Hypersensitivity to nitrates Hypotension; hypovolaemia Aortic stenosis Cardiomyopathy Cardiac tamponade Anaemia; hypothyroidism	Postural hypotension Sinus tachycardia Headache Dizziness	IV infusion Aerosol spray Orally	2–10mg per hour via IV infusion

		Rarely—nausea, vomiting, heartburn, flushing, rash
Malnutrition, hypothermia		
Head trauma		
Cerebral haemorrhage		
Recent MI, hypoxaemia		
Hepatic impairment		
Pregnancy, breastfeeding		
Susceptible to angle-closure glaucoma		

References

Allman KG and Wilson IH (eds) (2006). *Oxford Handbook of Anaesthesia* (2nd edn). Oxford University Press: Oxford.

British National Formulary. Available at: 🖳 http://bnf.org/bnf/

Sasada M and Smith S (2003). *Drugs in anaesthesia and intensive care* (3rd edn). Oxford University Press: Oxford.

Calcium channel blockers

Drug	Indications	Contraindications/cautions	Side effects	Drug route	Drug dose
Amlodipine	Prophylaxis of angina; Hypertension	Unstable angina; Cardiogenic shock; Aortic stenosis; Breast feeding; Hepatic impairment; Pregnancy	Nausea; dry mouth; fatigue; headache; dizziness; palpitations; flushing; abdominal pain	Orally	5mg orally (daily)
Nifedipine	Prophylaxis of angina; Hypertension	Unstable angina; Cardiogenic shock; Aortic stenosis; Heart failure; Hypotension; Diabetes; Pregnancy	Nausea; dry mouth; fatigue; headache; dizziness; palpitations; flushing; lethargy; abdominal pain; hypotension;	Orally	5mg orally (TDS)
Verapamil	Hypertension; Supraventricular arrhythmias	Bradycardia; Cardiogenic shock; Hypotension; heart failure; AV block; IV betablockers; Wolff–Parkinson–White syndrome; MI; First degree AV block; Hepatic impairment; Pregnancy; breastfeeding	Dry mouth; constipation; fatigue; headache; dizziness; palpitations; flushing; abdominal pain; hypotension; heart failure; heart block	IV injection; Orally	5–10mg slowly via IV injection

References

Allman KG and Wilson IH (eds) (2006). *Oxford Handbook of Anaesthesia* (2nd edn). Oxford University Press: Oxford.

British National Formulary. Available at: 🖥 http://bnf.org/bnf/

Sasada M and Smith S (2003). *Drugs in anaesthesia and intensive care* (3rd edn). Oxford University Press: Oxford.

Inotropic sympathomimetics

Drug	Indications	Contraindications/cautions	Side effects	Drug route	Drug dose
Adrenaline (epinephrine)	Emergency treatment of acute anaphylaxis Cardiopulmonary resuscitation	Hypertension Heart disease Diabetes mellitus Elderly Arrhythmias Cerebrovascular disease Caution with IV route of administration	Nausea and vomiting Arrhythmias; palpitation Tachycardia; dyspnoea Anxiety; restlessness Weakness Headache Hypertension	IV injection IM injection SC	*Adult dose:* Anaphylaxis: 1 in 10000 solution via slow IV injection Paediatric dose: Anaphylaxis: 150mcg via IM injection (15–30kg in weight) *See emergency care chapter for CPR drug dosages*
Dobutamine	Cardiac surgery Inotropic support following MI Cardiomyopathy Septic shock Cardiogenic shock *Dobutamine should be avoided with cardiac tamponade and aortic stenosis*	Tachyarrhythmia Phaeochromocytoma Aortic stenosis Caution in pregnancy	Dysrhythmias; tachycardia Hypertension Phlebitis Headache; chest pain Thrombocytopenia is rare	IV infusion	2.5–10mcg/kg per minute by IV infusion and titrated according to response

Dopamine	Cardiac surgery Cardiogenic shock following MI	Low dose in shock due to MI Correct hypovolaemia Renal impairment Caution in pregnancy	Nausea and vomiting Dysrhythmias Tachycardia; hypotension Hypertension Extravasation may cause necrosis	IV infusion	2.5–5mcg/kg per minute by IV infusion via central line and titrated according to response
Dopexamine	Acute heart failure Inotropic support in chronic heart failure *Dopexamine should be avoided with aortic stenosis, phaeochromocytoma and uncorrected hypovolaemia*	Hypertrophic cardiomyopathy Aortic stenosis Phaeochromocytoma Thrombocytopenia MI Correct hypovolaemia Angina; pregnancy	Nausea and vomiting Bradycardia; tachycardia Angina; arrhythmias Dyspnoea, headache Sweating; flushing MI	IV infusion	0.5–1mcg/kg per minute via IV infusion titrated according to response

References

Allman KG and Wilson IH (eds) (2006). *Oxford Handbook of Anaesthesia* (2nd edn). Oxford University Press: Oxford.

British National Formulary. Available at: 🖳 http://bnf.org/bnf/

Sasada M and Smith S (2003). *Drugs in anaesthesia and intensive care* (3rd edn). Oxford University Press: Oxford.

Vasoconstrictor sympathomimetic drugs

Drug	Indications	Contraindications/cautions	Side effects	Drug route	Dose
Ephedrine	Reversal of hypotension from general, spinal or epidural anaesthesia	Breastfeeding	Tachycardia (sometimes bradycardia)	Slow IV injection	3–6mg every 3–4 minutes
		Diabetes mellitus,	Arrhythmias		Maximum dose
		Ischaemic heart disease,	Nausea, vomiting		30mg
		Hyperthyroidism	Vasoconstriction with hypertension		
	Narcolepsy	Hypertension	Vasodilation with hypotension		
	Hiccups	Elderly	Anginal pain, Anorexia		
	Nasal decongestant	Pregnancy	Dizziness and flushing		
		Susceptibility to angle-closure glaucoma,	Headache confusion		
		Acute urine retention in prostatic hypertrophy	Anxiety, Dyspnoea		
			Difficulty in micturition		
			Urine retention		
			Restlessness		
			Psychoses, tremor		
			Sweating, hypersalivation		
			Changes in blood-glucose concentration		
			Very rarely angle-closure glaucoma		

Metaraminol	Acute hypotension during general/spinal anaesthesia	Hypertension	Tachycardia	IV injection	0.5–5mg by IV injection for emergencies
	Hypotension during cardiopulmonary bypass surgery	Pregnancy	Arrhythmias	IV infusion	
		Coronary, mesenteric, or peripheral vascular thrombosis	Hypertension		15–100mg via IV infusion
	Priapism	Cirrhosis, elderly	Headache, dizziness		
		Hypoxia	Bradycardia		
	Tissue necrosis may occur following extravascular injection	Hypercapnia	Peripheral ischaemia		
		pregnancy			
		Breastfeeding	*Excessive vasopressor response may cause a prolonged rise in BP*		
		Extravasation at injection site may cause necrosis			
Noradrenaline	Acute hypotension	Hypertension	Hypertension	IV injection	0.5–0.75 ml of a 200mcg/mL solution for cardiac arrest
	Cardiac arrest	Pregnancy	Headache	IV infusion	
		Coronary, mesenteric, or peripheral vascular thrombosis	Arrhythmias	Intracardiac injection	
		Uncorrected hypovolaemia	Bradycardia		
		Elderly	Peripheral ischaemia		
		Extravasation at injection site may cause necrosis			

References

Allman KG and Wilson IH (eds) (2006). *Oxford Handbook of Anaesthesia* (2nd edn). Oxford University Press: Oxford.

British National Formulary. Available at: 🖥 http://bnf.org/bnf

Sasada M and Smith S (2003). *Drugs in anaesthesia and intensive care* (3rd edn). Oxford University Press: Oxford

Fluid therapy and fluid replacement

Fluid therapy

Fluid compartment equilibrium may be disrupted by anaesthesia, surgery and illness.[1]

Perioperative considerations

- Patients undergoing surgery may need IV fluid to replace abnormal losses of fluid from bleeding or 'third space' loss. This usually amounts to approximately 10mL/kg/hour of surgery.
- Third space loss refers to fluid lost from the circulation during surgery.
  - Some of this fluid forms oedema in the area of the operation.
  - Some fluid may be lost into the bowel.
  - Fluid loss can also occur from evaporation.
- A general rule is that more replacement fluid will be required for major surgery.
- Measurement of pulse rate, CVP, and urine output will help to guide fluid therapy intraoperatively.
- These losses are usually replaced by balanced salt solutions e.g. Hartmann's solution.
- Preoperative fasting does not necessitate fluid replacement unless fasting has been prolonged.
- Perioperative hypovolaemia and dehydration are associated with morbidity.
- Warming fluid perioperatively can help to regulate temperature, particularly for infants and neonates.

Indications of fluid therapy

- Replacement and expansion of circulating volume.
- Replace existing fluid and electrolyte deficits.
- Maintain fluid and electrolyte balance.
- Replace surgical fluid and electrolyte losses.

General complications /side effects

- Fluid overload leading to oedema.
- Electrolyte imbalances.
- Coagulopathies.
- DVT.
- Patient discomfort.
- Infection.
- Air embolism.

Types of fluids

- *Colloids*: large-molecule fluids used primarily for short-term fluid expansion.
- *Crystalloids*: smaller-molecule fluids used for fluid, i.e. water, and electrolyte replacement.
- *Blood and blood products*: for long-term circulating volume and red cell replacement and treatment of coagulopathies.

Fluids after surgery

Whilst it is often indicated that caution should be exercised in the use of crystalloid fluids containing sodium in the immediate postoperative period, all fluid (and associated electrolyte) replacement should be determined on the basis of individual patient requirements.

📖 See also Colloids, p.540, for details of crystalloids commonly used in the perioperative environment.

References

1. Self R, Walker D, and Mythen M (2006). Blood products and fluid therapy. In Allman KG and Wilson IH (eds) *Oxford Handbook of Anaesthesia* (2nd edn). Oxford University Press: Oxford.

Green D, Ervine M, and White S (2003). *Fundamentals of Perioperative Management*. Greenwich Medical Media: London.

Law R (2003). Pre-operative management. *Update in Anaesthesia*. **13**, Article 14. Available at: 💾 http://www.nda.ox.ac.uk/wfsa/html/u17/u1714_01.htm

Crystalloids

Crystalloids are fluids comprising of water with either electrolytes and/or glucose used in the treatment or prevention of fluid, electrolyte, and small-scale calorific deficits. They are effective with few adverse side effects.[1]

Indications—general

For surgical patients in all perioperative phases:
- To meet normal fluid and electrolyte requirements.
- To replenish substantial deficits, e.g. from preoperative fasting, or continuing losses through surgical trauma.
- When adequate oral intake is not possible, e.g. nausea and vomiting.

When IV administration is not possible, fluid can be administered by SC infusion (hypodermoclysis), though this route is highly unlikely to be used in a perioperative setting. See Box 25.1 for 24-hour fluid replacements.

> ### Box 25.1 24-hour fluid requirements
>
> The following formula is commonly used to calculate the maintenance fluid requirements for a 24-hour period in adults:
> 1500mL for the first 20kg of body weight + 20mL/kg for each additional kg

The individual circumstances of each patient should be considered but as a general guide:
- Replace ECF depletion with saline.
- Rehydrate with glucose.

Perioperative considerations
- Balanced salt solutions (Hartmann's solution) are usually the first-line fluid replacement therapy within the perioperative period.
- Saline 0.9% is used for electrolyte replacement.
- Saline 0.9% is also used for hypovolaemic resuscitation.
- Glucose 5% is used for restore dehydration.
- Glucose 10%, 20%, and 50% can be used to promote normoglycaemia.[1]

Table 25.1 Serum and crystalloid electrolyte composition

		Na⁺	K⁺	Ca²⁺⁺	Cl⁻	HCO₃⁻	pH
Serum value		135–145 mmol/L	3.1–5.1 mmol/L	4.5–5.8 mmol/L	95–105 mmol/L	22–26 mmol/L	7.35–7.45
Fluid	**Indications**						
Hartmann's	In place of NaCl during surgery	131	5	4	112	129	6.5
0.9% saline	Sodium depletion	154	0	0	154	0	5.5
Dextrose-saline	Water and sodium depletion	31	0	0	31	0	4.5
5% glucose	Water depletion Emergency treatment of hyperkalaemia* Treatment of diabetic ketoacidosis**	0	0	0	0	0	4.1

*As part of a treatment regimen with calcium, bicarbonate, and insulin.

**Following correction of hyperglycaemia and must be accompanied by an ongoing insulin infusion.

References and further reading

1. Self R, Walker D, and Mythen M (2006). Blood products and fluid therapy. In Allman KG and Wilson IH (eds) *Oxford Handbook of Anaesthesia* (2nd edn). Oxford University Press: Oxford.

Green D, Ervine M, and White S (2003). Fundamentals of Perioperative management. Greenwich Medical Media: London.

British National Formulary (2008). Available at: 🖥 www.BNF.org

Colloids

Colloids are fluids that, because of their large molecular weight, remain within the vascular fluid compartment for extended periods of time and thus expand and maintain circulating volume. The duration of action of colloids is determined by physiochemical properties, integrity of capillary membrane and by metabolic and clearance pharmacokinetics.[1] Colloid solutions are sometimes used when losses are heavy.

Indications
- Immediate, short-term treatment of non-haemorrhagic hypovolaemia and shock.

Contraindications
- Long-term maintenance of plasma volume in burns or peritonitis.
- Known hypersensitivity to any constituents.

Cautions
- Cardiac disease.
- Liver disease.
- Renal impairment.
- Monitoring of urine output required.

Side effects
- Hypersensitivity reactions.
- Anaphylactoid reactions.
- Increased bleed times—transient.

Types of colloids (Table 25.2)
Colloids in general use fall into one of 3 groups:

Dextrans
- Hypertonic fluids exerting powerful osmotic effect.
- Can interfere with cross matching—blood samples should be taken before starting dextran infusions.

Gelatins
- Isotonic.
- 2–3 hours circulatory half-life.
- Associated with anaphylactoid reactions.

Starchs
- Hypertonic.
- Expand volume on approximate 1:1 ratio.
- Improved haemodynamic status for up to 24 hours.

Table 25.2 Colloid fluids overview

Fluid	Molecular weight	Dose
Dextrans		
Dextran 40 ®	40,000	Initially 500–1,000 ml
Dextran 70 ®	70,000	Initially 500–1000 ml rapidly, followed by 500 ml if necessary to a maximum total dosage of 20 ml/kg during initial 24 hours.
Gelatins		
e.g. Gelofusine ® Haemaccel ®	30,000–35,000	3.5–4% 500–1000 ml
Starches		
Hetastarch	450,000	1,500 ml (max 24 hours)
Pentastrach	200,000	6% 2,500 ml (max 24 hours) 10% 1,500 ml (max 24 hours)
Tetrastarch e.g. Venofundin ® Voluven ®	130,000	50 mg/kg

References and further reading

1. Self R, Walker D, and Mythen M (2006). Blood products and fluid therapy. In Allman KG and Wilson IH (eds) *Oxford Handbook of Anaesthesia* (2nd edn). Oxford University Press: Oxford.

Green D, Ervine M, and White S (2003). *Fundamentals of Perioperative Management.* Greenwich Medical Media: London.

Hudsmith J, Wheeler D, and Gupta A (2004). *Core Topics in Perioperative Medicine.* Greenwich Medical Media: London.

Blood

- Blood is a fluid, connective tissue comprising of cells and cell fragments—approximately 45% b/v (blood volume) suspended in a fluid medium (plasma approx 55% b/v).
- The primary purpose of blood is to ensure adequate oxygenation of tissue. Failure to perfuse tissue results in shock.

General indications for transfusion

- Restoration of circulating volume when a loss >30% of circulating blood volume has occurred—class 3 and class 4 shock.
- Where patients are symptomatic following blood loss of <30% and/or further blood loss is expected.
- Chronic anaemia.

Adverse effects

- Transfusion reactions.
- Haemolytic transfusion reaction—caused by ABO incompatibility.
- Delayed extravascular haemolysis—caused by Rh or non-ABO reactions.
- Non-haemolytic febrile reaction.
- Anaphylactoid reaction—caused by recipient reaction to plasma proteins in donor blood.
- Anaphylactic reaction—rare.
- Transmission of infection.
- Transfusion-related acute lung injury (TRALI).
- With massive transfusions, i.e. transfusion of entire circulating volume within 24 hours:
- Hyperkalaemia and acidosis.
- Coagulopathies including disseminated intravascular coagulation (DIC).
- Citrate toxicity ± citrate toxicity.
- Impaired tissue O_2 delivery.

Autologus transfusion

The re-transfusion of the patients own blood/blood products is collected in one of 4 ways:
- *Preoperative autologous donation (PAD):*
  - Blood donated in the weeks leading up to surgery.
  - Tested and stored as with allogenic blood, but is reserved for that patient alone.
  - Reinfused with the same safeguards for prescribed allogenic blood/products.
- *Acute normovolaemic haemodilution (ANH):*
  - Whole blood is taken from the patient (1–3 units) prior to the start of surgery (often post induction).
  - Blood volume restored with acellular fluid.
  - Blood is reinfused to the patient when needed or at the end of surgery.

- *Intraoperative cell salvage (ICS)* (□ also see Intraoperative cell salvage, p.544):
  - Blood lost during surgery is collected, red blood cells (RBCs) are separated from the whole blood and washed (with saline).
  - Resulting RBCs suspended in saline reinfused to the patient when needed or at the end of surgery.
- *Postoperative cell salvage (PCS)* (□ also see Postoperative cell salvage, p.546):
  - Post-operative blood loss is collected.
  - Depending on the system in use, salvaged blood is either filtered (unwashed system) or RBCs are separated out and washed as with ICS (washed system).
  - Resulting product reinfused as required.

Indications
- A clean operative field.
- Anticipated blood loss >1000mL or >20% EBV[1] (ICS).
- Anticipated postoperative blood loss >500mL for PCS.
- Low Hb/risk factors for bleeding.
- Rare blood type/multiple antibodies.
- Patients with objections to receiving allogenic blood.

Contraindications
- Contamination within the surgical field.
- Malignancy within the surgical field (where is no indication of metastatic spread).
- Non-IV materials should not be present within the surgical site.
- Sickle cell anaemia.

Cautions
- Use of leuco-depletion filters is recommended in obstetrics and malignancy.

Further reading

Green D, Ervine M, and White S (2003). *Fundamentals of Perioperative management*. Greenwich Medical Media: London.

Hudsmith J, Wheeler D, and Gupta A (2004). *Core Topics in Perioperative Medicine*. Greenwich Medical Media: London.

UK blood transfusion guidelines. Available at: 🖳 www.transfusionguidelines.org.uk/lcs

Intraoperative cell salvage

ICS is a technique whereby blood lost during a surgical procedure is collected and processed to produce autologous (the patients' own) RBCs for reinfusion. ICS can greatly reduce the need to transfuse allogeneic (donor) RBCs.

Indications

- Elective and emergency surgical procedures.
- Where there is a 'clean' surgical field.
- Anticipated blood loss of >1000mL or 20% of the patients' estimated total blood volume.

ICS may also be considered when the patient has:

- A low preoperative haemoglobin (Hb) level.
- Risk factors for bleeding, e.g. factor deficiencies.
- Rare blood groups or multiple antibodies.
- Objections to receiving allogeneic blood (and has consented to ICS).

Contraindications

- Contaminated surgical field e.g. bowel content.
- Non-IV substances within the surgical field (discontinue ICS and irrigate the wound with IV saline before resuming).
- Heparin induced thrombocytopenia when heparin is the anticoagulant (acid citrate dextrose (ACD) may be use as an alternative).

Warnings

The following have been identified as areas of concern when using ICS:

- The presence of the following contaminants within the surgical field:
  - Infection.
  - Gastric/pancreatic secretions.
  - Pleural effusions.
  - Amniotic fluid.
- Malignant disease (within the surgical field).
- Abnormal red blood cell disorders e.g. sickle cell disease.

In these circumstances, ICS should be carried out with caution, avoiding the aspiration of contaminants and at the direction of the lead clinician.

Equipment

In addition to the ICS machine, the equipment required for ICS includes:

- Anticoagulant: 30 000IU heparin/1000mL IV saline or ACD.
- Aspiration and anticoagulation line.
- Collection reservoir.
- Processing set.
- Blood giving set/filter (appropriate for the type of surgery).

The procedure also requires a vacuum (some ICS machines have an onboard vacuum) and other equipment generally available within the operating theatre department e.g. a wide bore plastic suction tip.

Procedure

The reinfusion bag should be labelled with an autologous transfusion label that includes handwritten patient details and the expiry time of the ICS blood (see local policy). Throughout the procedure it is important to:
- Maintain a low vacuum (−100 to −200mmHg) to minimise RBC damage (the vacuum may be increased during excessive bleeding).
- Ensure sufficient anticoagulant is flowing to prevent coagulation.
- Avoid aspirating non-IV substances into the system.

The ICS procedure can be divided into four main steps:

Collection

Blood is aspirated from the surgical field, anticoagulated and filtered (in the collection reservoir) to remove large debris e.g. bone fragments.

Separation

RBCs are separated from whole blood and waste products, e.g. anticoagulant, and concentrated to produce a high haematocrit (>50%).

Washing

The RBCs are washed with IV saline to remove residual waste products.

To prevent the reinfusion of potentially harmful contaminants, the minimum wash volume specified by the manufacturers should be used.

Reinfusion

The RBCs are pumped to a reinfusion bag. Upon reinfusion:
- Check the ICS blood has been prescribed by a clinician.
- Check the patient's identification against the label on the reinfusion bag.
- Check the expiry time of the blood—refer to local policy.
- Use a filter appropriate to the surgical procedure—refer to local policy.
- Monitor the patient for signs of reaction.
- Record the volume/time of the reinfusion in the patient's clinical record.

ICS blood should not be reinfused under pressure due to the presence of air in the reinfusion bag.

For consideration

- Staff should undergo appropriate training prior to using ICS (a UK ICS competency assessment framework is available).
- ICS should, where possible, be discussed with the patient prior to use.
- ICS only returns RBCs to the patient when massive blood loss occurs, it may also be necessary to transfuse allogeneic blood components.
- Local policy and manufacturers' guidelines should be adhered to.
- Some machines are designed to continue the cell salvage process by salvaging blood lost from the wound postoperatively.

Reference

UK Cell Salvage Action Group (2007). *Policy for the provision of Intraoperative Cell Salvage.* Available through the Better Blood Transfusion Toolkit at ⌨ http://www.transfusionguidelines.org.uk

Postoperative cell salvage

PCS is a technique whereby blood lost from the wound postoperatively is collected and reinfused. PCS involves either washed systems, which use a machine to produce autologous RBCs, or unwashed systems, which use an autologous wound drain to produce filtered autologous blood. This section relates to the use of unwashed systems (however the indications and contraindication are the same for washed systems). PCS can reduce the need to transfuse allogeneic RBCs.

Indications

- Elective and emergency orthopaedic surgical procedures.
- An uncontaminated wound.
- Anticipated post-operative blood loss of 500–1000mL.

PCS may also be considered when the patient has:
- A low preoperative haemoglobin (Hb) level.
- Risk factors for bleeding e.g. factor deficiencies.
- Rare blood groups or multiple antibodies.
- Objections to receiving allogeneic blood (and has consented to PCS).

Contraindications

- A contaminated wound, e.g., infection or malignancy.
- Non-IV substances within the wound e.g. antibiotics not licensed for IV use.

As with ICS, the use of PCS in patients with abnormal RBC disorders, e.g., sickle cell disease, should be carried out with caution at the direction of the lead clinician.

Equipment

The PCS system (autologous wound drain) normally comprises:
- Trocar and wound drain tubing.
- Collection set—including vacuum system and may include filters.
- Reinfusion set—this may be integral to the collection set or a separate reinfusion bag and normally includes filters.

Because PCS systems vary significantly it is vital that all staff involved in the process have received appropriate training and are competency-assessed for each of the devices they use.

Procedure

The PCS system (and where appropriate the reinfusion bag) should be labelled with an autologous transfusion label that includes handwritten patient details and the expiry time of the PCS blood (see local policy).

The PCS procedure begins within the operating theatre and continues into the recovery area and often onto the ward. The PCS system should be monitored throughout.

The PCS procedure can be divided into three main steps:

Insertion of the wound drain (within sterile field)

Prior to insertion of the drain, the surgical site should be irrigated with IV saline. The autologous drain is inserted prior to skin closure using the trocar and the collection set is attached to the drain. Most manufacturers recommend that the drain remain closed (clamped) for 20 minutes following skin closure (especially if a tourniquet has been used).

Collection

Following the release of the clamp, blood collects into the PCS system. Because clotting occurs within the wound, the blood that collects in the drain is defibrinated (i.e. depleted of fibrinogen). The lack of fibrinogen in the collected blood prevents coagulation, therefore, anticoagulant is not required for PCS. In some PCS systems, the blood is filtered in the collection set.

During the collection phase it may be necessary to:
- Reprime the vacuum on systems with an intermittent vacuum.
- Transfer the collected blood into the reinfusion bag on systems where the reinfusion set is not integral to the collection set.

Staff should be alert to large blood loss and contact the surgeon and/or anaesthetist under these circumstances.

Reinfusion

The collected blood is filtered prior to reinfusion. Depending on the system used, the individual responsible for the PCS system may need to attach a filter to the reinfusion set. Upon reinfusion:
- Check the PCS blood has been prescribed by a clinician.
- Check the patient's identification against the label on the PCS system.
- Check the expiry time of the blood (refer to local policy).
- Use the filter specified by the manufacturer.
- Monitor the patient for signs of reaction.
- Record the volume/time of the reinfusion in the patient's clinical record.

PCS blood should not be reinfused under pressure due to the presence of air in the reinfusion bag.

For consideration

- Staff should undergo appropriate training and be assessed as competent before using PCS.
- PCS should, where possible, be discussed with the patient prior to use.
- When massive blood loss occurs, it may also be necessary to transfuse allogeneic blood components.
- Local policy and manufacturers guidelines should be adhered to.

Reference

Department of Health (2007). *Better Blood Transfusion Toolkit. Effective Alternatives – Post-operative Cell Salvage*. Available at: http://www.transfusionguidelines.org.uk

Management principles of emergency care

Emergency care

Principles of emergency care

Prevention is better than cure: in a large number of in-hospital emergencies, critically-ill patients have presented with a history of physiological deterioration during the preceding hours.

Deterioration may be prevented by regular assessment and appropriate and timely interventions by suitably trained personnel.

If you have doubts about your patient's condition, call for senior help immediately, ensure the patient has patent venous access, administer high flow O_2, and observe continuously for changes to his/her condition.

The ABCDE approach

The **ABCDE** approach to assessment is now recommended to '*treat first that which kills first*' in all critically-ill and emergency patients.
- The ABCDE approach is identified as:
  - Airway.
  - Breathing.
  - Circulation.
  - Disability.
  - Exposure.
- Each stage of this approach must be assessed, treated as necessary, and re-evaluated before moving on to the next stage.
- If, during the course of treatment, any unexpected change occurs in the patient's condition, then assessment must begin again at 'A'.

Initial approach:
- Is it safe to approach the patient? Do not forget personal safety!
- Would you expect this patient to be responsive?
- The best immediate assessment of a patient is by talking with him/her.
- If the patient is unresponsive and not (for example) intubated and ventilated, call for help immediately and begin ABCDE assessment.

References and further reading

Cole E (ed) (2008). *Trauma Care: Initial assessment and management in the emergency department: essential clinical skills for nurses*. Wiley Blackwell: London.

Dougherty L and Lister S (eds) (2004). *The Royal Marsden Hospital Manual of Clinical Nursing Procedures* (6th edn). Blackwell Publishing: Oxford.

Evans C and Tippins E (2006). *The Foundations of Emergency Care*. Open University Press: Maidenhead.

Royal College of Anaesthetists (2004). *Guidelines for the Provision of Anaesthetic Services*. RCoA: London.

A: airway

- Is the patient's breathing normal/noisy/silent?
- Noise on inspiration generally indicates partial upper airway obstruction (including laryngospasm); noise on expiration may indicate bronchospasm/partial lower airway obstruction; silence may indicate complete airway obstruction!
- Check patient's mouth is clear of visible obstruction, e.g., vomitus, secretions, foreign bodies etc.
- Remove any secretions or foreign bodies safely (NB well-fitting dentures may enable effective airway maintenance in edentulous patients).
- Apply basic manoeuvres to open airway: head tilt/chin lift or jaw thrust (Figs. 26.1–3)—jaw thrust preferable in infants and trauma victims.
- Place own fingers **only** on bony parts of patient's face or jaw—pressing soft tissues may exacerbate airway obstruction.
- *Reassess.* If patient is unconscious or judged incapable of maintaining own airway, endotracheal intubation utilising RSI (☐ see Rapid sequence induction, p.202) should be considered.

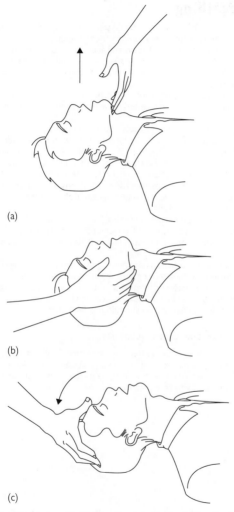

(a)

(b)

(c)

Fig. 26.1 (a) Performing a chin lift; (b) performing a jaw thrust; (c) performing a head tilt. Reproduced with permission from Thomas J and Monaghan T (2007). *Oxford Handbook of Clinical Examination and Practical Skills*, ISBN 9780198568384, Oxford University Press: Oxford.

B: breathing

- Assess patient's respiratory rate, O_2 saturation, end-tidal CO_2 values (in intubated patients), depth, symmetry, and equal, bilateral air entry (left–right) on auscultation, and appropriate chest/abdominal movement during respiration (NB 'see-saw' (paradoxical) respiration may indicate complete airway obstruction), and check for central cyanosis/pallor.
- Tachypnoea and dyspnoea are important signs of physiological disturbance and may indicate serious deterioration in the patient's condition.
- If atypical clinical signs or physiological measurements present, supportive interventions should be considered **urgently** e.g. administer high-flow O_2 via non-rebreathing face mask if rate and depth sufficient, if not assist ventilations using face mask with self-inflating resuscitator bag or Waters circuit (Mapleson C; 🕮 see Breathing systems, p.142);
- Consider *needle thoracocentesis* (Box 26.1) if tension pneumothorax suspected—asymmetric respiration, unilateral air entry, hyper-resonance and decreasing BP.
- If intubated patient exhibits adverse signs, also exclude *DOPES*: (displaced ETT, obstructed ETT, pneumothorax, equipment malfunction, stomach insufflation) and treat as required. Reassess patient following all interventions.
- If at this stage the patient is not breathing or exhibiting other signs of life, e.g., choking, coughing, moving limbs, etc. the *cardiac arrest team* should be called immediately and treatment protocols for adult or paediatric life support (🕮 see Principles of resuscitation in adults, p. 564, and 🕮 Principles of resuscitation in children, p. 568) followed.

Box 26.1 Needle thoracocentesis

Emergency treatment of tension pneuomothorax involving insertion of wide-bore cannula above third rib in mid-clavicular line into intra-pleural space of affected side. Chest drain to be inserted aseptically and chest x-rays taken following re-suscitation.

C: circulation

- Assess patient's pulse, BP, perfusion, urine output, and temperature.
- Homeostatic mechanisms normally maintain sufficient perfusion of tissues with O_2 and nutrients and the removal of waste products.
- This balance may be affected and hypoperfusion (shock) occur when circulating fluid volume is lost or when mechanical failure or obstruction impedes circulation.
- Tachycardia is a valuable sign of cardiovascular compensation for fluid volume loss but may also be caused by pain, anxiety, exercise, or infection, hence the patient's history along with other signs and parameters must always be considered during assessment.
- Bradycardia may be associated with respiratory insufficiency (hypoxia and hypercapnia), especially in the drowsy patient.
- Hypotension is a late sign of shock as BP is maintained by autonomic responses until decompensation occurs.
- Acute hypertension may be caused by untreated pain, thyroid toxicity, drug overdose, or autonomic dysreflexia in spinal injuries patients, and should be treated using appropriate medications.
- Urine output (≥ 1mg/kg/hour), centrally measured *capillary refill time* (Box 26.2), and colour of membranes (e.g. lips) are useful indicators of adequate tissue perfusion.
- Peripheral temperature, colour, and capillary refill (e.g. of nail beds) may be adversely affected by ambient temperature and hypothermia. Severe hypothermia (≤32°C) may also induce cardiac arrhythmias.

Box 26.2 Capillary refill time

Measurement of tissue perfusion achieved by pressing thumb on patient's sternum or nail bed for 5 seconds; blanched skin should reperfuse in the well hydrated patient within 2 seconds.

Types of shock

Hypovolaemic shock

- Loss of circulating volume caused by dehydration (e.g. through poor fluid balance, diarrhoea, and vomiting etc), burns, or haemorrhage.
- Characterised by cool, clammy peripheries, pallor, and fast, thready pulses.
- Hypotension is a late sign! Treatment of dehydration is by fluid and electrolyte replacement.
- Immediate fluid replacement in severe burns cases is calculated according to formulae, e.g. Muir and Barclay:

  [weight (kg) × %burn]/2 = mL colloid IV fluid (e.g. Gelofusine®) per time period (4 hours, 4 hours, 4 hours, 6 hours, 6 hours, 12 hours)

- Haemorrhage is treated with oxygenation (to optimise remaining O_2 carrying capacity), application of direct pressure (tamponade) where possible, moderate fluid and blood product replacement with urgent surgical intervention where required.
- The use of tourniquets is discouraged in most cases and rapid, large-volume infusions and transfusions are now viewed as being potentially counter-productive in the treatment of haemorrhage, especially following trauma.[1,2]

Distributive shock

Circulating volume is lost to the interstitial tissues through the capillary beds, as in anaphylactic and septic shock.

- Anaphylactic shock is characterised by a rapid fall in BP, tachycardia, dyspnoea, wheezing, skin rash. However, it is common for anaphylaxis to display some but not all of these symptoms.
- Recommended treatment of severe anaphylaxis involves removal of the offending allergen (e.g. blood transfusion), administration of IM adrenaline 0.5mg (1:1000 solution) repeated at 5-minute intervals as required, the administration of crystalloid IV fluids if severe hypotension is present, and also antihistamines.
- Advanced airway management (intubation ± ventilation) may also be required if oedema of the upper airway and bronchospasm are present.
- Sepsis is characterised by a steady fall in BP, tachycardia, tachypnoea, and hypo- or hyperthermia.
- Septic shock is a complex and potentially grave condition often requiring large-volume fluid infusion and multi-organ support in a level 3 ITU.

Cardiogenic shock

- Resulting from failure of the heart (due to arrhythmias or other dysfunction) to provide sufficient output to perfuse the tissues adequately.
- Characterised by falling BP, dyspnoea, raised CVP, and cool peripheries.
- The underlying heart condition should be treated urgently and IV fluids should only be given with extreme caution.

Obstructive shock

- Resulting from physical obstruction to the circulation, as in pulmonary embolus, tension pneumothorax, or cardiac tamponade.
- Successful treatment involves identification of and removal of the cause of the obstruction.
- In cases of tension pneumothorax this may be relatively simple (📖 see B: breathing, p. 556), and if cardiac tamponade is suspected in a trauma victim, needle pericadiocentesis may be effective.
- Otherwise it is not always possible to achieve this aim within the available time in cases of obstructive shock, and a poor outcome is common.

References

Anderson I D (2003). *Care of the Critically Ill Surgical Patient* (2nd edn). Arnold: London.

Pepe PE (2003). Shock in polytrauma. *British Medical Journal* **327**, 1119–20.

D: disability and E: exposure

Disability

- Assess patient's level of consciousness and pupil reactions to light stimulus. Immediate assessment of consciousness is best achieved using AVPU scale (patient is *a*lert, patient responds to *v*oice, patient responds to *p*ain, patient is *u*nresponsive), but a thorough neurological assessment requires repeated use of the Glasgow Coma Scale (GCS).
- An alert patient would normally be assessed as GCS 15; any patient with a GCS of 8 or below (corresponding with P on the AVPU scale) is cause for concern and maybe incapable of protecting his/her own airway.
- Urgent ET intubation should be considered in such cases. Remember also that in addition to hypoxia or ischaemia, changes in levels of consciousness may be due to hyper- or hypoglycaemia, so bedside glucose monitoring with corrective treatment as necessary is recommended at this stage.

Glasgow Coma Score

The GCS is scored between 3 and 15, 3 being the worst, and 15 the best. It is composed of three parameters: best eye response, best verbal response, best motor response, as shown

Best eye response (4)
1 No eye opening.
2 Eye opening to pain.
3 Eye opening to verbal command.
4 Eyes open spontaneously.

Best verbal response (5)
1 No verbal response.
2 Incomprehensible sounds.
3 Inappropriate words.
4 Confused.
5 Orientated.

Best motor response (6)
1 No motor response.
2 Extension to pain.
3 Flexion to pain.
4 Withdrawal from pain.
5 Localising pain.
6 Obeys Commands.

A GCS of 13 or higher correlates with a mild brain injury; 9 to 12 is a moderate injury; and 8 or less a severe brain injury. See also Assessing levels of consciousness, p.574.

Exposure

- Perform systematic examination of patient's body, removing wet clothes as necessary to prevent unnecessary cooling, but ensuring maintenance of dignity as far as possible.
- Signs such as bleeding from orifices, distended abdomen, possible fractures, surgical wounds, lacerations, and bruising should all be noted and taken into account, along with a detailed history and case note examination when planning further care.

References and further reading

Association of Anaesthetists of Great Britain and Ireland (2004). *Catastrophes in Anaesthetic Practice – dealing with the aftermath.* AAGBI: London.

Cole E (ed) (2008). *Trauma Care: Initial assessment and management in the emergency department: essential clinical skills for nurses.* Wiley Blackwell: London.

Evans C and Tippins E (2006). *The Foundations of Emergency Care.* Open University Press: Maidenhead.

Teasdale G and Jennett B (1974). Assessment of coma and impaired consciousness: a practical scale. *Lancet* **ii** 81–3.

Professional, ethical, and legal considerations of emergency care

Legal considerations

- It is not always possible, or even ethically appropriate, to try and gain informed consent from critically ill or injured patients.
- Do Not Attempt Resuscitation (*DNAR*) orders are signed and *regularly updated* by the consultant in charge of that patient's care, and are based on a considered decision that any attempt at resuscitation of that patient would not lead to prolonging his or her life at an acceptable quality (futility of treatment).
- This decision is taken by the senior clinician, but good practice recommends that the views of the patient, or relatives, should be sought before the decision is made.
- Unless lasting power of attorney has been appointed under the Mental Capacity Act 2005,[1] no person may give or withhold consent on behalf of another

Mental Capacity Act 2005[1]

Assessing lack of capacity

- The Mental Capacity Act 2005 identifies a single test for assessing whether a person lacks capacity to take a particular decision at a particular time.
- It is a 'decision-specific' and time-specific test.
- No person can be labelled 'incapable' because of a medical condition or diagnosis.

Best interests

- A decision made for, or on behalf of, a person who lacks capacity must be in that person's best interests.
- A checklist of factors that decision-makers must work through in deciding what is in a person's best interests is identified in the Act.
- A person making the decision must consider the patient's wishes and feelings explained in a previously written statement.
- People involved in caring for the person lacking capacity have a right to be consulted concerning a person's best interests.

Acts in connection with care or treatment

- A person performing an act in connection with the care or treatment of someone who lacks capacity is offered statutory protection from liability.
- This might cover actions that might otherwise attract criminal prosecution or civil liability if someone has to interfere with the person's body or property in the course of providing care or treatment.[1]

Independent mental capacity advocate (IMCA)

- An IMCA can be appointed to support a patient who lacks capacity but has no one to speak for them; this can include family or friends.
- An IMCA is only involved when decisions are being made about serious medical treatment and can make representations about the person's wishes, feelings, beliefs, and values.

- The IMCA can challenge the decision-maker on behalf of the person lacking capacity.

Advance decisions to refuse treatment
- The Act enables people to make a decision in advance to refuse treatment if they should lack capacity in the future.
- When an advance decision concerns treatment necessary to sustain life, the decision must be in writing, signed, and witnessed. There must also be an express statement that the decision stands 'even if life is at risk' which must also be in writing, signed, and witnessed.

'A lack of capacity cannot be established by reference to a person's age, appearance, or any condition or aspect of a person's behaviour which might lead others to make unjustified assumptions about capacity'.[1]

Professional and ethical considerations
- While it may seem obvious, it is always worth remembering that the experience of life-threatening illness or injury may cause intense emotional distress in patients and their relatives, as well as staff, and the behaviour of healthcare practitioners at such times frequently leaves a lasting impression.
- For this reason it is particularly important to ensure that all communications are clear and unambiguous, that one behaves in a calm and professional manner at all times, and that the rights and sensibilities of the patient and relatives are respected as far as is practicable under the circumstances.

Reference and further reading

1. Mental Capacity Act 2005. Available at: 🖳 www.opsi.gov.uk/acts/acts2005/ukpga_20050009 _en_1.htm

Anderson I D (2003). *Care of the Critically Ill Surgical Patient* (2nd edn). Arnold: London.

Pepe PE (2003). Shock in polytrauma. *British Medical Journal* **327**, 1119–20.

Resuscitation Council (UK) (2006). *Advanced Life Support Provider Manual* (5th edn). Resuscitation Council (UK): London.

Resuscitation Council (UK) (2006). *European Paediatric Life Support Provider Manual* (2nd edn). London: Resuscitation Council (UK): London.

Smith G (2003). *ALERTTM: Acute Life-threatening Events, Recognition and Treatment* (2nd edn). Portsmouth Institute of Medicine, Health and Social Care: Portsmouth.

Principles of resuscitation in adults

Cardiac arrest in adults

Cardiac arrest can be defined as the failure of the heart to perfuse the body's tissues, especially those essential to life. In those patients who have suffered cardiac arrest and for whom resuscitation is indicated, *basic life support* (BLS) must be initiated and the cardiac arrest team called *immediately*.

Basic life support

On finding a collapsed patient:
- Ensure personal safety.
- Gently shake patient; if unresponsive call for help.
- *A*: open patient's mouth and check for foreign bodies; perform head tilt/chin lift or jaw thrust manoeuvre (see Fig. 26.1, p551).
- *B*: look, listen, and feel for breathing (up to 10 seconds); if not breathing send for cardiac arrest team immediately. Where signs of life are present, support respiration until skilled help arrives.
- *C*: assess for circulation (carotid pulse) or signs of life (coughing, purposeful movement etc.).
- If none present commence **cardiopulmonary resuscitation (CPR)**—*cycles of 2 ventilations* (using high-flow O_2, self-inflating resuscitator bag and mask or pocket mask, plus oropharyngeal airway if available) **followed by 30 compressions** of the lower half of victim's sternum (approximately 1/3 depth of chest) at a **rate of 100 per minute**. If the patient is intubated, compressions should be continuous.

Attach cardiac monitor or adhesive defibrillator pads when available and initiate defibrillation if appropriate.

The ECG rhythms associated with cardiac arrest are pulseless *ventricular tachycardia* (VT, broad complex rhythm with a rate >100bpm) or *ventricular fibrillation* (VF, uncoordinated, coarse, or fine, 'bizarre' waveform with no recognisable complexes), *pulseless electrical activity* (PEA, electrical activity of the heart might otherwise be compatible with life but no effective pulse (cardiac output) is present) or *asystole*, (normally a shallow wavy line on the ECG indicating an absence of electrical activity). VF and pulseless VT are classified as the '*shockable*' rhythms, while PEA and asystole are classed as '*non-shockable*'. See Fig. 26.2.

In out of hospital settings, approximately 70% of adult cardiac arrests are due to primary cardiac events (usually MI), and the presenting rhythm is, initially, pulseless VT or VF. These respond well to *early defibrillation* and CPR, although it has been suggested that for every minute defibrillation is delayed, the mortality rate increases by 7–10%.[1,2]

In hospital settings the incidence of VF/VT arrests is decreased (<25%), but survival rates of >40% have been reported.[3] The survival rate of those presenting with PEA or asystolic arrest is considerably less, however, and in such cases it is particularly important to treat the *potentially reversible causes* (4Hs and 4Ts; 📖 see Potentially reversible causes, p.566) while performing CPR and administering *10mL (1mg) 1:10 000 adrenaline (IV) every 3–5 minutes*.

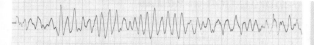

Fig. 26.2 Ventricular fibrillation. Reproduced from Myerson S, Choudhury P, and Mitchell A, *Emergencies in Cardiology*, 2005, ISBN 9780198569596, with permission from Oxford University Press: Oxford.

References and further reading

1. Resuscitation Council (UK) (2006). *Advanced Life Support Provider Manual* (5th edn). Resuscitation Council (UK): London.

2. Resuscitation Council (UK) (2006). *European Paediatric Life Support Provider Manual* (2nd edn). London: Resuscitation Council (UK): London.

3. Gwinnutt CL, Columb M, and Harris R (2000). Outcomes after cardiac arrest in adults in UK hospitals: effect of the 1997 guidelines. *Resuscitation* **47**: 125–35.

Anderson I D (2003). *Care of the Critically Ill Surgical Patient* (2nd edn). Arnold: London.

Pepe PE (2003). Shock in polytrauma. *British Medical Journal* **327**: 1119–20.

Smith G. (2003). *ALERTTM: Acute Life-threatening Events, Recognition and Treatment* (2nd edn). Portsmouth Institute of Medicine, Health and Social Care: Portsmouth.

Defibrillation in adults

- Safety is paramount when defibrillators are used and so these must only be used by suitably trained personnel.
- Successful defibrillation requires sufficient electric current to pass through the heart to depolarise the myocardium, thereby terminating unco-ordinated activity (fibrillation) and allowing the heart's natural pacemaker to instigate a normal, perfusing rhythm.
- Most defibrillators found in hospitals are of the manual variety and require the operator to analyse the patient's rhythm, then set and deliver the appropriate output charge. Automated external defibrillators (AEDs) are becoming increasingly common in public access areas.
- With the introduction of sophisticated biphasic defibrllators, current guidelines now recommend the delivery of a single, maximum power shock in VF/pulseless VT arrests, followed by 2 minutes of CPR, the cycle then being repeated as necessary with 10mL(1mg) 1:10 000 adrenaline (IV) being administered before the third shock.
- Following successful return of spontaneous circulation, the patient may be referred for *reperfusion therapy* —thrombolysis, coronary artery, stenting, or angioplasty.

Potentially reversible causes

- *Hypoxia*: ensure adequate and effective ventilation with high-flow O_2.
- *Hypovolaemia*: establish IV access and administer at least 500mL bolus of 0.9% sodium chloride or Hartmann's solution ('fluid challenge') and seek surgical opinion if haemorrhage is suspected.
- *Hyper/hypokalaemia*: following biochemical testing, correct with potassium supplement (hypo) or insulin/dextrose infusion (hyper) as necessary. Electrolyte and hydrogen ion (acid:base) levels can be measured swiftly in electronic blood-gas analysers. Blood glucose levels should also be measured and treated as necessary.
- *Hypothermia*: rare in hospital in-patients but common in patients brought into ED by ambulance (especially cases of trauma, overdose, drowning etc.). If moderate or severe hypothermia present (<32°C), warm air blankets, warmed ventilator gases and IV fluids should be employed to gradually re-warm the victim. CPR should be continued until the patient is re-warmed
- *Tension pneumothorax*: characterised by asymmetrical chest movement, hyper-resonance, and absent breath sounds on affected side and symptoms of shock; must be treated by urgent needle thoracocentesis (insertion of wide-bore cannula above third rib in mid-clavicular line) followed by chest drain insertion.
- *Tamponade*: suspect in cases of penetrating chest trauma; treat with needle pericardiocentesis or emergency thoracotomy.
- *Toxicity*: reactions to or overdose of therapeutic agents must be excluded or treated as required; in cases of poisoning supportive treatment (CPR, ventilation) should be employed—contact with toxins centre (TOXBASE[1]) may be required to identify suitable antidote once agent identified.

- *Thrombo-embolic*: high index of suspicion of PE in surgical cases complicated by contra-indication of thrombolysis following major surgery, haemorrhagic strokes etc.

Following successful resuscitation, care should include continuing O_2 therapy and physiological monitoring (ECG monitoring (12-lead and continuous 3-lead), BP, O_2 saturation, cardiac enzymes, blood gases).

The induction of mild hypothermia following resuscitation may demonstrate improved neurological outcomes.

Reference and further reading

1. TOXBASE. Available at: ⬚ http://www.toxbase.org/

Gwinnutt CL, Columb M, and Harris R (2000). Outcomes after cardiac arrest in adults in UK hospitals: effect of the 1997 guidelines. *Resuscitation* **47**, 125–35.

Resuscitation Council (UK) (2006). *Advanced Life Support Providers Manual* (5th edition). Resuscitation Council (UK): London.

Principles of resuscitation in children

Cardiac arrest in children

Cardiorespiratory arrest in children is rarely due to a primary cardiac event, as in adults, but more usually secondary to *hypoxia* or *hypovolaemia*. Trauma and infection are common causes of hypovolaemia and airway obstruction, while choking is a common occurrence in young children.

Paediatric physiology readily compensates for respiratory and circulatory failure, so signs such as decreased level of consciousness, bradypnoea, bradycardia, and hypotension indicate that the child is in extremis. It is imperative therefore that clinical signs indicating serious illness in children are recognised and treated promptly to prevent further deterioration.

Signs of serious illness

- *A*: noisy (inspiratory stridor, expiratory wheeze) or silent breathing indicate partial or complete airway obstruction.
- *B*: tachypnoea, bradypnoea (late sign), decreased level of consciousness, increased effort of breathing including grunting, intercostals/subcostal/sternal recession, use of accessory muscles (neck and abdominal muscles, nasal flaring), asymmetrical breathing; NB young children are diaphragmatic breathers so care is necessary to differentiate normal abdominal movement from obstructive 'see-saw' respiration.
- *C*: tachycardia, hypotension (late sign), bradycardia, pale or mottled skin, cool peripheries, central capillary refill time >2 seconds.

Basic life support—on finding a collapsed child:

- *Ensure safety and gently stimulate.*
- *Shout for help if no response from child.*
- *A*: place head in neutral position (<1 year old) or head tilt (older children), open airway with chin lift or jaw thrust; check for foreign bodies or excessive secretions and remove if possible N.B. do not 'finger sweep'. Administer high-flow O_2.
- *B*: look, listen and feel for breathing (10 seconds). If absent or inadequate, give 5 rescue breaths using appropriate size self-inflating bag and mask attached to high-flow O_2 where available (use oropharyngeal airways as required); each breath should be delivered slowly (1–1.5 seconds) to avoid gastric distension and diaphragmatic splinting. If adequate respiration present place child in recovery position.
- *C*: check for central pulse (brachial <1 year old, otherwise carotid or femoral) or signs of life (coughing, purposeful movement etc.); if *pulse absent or <60/min* commence *CPR* (ratio *2 breaths* (see above) to *15 chest compressions* (approximately 1/3 depth of chest, <1 year old, two fingers on lower half of sternum; 1–8 years old, one hand on lower half of sternum; two if larger child). Attach cardiac monitor when available to identify rhythm.

Advanced airway management

ET intubation of seriously ill young children requires great skill to avoid damaging an easily compromised airway and is consequently best left to experienced paediatricians or anaesthetists. The formula

[Age in years]/4 +4 is used when sizing ET tube internal diameters for children, but experience suggests that at least one tube size either side of the resulting figure should be at hand when intubating children.

Calculating child weights

If the weight of a child is not known, measuring systems that indicate drug dosages and ET tube sizes etc. based on the child's height are commercially available (e.g. Brownslow system). In the absence of these, the following formula is recommended:

Under 1 year old: birth weight (full term) = 3.5kg, weight at 6 months = 7kg, weight at 1 year old = 10kg;

Over 1 year old = [age in years + 4] × 2kg.

Venous access

Prompt and reliable venous access is a vital component in the successful resuscitation of children; venous cannulation should be attempted no more than three times in seriously ill children, after which the *intraosseus* (IO) route is recommended. This involves the insertion of a specialised needle into the marrow cavity of a long bone, usually medial and inferior to the tibial tubercle (avoiding growth plate). This route is effective for drug and fluid administration, though fluids are most effectively administered with a syringe and 3-way tap.

Fluid resuscitation

Boluses of 20ml/kg of warmed 0.9% saline or Hartmann's IV solutions should be administered to the shocked child. The normal circulating volume for a child is in the region of 80mL/kg, so after the second bolus of crystalloid fluids the use of blood products should be considered as should ET intubation and controlled ventilation to counteract the risks of any pulmonary oedema resulting from fluid replacement. Children are also at serious risk from hypoglycaemia, so bedside glucose monitoring should be conducted regularly and treatment with boluses of 5mL/kg of 10% glucose solution initiated as necessary.

Adrenaline

During cardiopulmonary resuscitation the dosage of adrenaline is calculated as 10 mcg/kg or 0.1ml/kg of 1:10 000 solution by the IV or IO route

Defibrillation

If a rhythm of ventricular fibrillation or pulseless ventricular tachycardia is identified, defibrillator shocks should be administered by a suitably trained practitioner once every 2 minutes as required. The defibrillator power setting for children is calculated using the formula 4J/kg.

Reference

Resuscitation Council (UK) (2006). *European Paediatric Life Support: Providers Manual*. Resuscitation Council (UK): London.

Choking in children

<1 year old (or small toddler): if coughing is ineffective place child prone on lap with head supported in downwards position and deliver up to 5 sharp blows with the heel of hand between shoulder blades, followed by sharp compressions with two fingers to lower half of sternum; repeat cycle until foreign body displaced or child loses consciousness, in which event BLS protocol should be followed.

In the larger child encourage coughing and deliver up to 5 slaps between shoulder blades followed by up to 5 abdominal thrusts (stand/kneel behind child and place clenched fist between xiphisternum and umbilicus, grasp fist with other hand and pull sharply inwards and upwards). Repeat cycle if ineffective or proceed to BLS if child loses consciousness.

Reference

Resuscitation Council (UK) (2006). *European Paediatric Life Support: Providers Manual.* Resuscitation Council (UK): London.

Death in the operating theatre

Unexpected death

This happens much less than might be thought even in emergency surgery; however, when patients do die in the operating theatre it can be especially upsetting for those staff present. Consideration should be given to providing support for staff who witness it and are involved with a deceased patient in the perioperative environment. It is particularly important to support junior and unqualified staff who may not have witnessed such an event previously. A referral to the appropriate support services may also be considered for some staff who may be more affected by an unexpected death in the operating theatre.

The bereaved relatives may wish to view the body and their wishes to do so must be respected. This will include respect of the patient and their family's religion which must be taken into consideration as certain faiths require the dead body to be treated in a certain way. The local policy should provide guidance on this matter.

Brain-stem death

This may typically occur when organs are to be removed from a patient who has been diagnosed as brain-stem dead and who has previously given consent (either themselves or by their relatives) to donate their organs to another person. Despite the predicable nature of this death it may still be upsetting for certain members of staff as already described. In these situations the transplant coordinator may be utilised to provide support for staff who might require it.

Care of the deceased

The body should be removed from the operating theatre to a place where the family can view it in some privacy. The following is a guide as practitioners should follow their local policy.

- The closed wound should be dressed to prevent leakage.
- Drains, IV cannulas, arterial and CVP lines, ET tubes, and catheters should be secured and closed with a spigot where appropriate.
- Last offices should be carried out with respect and dignity.
- The body should be dressed in a shroud and placed in a body bag and labelled in accordance with local policy and the required documentation completed.
- Arrangements must then be made to transfer the body to the mortuary and accompanied by a member of the operating theatre team.

Further reading

Association of Anaesthetists of Great Britain and Ireland (2004) *Catastrophes in Anaesthetic Practice – dealing with the aftermath*. AAGBI: London.

Levels of consciousness

- Consciousness depends on a patient's arousability and awareness.
- Causes of unconsciousness are numerous and may dictate the length of the coma period.
- It is appropriate to determine the cause of the coma so that appropriate treatment can be provided.
- Alterations in level of consciousness vary from slight to severe changes, indicating the degree of brain dysfunction.[1]
- Previous or pre-existing conditions should be noted when assessing level of consciousness e.g. hemiplegia, deafness.[1]

Causes of unconsciousness can be classed into the categories identified in Box 26.3.

Assessment of vital signs is essential to monitor a patient's condition and should include pulse, BP, respiratory rate, temperature, O_2 saturation, and level of consciousness. Changes in vital signs may indicate:

- Shock.
- Haemorrhage.
- Electrolyte imbalance.
- Raise intracranial pressure.

Raised intracranial pressure (ICP)

Signs of raised ICP that must be reported to an anaesthetist and neuro-surgeon:[2]

- Deterioration of level of consciousness.
- Changes in respiratory rate or breathing pattern.
- Dilated pupil that indicates transtentorial herniation of the brain.
- Decreased movement and muscle power down one side of the body.

Complications associated with unconsciousness

The unconsciousness patient is subject to many complications:

- Respiratory failure may develop shortly after the patient becomes unconscious.
- Pneumonia is common in patients receiving mechanical ventilation or in those who cannot maintain and clear their airway.
- Pressure ulcers may become infected and therefore become a source of sepsis.

Box 26.3 Causes of unconsciousness

Poisons or drugs
- Alcohol.
- Overdose of solvents.
- General anaesthesia.
- Heavy metals e.g. lead poisoning.
- Gases e.g. carbon monoxide.

Vascular causes
- Post-cardiac arrest.
- Haemorrhage.
- Anaphylaxis.

Infections
- Septicaemia.
- Meningitis.
- Viruses e.g. HIV, encephalitis.

Neurological disorders
- Epilepsy.
- Head injury.
- Pre-eclampsia
- Hypoglycaemia.

Metabolic disorders
- Hypoxia.
- Renal failure.
- Hepatic encephalopathy.

References and further reading

1. Crawford B, Guerrero D (2004). Observations: neurological. In Dougherty L and Lister S (eds) *The Royal Marsden Hospital Manual of Clinical Nursing Procedures* (6th edn). Blackwell Publishing: Oxford.

2. Hatfield A and Tronson M (2008). *The Complete Recovery Room Book* (4th edn). Oxford University Press: Oxford.

Drain CB and Odom-Forren J (2008). *Perianaesthesia Nursing: A Critical Care Approach* (5th edn). Saunders: Philadelphia, PA.

Evans C and Tippins E (2006). *The Foundations of Emergency Care*. Open University Press: Maidenhead.

Pudner R (ed) (2005). *Nursing the surgical patient* (2nd edn). Elsevier: Edinburgh.

Assessing levels of consciousness

The assessment of level of consciousness involves three phases:[1]
- Eye opening indicates that arousal mechanisms in the brain are active.
- Evaluation of verbal response may be orientated, confused, incomprehensible or absent.
- Evaluation of motor response is used to assess brain function.

Glasgow Coma Scale (GCS) (Table 26.1)

The GCS was first developed by the Institute of Neurological Sciences in Glasgow and was originally used to assess head injury. It is also used to assess conscious state during the postoperative period. Assessment of consciousness:
- *Awake*: alert, conscious, eyes open.
- *Drowsy*: eyes are shut except when spoken to; patient will cooperate on request.
- *Rousable*: the patient opens his/her eyes and also responds to stimulus.
- *Coma*: the patient does not respond to stimulus.

Unconscious patient present a score of 8 or less on the GCS, fail to obey commands, express no sounds and do not open eyes.

Table 26.1 Glasgow Coma Scale[2]

		Score
Eye opening	Nil	1
	To pain	2
	To commands	3
	Spontaneously	4
Motor response	Nil	1
	Extends	2
	Abnormal flexion	3
	Withdraws	4
	Localises	5
	Obeys commands	6
Verbal response	Nil	1
	Incomprehensible	2
	Inappropriate	3
	Confused	4
	Orientated	5

Note: the lower the score the more deeply unconscious the patient is. Patients presenting with a GCS score of less than 8 are in danger of a compromised airway.

AVPU scoring system (Table 26.2)

- The AVPU scale is a system used to measure and record a person's level of consciousness.
- The AVPU scale has only 4 possible outcomes for recording.
- The patient is assessed from best (A) to worst (U) to avoid unnecessary tests on conscious.
- It is a simplified GCS , which assesses a patient response in relation to:
  - Eyes.
  - Voice.
  - Motor skills.
- The AVPU scale should be assessed using three identifiable traits above, identifying the best response of each.
- The scale is generally used as a first aid mechanism and may be followed with a more extensive assessment using the GCS.
- Note that the scale is not suitable for long-term neurological use.

Table 26.2 The AVPU scale

A	Alert	Patient is fully responsive and lucid
		Patient answers questions
V	Voice	Patient is responsive to voice
		Patient may be drowsy with eyes closed
		Patient may not speak coherently
P	Pain	Patient is not alert and does not respond to voice
		Patient may respond to painful stimulus e.g. shaking the shoulders or pinching an ear lobe
U	Unresponsive	Patient is unresponsive to any of the above
		Patient is unconscious

References and further reading

1. Crawford B, Guerrero D (2004). Observations: neurological. In Dougherty L and Lister S (eds) *The Royal Marsden Hospital Manual of Clinical Nursing Procedures* (6th edn). Blackwell Publishing: Oxford.

2. Teasdale G and Jennett B (1974). Assessment of coma and impaired consciousness: a practical scale. *Lancet* ii 81–3.

Drain CB and Odom-Forren J (2008). *Perianaesthesia Nursing: A Critical Care Approach* (5th edn). Saunders: Philadelphia, PA.

Ruptured abdominal aortic aneurysm repair

This is arguably the operation about which novice practitioners that work in departments that undertake emergency surgery feel most anxious about. It should be remembered that patient with a ruptured (leaking) aneurysm will almost certainly be admitted via the ED and would not often be brought straight to the operating theatre.

Presentation

An abdominal aortic aneurysm (AAA) is defined as an increase in the diameter of the aorta by 50% usually regarded as greater than a diameter of 3cm. There is a higher incidence of AAA in elderly men with a ratio of 1:4 men to women. The mortality rate for an emergency repair of AAA is >50%.

Anaesthesia management

- IV access as soon as possible.
- Patient is usually anaesthetised in theatre using rapid sequence induction.
- Close patient monitoring is essential during the perioperative period
- Invasive monitoring including arterial BP, and triple lumen CVP ± cardiac output if necessary.
- Attention to temperature regulation is vital during long surgical procedures.
- Hypertension, coughing, and straining should be avoided as this may precipitate further bleeding.
- Warm fluids and blood if possible.
- IV Hartmann's is a balanced solution and will help to prevent metabolic acidosis.
- Close monitoring of fluid balance is essential.
- Surgery can proceed once ET intubation is confirmed
- Ensure availability of intensive care bed.

Surgical requirements

General laparotomy set, arterial clamp set, two suction sets, large self-retaining abdominal retractor, selection of aortic grafts and sutures.

- To minimise the risk of the aneurysm further rupturing the patient may be brought straight into the operating theatre and the IV access secured, CVP, arterial line and urinary catheter inserted and the skin prepped and the patient draped prior to the administration of the general anaesthetic.
- It will be necessary to explain carefully to the patient what is to happen to them as they are likely to be extremely anxious.
- Any accompanying relatives or friends must also be cared for and provided with the appropriate information, and this may fall to the perioperative staff since the medical staff may not have the opportunity to undertake this until after the procedure.

Surgical approach

- The surgical approach is via a routine laparotomy and the intestines mobilised and pushed out of the way.
- The posterior peritoneum is incised to expose the aorta.
- In a ruptured AAA the aorta must be crossed-clamped as soon as possible.
- Patients are then heparinised as bleeding is not controlled until the cross clamp is on.
- Once this has occurred then there is time and opportunity to take stock and continue to stabilise the patient before proceeding to repairing the aorta.
- Once the aorta is clamped, the aneurysm is then incised and repaired using a graft which is anastomosed using the vascular sutures
- The clamp is then removed and the abdomen closed in the normal way.

References and further reading

Allman KG and Wilson IH (eds) (2006). *Oxford Handbook of Anaesthesia* (2nd edn). Oxford University Press: Oxford.

Association of Anaesthetists of Great Britain and Ireland (2007). *Recommendations for standards of monitoring during anaesthesia and recovery* (4th edn). AAGBI: London.

Association of Anaesthetists of Great Britain and Ireland (2004). *Catastrophes in Anaesthetic Practice – dealing with the aftermath*. AAGBI: London.

Evans C and Tippins E (2006). *The Foundations of Emergency Care*. Open University Press: Maidenhead.

Nicholls A and Wilson I (2000). *Perioperative Medicine: Managing Surgical Patients with Medical Problems*. Oxford University Press: Oxford.

Pudner R (ed) (2005). *Nursing the surgical patient* (2nd edn). Elsevier: Edinburgh.

Royal College of Anaesthetists (2004). *Guidelines for the Provision of Anaesthetic Services*. RCoA: London.

Royal College of Surgeons of England (2008). *Good surgical practice*. Available at: 🖳 www.rcseng.ac.uk/publications/docs/good-surgical-practice-1

Appendicectomy

Presentation

The patient will be admitted with central lower abdominal pain which may then move to the right lower quadrant and the patient may present with vomiting, anorexia, and low-grade pyrexia. Acute appendicitis is more common in children than in adults and the abdominal pain may be due to:

- Urinary tract infection.
- Non-specific abdominal pain.
- Pelvic inflammatory disease.
- Renal colic.
- Ectopic pregnancy.
- Constipation.

Diagnosis of acute appendicitis is largely a clinical one and 10–20% of appendixes removed are normal.

Anaesthesia management

- General anaesthesia with rapid sequence induction and muscle relaxation.
- Patient monitoring should include:
  - BP.
  - ECG.
  - Capnography.
  - SpO_2.
  - Temperature.
- IV fluid therapy.
- Analgesia can include:
  - NSAIDS administered PR if consent provided.
  - Local infiltration to wound site or right inguinal nerve block.
- Patient should be extubated awake in left lateral position.

Main requirements

- Laparotomy or a minor intestinal tray.
- Suction.
- Abdominal lavage.
- Absorbable sutures 2/0 for purse string and 3/0 or 2/0 for closure of the muscle layer and then the desired skin closure.

Operation

- The operation may be carried out as either an open procedure or laparoscopically.
- For the open procedure a transversely oblique incision (Lanz incision) is made in the right lower abdomen.
- A culture swab may also be taken.
- Care should be taken not to reuse instruments that have been in contact with the mucosal side of the bowel or the infected appendix.
- A washout using normal saline may be performed and the appendix is sent for pathological examination.
- While the laparoscopic technique will be carried out in the standard manner (see Laparoscopy, p.352).

Reference and further reading

Association of Anaesthetists of Great Britain and Ireland (2007). *Recommendations for standards of monitoring during anaesthesia and recovery* (4th edn). AAGBI: London.

Evans C and Tippins E (2006). *The Foundations of Emergency Care*. Open University Press: Maidenhead.

Nicholls A and Wilson I (2000). *Perioperative Medicine: Managing Surgical Patients with Medical Problems*. Oxford University Press: Oxford.

Pudner R (ed) (2005). *Nursing the surgical patient* (2nd edn). Elsevier: Edinburgh.

Royal College of Surgeons of England (2008). *Good surgical practice*. Available at: 🖳 www.rcseng. ac.uk/publications/docs/good-surgical-practice-1

Rucklidge M (2006). General surgery. In Allman KG and Wilson IH (eds) *Oxford Handbook of Anaesthesia* (2nd edn). Oxford University Press: Oxford.

Splenectomy

Presentation

The usual reason for removing the spleen is because of blunt trauma often occurs along with lower rib fractures. The spleen can sometimes be damaged inadvertently during other abdominal operations. The patient may have lost blood and may be hypovolaemic and apart from the usual IV access is likely to require, CVP, and arterial lines. Fluid replacement with crystalloid, colloid fluid or cross-matched blood may be required.

Main requirements

Laparotomy tray, intestinal tray, arterial clamp set, abdominal closure sutures and ties for ligation (surgeon's preference), suction, cell salvage equipment (optional).

Operation

The normal approach is by a mid-line incision. The surgeon will explore the surrounding area and the abdominal contents. Having identified and mobilised the spleen the splenic artery and vein are identified, clamped and ligated, and then severed. Due to the internal bleeding it may prove necessary to evacuate clots ftrom the abdomen so a large bowl will be required to receive these. The abdominal cavity may be irrigated with warm saline prior to the routine abdominal closure.

The patient is likely to require a HDU or ITU bed postoperatively.

Reference and further reading

Allman KG and Wilson IH (eds) (2006). *Oxford Handbook of Anaesthesia* (2nd edn). Oxford University Press: Oxford.

Evans C and Tippins E (2006). *The Foundations of Emergency Care*. Open University Press: Maidenhead.

Nicholls A and Wilson I (2000). *Perioperative Medicine: Managing Surgical Patients with Medical Problems*. Oxford University Press: Oxford.

Pudner R (ed) (2005). *Nursing the surgical patient* (2nd edn). Elsevier: Edinburgh.

Royal College of Anaesthetists (2004) *Guidelines for the Provision of Anaesthetic Services*. RCoA: London.

Royal College of Surgeons of England (2008). *Good surgical practice*. Available at: 🖫 www.rcseng. ac.uk/publications/docs/good-surgical-practice-1

Rucklidge M (2006). General surgery. In Allman KG and Wilson IH (eds) *Oxford Handbook of Anaesthesia* (2nd edn). Oxford University Press: Oxford.

Bowel obstruction

Small bowel

Small bowel obstructions account for approximately 5% of surgical admissions and in the UK the commonest causes are

- Adhesions.
- Strangulated hernia.
- Malignancy.
- Volvulus.

In the newborn, intestinal obstruction is the commonest GI surgical emergency intervention.

Presentation

The patient may present with

- Colicky abdominal pain.
- Vomiting.
- Abdominal distension.
- Constipation.

Anaesthesia management

- The patient is likely to require fluid resuscitation, arterial and CVP lines, and anaesthetic preparation for a major procedure supported with neuraxial blockade for postoperative analgesia.
- General anaesthesia with rapid sequence induction.
- Close patient monitoring is essential during the perioperative period.
- Attention to temperature regulation is vital during long surgical procedures.
- Warm fluids and blood if possible.
- Close monitoring of fluid balance is essential.

Main requirements

Laparotomy (or paediatric) tray, intestinal set, suction, intestinal surgical anastomosis set, normal saline for abdominal lavage, abdominal closure and skin closing sutures or clips. Gloves and gowns (as per local procedure) for surgical team to change in to following bowel resection.

Operation

The repair of the intestinal obstruction may include:

- The division of an intestinal band.
- Release of an intestinal hernia.
- Resection of the bowel with anastomosis or creation of a stoma.
- Untwisting of a volvulus.

A 'clean and dirty' or bowel technique should be utilised and instruments used while the bowel is opened not used during the abdominal closure. In many units the 'clean' period is following abdominal lavage where gloves and gowns are changed.

Large bowel

Large bowel obstruction is usually caused by tumour with most patients being >70 years old. The risk of obstruction is greater in left-sided lesions and patients tend to present at a more advanced stage with 15% presenting with obstruction; patient may require fluid resuscitation and should be prepared.

Presentation

Caecal tumours present with small bowel obstruction and the symptoms include
- Colicky abdominal pain.
- Early vomiting.
- Constipation.
- Variable extent of constipation.

Left-sided tumours present with large bowel obstruction and symptoms include:
- Change in bowel habit.
- Constipation.
- Abdominal distention.
- Early vomiting.

The patient is likely to require fluid resuscitation, arterial and CVP lines and anaesthetic preparation for a major procedure.

Main requirements

Laprorotomy tray, intestinal set, suction, intestinal surgical anastomosis set, stoma sutures, normal saline for abdominal lavage, linear cutter stapler, Gloves and gowns (as per local procedure) for surgical team to change in to following resection, abdominal closure and skin closing sutures or clips.

Operation

A full laparotomy is carried out and the liver palpated for metastases and the colon inspected for tumour. Depending on the location of the tumour mass one of the following procedures may be carried out.
- Right hemicolectomy (right-sided lesions).
- Extended right hemicolectomy (transverse colon lesions).
- Various operations for left-sided lesions such as:

Three-stage procedure
- Defunctioning colostomy.
- Resection and anastomosis.
- Closure of colostomy.

Two-stage procedure
- Hartmann's procedure.
- Closure of colostomy.

One-stage procedure
- Resection and primary anastomosis (no colostomy).

Patients undergoing surgery for bowel obstruction may require a HDU or ITU bed postoperatively.

Reference and further reading

Evans C and Tippins E (2006). *The Foundations of Emergency Care*. Open University Press: Maidenhead.

Nicholls A and Wilson I (2000). *Perioperative Medicine: Managing Surgical Patients with Medical Problems*. Oxford University Press: Oxford.

Pudner R (ed) (2005). *Nursing the surgical patient* (2nd edn). Elsevier: Edinburgh.

Royal College of Anaesthetists (2004) *Guidelines for the Provision of Anaesthetic Services*. RCoA: London.

Royal College of Surgeons of England (2008). *Good surgical practice*. Available at: ▣ www.rcseng. ac.uk/publications/docs/good-surgical-practice-1

Gastrointestinal bleed

Presentation

Upper GI bleeding may be caused by:
- Peptic ulcer.
- Gastric erosions.
- Oesophageal or gastric varices.
- Mallory–Weiss tear (caused by violent vomiting).
- Gastric neoplasia.

Patients will be likely to present with haematemisis and will require an early endoscopy to determine the site of the bleeding. There are several endoscopic therapies that can be utilised to stop the bleeding:
- Laser photocoagulation.
- Bipolar electrocautery.
- Heat probes.
- Adrenaline or scleresent injection.

Should endoscopic therapy prove unsuccessful or there is recurrent bleeding the patient will require a surgical intervention. The chosen operation is performed via a laporatomy

Anaesthesia management
- The patient may require fluid resuscitation, arterial and CVP lines and anaesthetic preparation for a major procedure.
- General anaesthesia with RSI.
- Close patient monitoring is essential during the perioperative period.
- Attention to temperature regulation is vital during long surgical procedures.
- Warm fluids and blood if possible.
- Close monitoring of fluid balance is essential.

Main requirements
- Laparotomy tray.
- Intestinal set.
- Suction.
- Intestinal surgical anastomosis set.
- Anasotomsis or undersewing sutures.
- Normal saline for abdominal lavage.
- Abdominal closure and skin closing sutures or clips.
- A 'clean and dirty' technique should be utilised when the stomach or duodenum is open.
- NG or feeding tube.

Operation
- For a duodenal ulcer a gastroduodenotomy with the ulcer under-sewn with a 2/0 absorbable suture.
- For a gastric ulcer a local resection or total or partial gastrectomy.

Reference and further reading

Allman KG and Wilson IH (eds) (2006). *Oxford Handbook of Anaesthesia* (2nd edn). Oxford University Press: Oxford.

Evans C and Tippins E (2006). *The Foundations of Emergency Care*. Open University Press: Maidenhead.

Nicholls A and Wilson I (2000). *Perioperative Medicine: Managing Surgical Patients with Medical Problems*. Oxford University Press: Oxford.

Pudner R (ed) (2005). *Nursing the surgical patient* (2nd edn). Elsevier: Edinburgh.

Royal College of Anaesthetists (2004). *Guidelines for the Provision of Anaesthetic Services*. RCoA: London.

Royal College of Surgeons of England (2008). *Good surgical practice*. Available at: www.rcseng. ac.uk/publications/docs/good-surgical-practice-1

Obstetric surgery

Emergency obstetric surgery can include Caesarean section, vaginal delivery, and removal of retained products of conception. Caesarean section is generally performed for the benefit of the mother, foetus or both (Box 26.4). Although Caesarean section was traditionally classified as elective surgery, this procedure is now classified into four grades:

- Immediate threat to the life of the mother or foetus.
- Maternal or foetal compromise but not immediately life-threatening.
- No maternal or foetal compromise but early delivery required.
- Elective delivery to suit the mother and maternity team.

Box 26.4 Indications for Caesarean section

- Previous Caesarean section.
- Maternal exhaustion.
- Multiple pregnancy.
- Malposition.
- Pre-existing maternal disease.
- Placenta praevia.
- Placental abruption.
- Cord prolapse.
- Obstructed labour.
- Foetal compromise.

Anaesthetic management of obstetric surgery and the choice of anaesthetic technique are dependent on a number of factors:

- Degree of urgency.
- Anticipated obstetric complications.
- Anaesthetic history or anticipated anaesthetic complications.
- Whether an epidural catheter is in situ.
- To a lesser degree, anaesthetist's and patient's' choice.

The AAGBI make recommendations regarding obstetric services that include:[1]

- A duty anaesthetist should be immediately available for the obstetric delivery suite 24 hours per day.
- A nominated consultant should be in charge of obstetric anaesthesia.
- There should be a clear line of communication from the duty anaesthetist to the supervising consultant at all times.
- Increasing workload in the modern obstetric unit requires an increase in anaesthetic staffing above currently accepted levels.
- When obstetric units are small, or workload is sporadic, that provision of the basic minimum staffing levels is not cost effective, consideration should be given to amalgamation with other local units.
- Women should have antenatal access to information about the availability and provision of all types of analgesia and anaesthesia.
- An agreed system whereby the anaesthetist is given sufficient advance notice of all potential high-risk patients should be in place.

- Where a 24-hour epidural service is offered, the time from the anaesthetist being informed about an epidural until being able to attend the mother should not normally exceed 30 minutes, and must be within one hour except in exceptional circumstances.
- Provision should be made for those who cover the delivery suite on-call, but do not have regular sessions there, to spend time in the delivery suite in a supernumerary capacity with one of the regular obstetric anaesthetic consultants.
- Separate staffing and resources should be allocated to elective Caesarean section lists to prevent delays due to emergency procedures and provision of regional analgesia in labour.
- The anaesthetic assistant must have no other conflicting duties, must be trained to a recognised national standard, and must work regularly in the obstetric unit.
- The training undergone by staff in the maternity recovery unit and the facilities provided must be to the same standard as for general recovery facilities.
- Appropriate facilities should be available for the antenatal and peripartum management of the sick obstetric patient.

The AAGBI also make a list of recommended protocols that should be readily available in all obstetric departments:[1]
- Conditions requiring antenatal referral to the anaesthetist.
- Management of major haemorrhage, pre-eclampsia and eclampsia.
- Management of failed/difficult intubation.
- Management of regional anaesthesia, high regional block, and hypotension during regional block.
- Management of accidental dural puncture and post-dural puncture headache.
- Admission and discharge criteria from/to HDU.
- Management of regional techniques in patients on thromboprophylaxis.
- Antacid prophylaxis for labour and delivery.
- Oral intake during labour.
- Resuscitation of the pregnant patient.

References
1. Association of Anaesthetists for Great Britain and Ireland (2005). *Guidelines for Obstetric Anaesthetic Services. Revised Edition 2005*. AAGBI: London.

National Institute for Clinical Excellence (2004). *Clinical Guideline 13: Caesarean section*. NICE: London.

Gynaecology surgery

Emergency gynaecology surgery can include:
- Suspected ectopic pregnancy.
- Ruptured ectopic pregnancy.
- Evacuation of retained products of conception.
- Incision and drainage of Bartholin's abscess (although this is sometimes performed at ward level).

Ectopic pregnancy

Ectopic or tubal pregnancy can be managed surgically or medically and this management should be tailored to the clinical condition and future fertility requirements of the woman.[1]
- RCOG advise that laparoscopic approach as opposed to an open approach to the surgical management of ectopic pregnancy, is preferable in a patient who is haemodynamically stable.[1]
- Surgical procedures undertaken laparoscopically are often associated with decreased operation times, reduced blood loss, and lower analgesic requirements.
- If a patient is haemodynamically instable, a laparotomy is the preferred method of management of ectopic pregnancy.
- Intra-muscular methotrexate is advocated for medical management of ectopic pregnancy although surgical laparoscopy is often used to confirm its presence.
- RCOG[1] advise against medical management of ectopic pregnancy if hypovolaemic shock is suspected.
- Anti-D immunoglobulin should be given to all non-sensitised women who are Rh negative with a confirmed ectopic pregnancy.

Early pregnancy loss

- Early pregnancy loss is defined by RCOG as a loss within the first 12 completed weeks of pregnancy.[2]
- Early pregnancy loss can be managed surgically or medically.
- Surgical evacuation of retained products of conception (ERPC) for early pregnancy loss used to be the main treatment for patients due to possible risks that include haemorrhage and infection.
- Treatment is now available on an outpatient basis.
- If a patient presents with excessive bleeding, unstable vital signs, or retained, infected tissue, then surgical evacuation via suction curettage is considered the treatment of choice.
- Complications of ERPC can include perforated uterus, haemorrhage, intra-abdominal trauma, intrauterine adhesions, and cervical tears.
- Medical management of early pregnancy loss involves the use of prostaglandin drugs but vaginal bleeding can occur for up to 3 weeks following miscarriage.
- Prophylactic antibiotic therapy should be administered according to individual need.
- RCOG[2] recommend that anti-D immunoglobulin should only be given for threatened miscarriage under 12 weeks' gestation when bleeding is heavy or associated with pain. They state it is not required for complete miscarriage under 12 weeks of gestation when there has been no formal intervention to evacuate the uterus.

Anaesthetic management:

The majority of gynaecology patients presenting for emergency surgery are fit. Anaesthetic management of gynaecology surgery and the choice of anaesthetic technique are dependent on a number of factors: degree of urgency; anticipated complications; anaesthetic history or anticipated anaesthetic complications; and to a lesser degree, anaesthetists' and patients' choice.

- All professionals should be sensitive to the needs of patients as some may require considerable psychological support.
- Prophylactic anti-emetic therapy should be considered as nausea and vomiting can be problematic postoperatively.
- Vagal stimulation can occur intraoperatively when dilating the cervix or during laparoscopic procedures.
- Attention to temperature regulation is vital during long surgical procedures.
- Intubation with ranitidine premedication is recommended where there are symptoms of reflux.
- Rapid sequence induction is advocated for ectopic pregnancy.

References and further reading

1. Royal College of Obstetricians and Gynaecologists (2004). *The management of tubal pregnancy*. RCOG: London.

2. Royal College of Obstetricians and Gynaecologists (2006). *The management of early pregnancy loss*. RCOG: London.

Association of Anaesthetists for Great Britain and Ireland (2005). *Guidelines for Obstetric Anaesthetic Services. Revised Edition 2005*. AAGBI: London.

National Institute for Clinical Excellence (2004). *Clinical Guideline 13: Caesarean section*. NICE: London.

NICE Gynaecology Guidelines. Available at: 🖳 www.nice.org.uk/guidance/index.jsp?action=by Topic&o=7258

Saddler J (2006). Gynaecological surgery. In Allman KG and Wilson IH (eds) *Oxford Handbook of Anaesthesia* (2nd edn). Oxford University Press: Oxford.

Neurosurgery

Patients requiring emergency neurosurgical procedures will normally be transferred to a specialist regional centre for their treatment. Emergency operations can be carried out for:
- Intracranial haematoma.
- Sub arachnoid haemorrhage.
- Hydrocephalus.

Types of intracranial haematomas
- Extradural.
- Subdural.

Extra dural haematoma can be the result of a low velocity injury and the patient may experience
- A transient loss of consciousness that can rapidly recover.
- A period of lucidity.
- Rapid deterioration in their level of consciousness.
- Increase in BP and fall in HR.
- Limb weakness.
- Dilatation of pupils.

The treatment of choice will be to carry out an emergency decompression operation, such as burr holes, to evacuate the clot and reduce the intracranial pressure. See Fig. 26.3.

Subdural haematoma can be a complication of a high velocity injury and the patient will usually:
- Be unconscious from the time of injury.
- Exhibit a deteriorating level of consciousness.

The patient will require a de-compressive craniotomy.

Causes of sub arachnoid haemorrhage may be:
- Intracranial aneurysm.
- Arteriovenous malformation.
- Hypertension.
- Idiopathic.

Common symptoms include:
- Sudden onset severe headache.
- Nausea.
- Photophobia.
- Vomiting.
- Neck stiffness.

If the patient is fit enough they may undergo a craniotomy to clip the aneurysm at its neck while maintaining the blood flow in the native vessel. The timing of surgical intervention is controversial with some cases being delayed for 10 days after the initial haemorrhage. Early surgery may be associated with reduced mortality and no increased morbidity.

Hydrocephalus is condition in which there is an increase in CSF in the cranial cavity. This may be due to:
- Excessive production.
- Inadequate absorption.
- An obstruction that impedes flow through the ventricular system.

The surgical treatment may involve the insertion of a ventriculopertoneal (VP) shunt where a catheter is placed in the lateral ventricle, connected via a valve and a long tunnelled catheter to the peritoneum. The valve is located under the scalp and can be compressed digitally to flush CSF from the ventricle to the peritoneum.

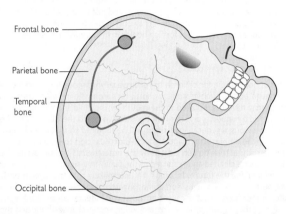

Frontal bone

Parietal bone

Temporal bone

Occipital bone

Fig. 26.3 Emergency burr holes. Adapted with permission from Gardiner M and Borley N (2009). *Training in Surgery*, ISBN 9780199204755, Oxford University Press, Oxford.

References and further reading

Allman KG and Wilson IH (eds) (2006). *Oxford Handbook of Anaesthesia* (2nd edn). Oxford University Press: Oxford.

Dougherty L and Lister S (eds) (2008). *The Royal Marsden Hospital Manual of Clinical Nursing Procedures* (7th edn). Wiley Blackwell: Oxford.

Evans C and Tippins E (2006). *The Foundations of Emergency Care*. Open University Press: Maidenhead.

Nicholls A and Wilson I (2000). *Perioperative Medicine: Managing Surgical Patients with Medical Problems*. Oxford University Press: Oxford.

Pudner R (ed) (2005). *Nursing the surgical patient* (2nd edn). Elsevier: Edinburgh.

Royal College of Anaesthetists (2004) *Guidelines for the Provision of Anaesthetic Services*. RCoA: London.

Royal College of Surgeons of England (2008). *Good surgical practice*. Available at: ⌨ www.rcseng. ac.uk/publications/docs/good-surgical-practice-1

Ear, nose, and throat

ENT surgery is a speciality that is performed in most UK hospitals and compared with many specialities has relatively few emergency cases. This can make it more difficult for practitioners to maintain their skill level. It is therefore advisable that practitioners spend some time familiarising themselves with elective ENT procedures and noting the whereabouts of instruments and equipment. Emergency ENT procedures include:

• Endoscopy for removal of foreign bodies in the airway or oesophagus.
• Tracheostomy.
• Mastoidectomy.
• Treatment for epistaxis.

It is not uncommon for children to require a laryngoscopy for the removal of foreign bodies such as coins or small toys from their cricopharyngeus which may have been placed in the mouth by the child themselves. Once confirmed by an x-ray, and if it is not possible to reach the object with the child conscious, a general anaesthetic will be required so that a rigid laryngoscopy can be performed and a grasping forceps used to grab the object. This can sometimes be carried out by the anaesthetist! If appropriate the object can be cleaned and returned to the family in a suitable container as a reminder for the future. In adults it is more likely that the foreign body will be in the oesophagus sometimes ingested when intoxicated and is often a food bolus that is caught at the aortic indentation or diaphragm. A rigid oesophogoscopy is performed under a general anaesthetic and the foreign body removed or occasionally advanced into the stomach.

Tracheostomy may be performed to relieve an upper airway obstruction or to replace an ET tube for a mechanically ventilated patient. Requirements include:

• Tracheostomy set.
• Selection of appropriate sized tracheostomy tubes.
• Syringe to inflate tracheostomy tube cuff.
• Suction and suction catheter.
• Cotton tape to secure tracheostomy tube.

Mastoidectomy is occasionally performed as an emergency in the presence of a mastoid abscess. The condition is painful but not life threatening and the operation is carried in the same as the elective procedure.

Epistaxis can sometimes require a surgical intervention if the haemorrhage cannot be stemmed. Surgical techniques include:

• The insertion of a nasal balloon or posterior nasal pack.
• Electrocautery to the affected area.
• Ligation of maxillary and anterior ethmoidal artery.

References and further reading

Dougherty L and Lister S (eds) (2008). *The Royal Marsden Hospital Manual of Clinical Nursing Procedures* (7th edn). Wiley Blackwell: Oxford.

Evans C and Tippins E (2006). *The Foundations of Emergency Care*. Open University Press: Maidenhead.

Nicholls A and Wilson I (2000). *Perioperative Medicine: Managing Surgical Patients with Medical Problems*. Oxford University Press: Oxford.

Pudner R (ed) (2005). *Nursing the surgical patient* (2nd edn). Elsevier: Edinburgh.

Royal College of Anaesthetists (2004) *Guidelines for the Provision of Anaesthetic Services*. RCoA: London.

Royal College of Surgeons of England (2008). *Good surgical practice*. Available at: 🖥 www.rcseng. ac.uk/publications/docs/good-surgical-practice-1

Ophthalmology surgery

Retinal detachment

Retinal detachment is a rare but serious and sight-threatening event and affects about one person per 10 000. Not all cases of retinal detachment require urgent surgery but a delay in treatment should be avoided.

- A retinal detachment usually happens naturally and occurs when the retina becomes separated from the underlying tissue. This may be caused by a hole or tear in the retina which allows fluid to get underneath, weakening the attachment of the retina which then becomes detached.[1]
- Without treatment, this condition can lead to blindness in the affected eye.
- Symptoms are not generally painful but can include a shadow or curtain spreading across the vision of one eye, bright flashes of light, and/or showers of dark spots called floaters.
- Those at a higher risk of developing a retinal detachment include people who are or have:
  - Short-sighted.
  - Previous cataract surgery.
  - A recent severe direct blow to the eye.
  - Ocular tumours.
  - Diabetic eye disease.
  - Some are familial but these are rare.

Complications are rare and very rarely blindness can occur. Possible complications during the operation can include:

- Bleeding inside the eye.
- The surgery producing more holes in the retina.

Anaesthetic management

- Ophthalmic surgery is often required for ocular manifestations of systemic disease and there is a relatively high incidence of patients with uncommon medical conditions.[2]
- General anaesthesia should be considered if a patient cannot lie flat and still for up to 1 hour.
- A laryngeal mask is recommended unless contraindicated.
- Administration of glycopyrronium can reduce salivary function and avoid pooling behind an LMA.[3]
- Sub-Tenon's block complements general anaesthesia and improves intraoperative stability and reduces postoperative pain.

Anaesthetic factors increasing IOP[3]

- Laryngoscopy.
- Suxamethonium.
- Large volumes of local anaesthesia drugs.
- External compression of the globe by tightly applied face mask.

The following should be considered emergency surgery, especially when outside of normal working hours:

- The eye condition.
- ASA grade.
- Age of patients.

The RCoA[2] advise that all ophthalmic theatre nurses, anaesthetic nurses and ODPs must have up-to-date BLS training and ophthalmic nurses should be trained in cardiopulmonary resuscitation:

'There must be a robust procedure for checking the laterality of the eye to be operated on prior to local anaesthetic block. This should include the eye being marked by the responsible surgical team prior to admission to the surgical suite. On arrival in the anaesthetic room the consent form must be checked. This must be done by the anaesthetist or surgeon performing the block and an ODP or theatre nurse. The patient must be asked to confirm on which eye they expect to have the operation'.[2]

References and further reading

1. RCOPHTH (2003). *Management of retinal detachment.* Available at: ▣ www.rcophth.ac.uk/docs/profstands/ophthalmic-services/ManagementRetinalDetachment.pdf

2. Royal College of Anaesthetists (2004). *Guidance on the provision of Ophthalmic Anaesthesia Services.* Available at: ▣ www.rcoa.ac.uk/docs/GPAS-Ophth.pdf

3. Farmery A (2006). Ophthalmic surgery. In Allman KG and Wilson IH (eds) *Oxford Handbook of Anaesthesia* (2nd edn). Oxford University Press: Oxford.

NICE Ophthalmic Guidance. Available from: ▣ www.nice.org.uk/guidance/index.jsp?action=by Topic&o=7247&set=true

Royal College of Optometrists. Available at: ▣ www.college-optometrists.org/index.aspx/pcms/site.home

Royal National Institute for the Blind. Available at: ▣ www.rnib.org.uk/xpedio/groups/public/documents/code/InternetHome.hcsp

Orthopaedic trauma surgery

Trauma is an injury to the body caused by the application of external energy. The type and amount of energy exerted will result in a variety of injuries. The severity of the injuries is influenced by the violence of the impact.

Trauma and fractures are not the same; however the majority of trauma surgery is related to damage of bones, muscles and joints.

The aim of fracture treatment is to restore function and normal anatomical position, with function being the priority.

Principles of fracture treatment (see Figure 26.4)
Summarised as the 5 Rs:
- Resuscitation: shock, blood loss, pain.
- Reduction: realignment of the bone.
- Restriction: plaster cast, traction, open reduction/internal fixation, external fixation.
- Restoration.
- Rehabilitation.

Diagnosis of fracture
- Deformity: may not always be obvious.
- Pain at site of injury.
- Bruising at site of injury.
- Impaired function.
- Swelling.

Investigations
- Radiological examination of the injured part, including the joint above and below; should be x-rayed in two views.

Anaesthetic management
- General anaesthesia is usually advocated for major trauma patients with RSI .
- Care should be taken when moving, handling, and transferring trauma patients.
- Patients should be positioned carefully with appropriate protection and padding of pressure areas.
- IV antibiotics prophylactically.
- Invasive monitoring maybe necessary for patient with CVS disease.
- Intracranial pressure monitoring with head injury patients.
- Urinary catheter for long procedures.
- Blood loss may be extensive so monitor carefully.
- A tourniquet is used to reduce bleeding but maybe contraindicated due to fracture site.[1]
- Intraoperative cell salvage and drain salvage may be considered.
- Patients should be actively warmed intraoperatively.
- Patients with limb fractures are at risk of fat embolism.

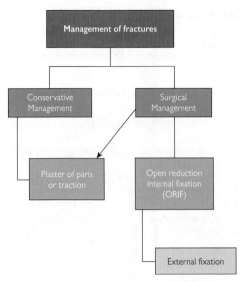

Fig. 26.4 Management of fractures.

Reference

1. Worms R and Griffiths R (2006). Orthopaedic surgery. In Allman KG and Wilson IH (eds) *Oxford Handbook of Anaesthesia* (2nd edn). Oxford University Press: Oxford.

Further reading

Dougherty L and Lister S (eds) (2008). *The Royal Marsden Hospital Manual of Clinical Nursing Procedures* (7th edn). Wiley Blackwell: Oxford.

Evans C and Tippins E (2006). *The Foundations of Emergency Care*. Open University Press: Maidenhead.

Nicholls A and Wilson I (2000). *Perioperative Medicine: Managing Surgical Patients with Medical Problems*. Oxford University Press: Oxford.

Pudner R (ed) (2005). *Nursing the surgical patient* (2nd edn). Elsevier: Edinburgh.

Royal College of Anaesthetists (2004). *Guidelines for the Provision of Anaesthetic Services*. RCoA: London.

Royal College of Surgeons of England (2008). *Good surgical practice*. Available at: 🖳 www.rcseng. ac.uk/publications/docs/good-surgical-practice-1

Postoperative emergencies

Postoperative emergencies are uncommon and an incidence of between 0.8–5% is suggested.[1] Emergency situations can occur spontaneously but in most cases postoperatively, can be prevented. Emergency situations can be classified into two groups: *anaesthetic-related emergencies* and *general emergencies*.

These emergencies are specific to anaesthesia and post-anaesthetic care.

Table 26.3 Anaesthetic-related emergencies.

• Atelactasis.	• Laryngospasm.
• Compartment syndrome.	• Malignant hyperpyrexia scoline apnoea.
• Delayed emergence and inadequate reversal.	• Stridor.
• Dehiscence.	• Thyroid storm.
• Disseminated intravascular coagulation (DIC).	• Upper airway obstruction.
• Hypoxaemia.	

General emergencies[1,2]

Table 26.4 General emergencies[1,2]

• Allergy and anaphylaxis.	• Pneumothorax.
• Arrhythmias.	• Respiratory arrest.
• Cardiac arrest.	• Seizures.
• Cardiac tamponade.	• Sepsis.
• Chest pain.	• Severe hypo/hyperglycaemia.
• Convulsions.	• Shock (normovolaemic/ hypovolaemic).
• Extravasation.	• Sinus tachycardia.
• Malignant hypo/hypertension.	• Status epilepticus.
• Myocardial infarction.	• SVT.
• Metabolic disturbances.	• Tension pneumothorax.
• PE.	• VT.

Management of postoperative emergencies

Irrespective of the emergency, a universally methodical approach should be adopted by the practitioner. The ABCDE (primary survey) approach is an effective method in which to achieve this:

- A: airway.
- B: breathing.
- C: circulation.
- D: disability.
- E: exposure.

Airway

The airway is the priority in any emergency. The absence of a patent airway can lead to a quick death without intervention. The airway should be inspected, suctioned (if necessary), and appropriate adjuncts and techniques used to preserve its patency, such as oropharyngeal airways, jaw thrust/chin lift.

Breathing and ventilation

The patient's chest rise/fall and pattern of breathing should be observed. Use of accessory muscles, bilateral or unilateral rise/fall, evidence of pain on inspiration/expiration, breath-holding, and alternative breathing patterns, such as Kussmaul's and Cheyne-Stokes should be noted.

Sp/SaO$_2$ levels should be observed and measured alongside peripheral/ central perfusion (capillary refill, ashen/cyanosed appearance).

Circulation

BP and circulating blood volume should be noted. The mean arterial pressure (MAP) is a principal indicator of organ perfusion and should be kept above 60mmHg; any decrease below this can lead to renal, coronary artery and brain tissue ischaemia. Malignant ↑ or ↓BP are concerning and require prompt treatment; these are often signs of an underlying cause, such as hypovolaemia. HR should be observed in conjunction with BP, as both are interrelated. Tachycardias/bradycardias often correspond to a ↓ and ↑BP respectively. Compensatory mechanisms, such as this, are a principal indicator of shock. Rhythm should be analysed and any major abnormalities should be investigated further with a 12-lead ECG. VTs are an example and require prompt anaesthetic input. An unmanaged VT can quickly lead to cardiac arrest.

Fluid balance and urine output can be used as additional markers. Oliguria and anuria in postoperative patients can be initial signs of complication. Urine output should always exceed 1mL/kg/hour (this calculation is negated when patients are administered diuretics).

Disability (neurological assessment)

Neurological status should be assessed. The use of an assessment tool such as GCS is of significant benefit here. Consciousness level, responsiveness and coherence, sensory/motor weaknesses, visual acuity, and pupil reaction are all methods which can be used to assess and diagnose deficit. Neurological deficit can be expected with some types of surgery (neurosurgery) and preoperative status should always be noted (dementia, psychiatric disorders).

Exposure (everything else)

This part of the assessment should cover 'everything else'. Full exposure of the patient should occur: inspection of the wound site and surrounding tissue, palpation of the abdomen, and attention made to 'additionals', such as temperature and blood sugar, can assist the practitioner with diagnosis.

Always turn the patient as haemorrhage can occur in a site, which is non-evident whilst a patient is supine.

Patient dignity must be fully observed during this part of the assessment.

(Adapted from Resuscitation Council UK, 2006.[3])

References

1. Lee A, Lum ME, O'Regan WJ, *et al.* (1998). Early postoperative emergencies requiring intensive care team intervention. The role of ASA physical status and after-hours surgery. *Anaesthesia* **53**(6), 529–35

2. Hatfield A and Tronson M (2008). *The Complete Recovery Room Book* (4th edn). Oxford University Press: Oxford.

3. Resuscitation Council UK (2006). *Advanced Life Support* (5th edn). Resuscitation Council (UK): London.

Respiratory disorders

Respiratory disorders are common within the post-anaesthetic setting. An incidence of between 1–30% is suggested, depending upon the complication and its severity.[1,2] They can occur as a direct result of the surgery or anaesthesia and are the most common cause of life-threatening incidents in the recovery room. Respiratory disorders can be classified as being either *airway* or *breathing* in nature and an early diagnosis and resolve of the cause can prevent further deterioration and death.

Airway

Airway compromise is the principal cause of all respiratory complications. In most instances, compromise is due to airway obstruction, which can arise from either the upper (nose/lips to bronchus) or lower bronchioles to alveoli) part of the airway. Airway sounds emitted by the patient are usually the first indicators of obstruction. Stridor and snoring are indicative of upper airway obstruction whilst wheezing and excessive coughing denote the presence of obstruction in the bronchioles and lower airway.

Stridor: stridor is always a medical emergency and presents as a 'crowing' noise, which is most often caused by partial airway obstruction in the larynx. Stridor can occur on inspiration or expiration; postoperatively, inspiratory stridor is most common, occurring as a result of laryngospasm. The management of stridor should follow a systematic approach:

- Open and inspect the airway by use of jaw thrust or chin lift manoeuvres.
- If airway difficult to visualise, use laryngoscope.
- Clear the airway of any secretions or foreign bodies via suction.
- Administer 100% O_2 via high concentration non-rebreather mask.

If these methods do not improve the patient's condition:

- Call for assistance.
- Insert an oropharyngeal/nasopharyngeal airway (if patient is not fully conscious).
- Fully extend jaw (not possible with confirmed/?C-spine #).
- Hand-ventilate airway using bag and mask, ensure that the seal between the airway and mask is effective—the aim of hand ventilation is the application of positive pressure.

In worst case scenarios, if the above measures have failed:

- Suxamethonium and an induction agent e.g. propofol should be readily available in cases of stridor.
- Administer a small bolus dose of suxamethonium or propofol.
- Prepare for emergency ET intubation and/or cricothyroidotomy.[3,4]

Wheezing and bronchospasm: wheezing is a principal sign of bronchial irritation, inflammation and/or oedema and predominantly indicates bronchospasm.[1] The risk of a patient developing a bronchospasm postoperatively is greatly affected by their preoperative respiratory physiology. ↑ incidence in asthmatics, smokers, and patients with COPD.[5]

Wheezing is an initial sign of complication and should never be ignored, it is often accompanied by:

- Dyspnoea and tachypnoea.
- ↓BP.

- Paradoxical ('see-saw') breathing.
- Cyanosis.[1]

When bronchospasm is detected, it should be managed with high-flow O_2 (100%) administered via a non-rebreather mask. The patient should be closely monitored and if the wheeze persists, the anaesthetist consulted. Reassurance is often beneficial if the patient is conscious. A continuous wheeze can indicate allergy, aspiration, or pulmonary oedema.[5]

Breathing

Several conditions directly influencing the respiratory drive can cause postoperative complication. These include: scoline apnoea, respiratory paralysis (inadequate reversal of neuromuscular blockade), hypoventilation, and aspiration pneumonitis (⧠ see Chapter 11, p.207)

Hypoxia

The eventual consequence of any airway/breathing event is hypoxia and the principal function of the recovery room is to prevent its occurrence. Cyanosis is an intermediary sign; peripheral cyanosis usually indicates a SpO_2 of ≤85%. Hypoxia can cause death quickly and subtly and the most effective treatment is prompt recognition.[1]

Patients who develop cyanosis should be given 100% O_2 via a non-rebreather mask. Airway patency and efficiency of breathing should then be assessed. Once the cause of hypoxia is ascertained, appropriate methods should be taken to correct it. If left untreated, hypoxia leads to cardiac arrest.

Risk factors

Several factors increase the risk of developing airway/breathing events postoperatively, these are:
- Age: ≤1 year or ≥60 years.
- Obesity: 120kg+ in men/100kg+ in women.
- ASA grading: ↑grading = ↑risk.
- Pre-existing Illness and lifestyle: COPD, renal disease.
- Cardiovascular disease, diabetes mellitus, smoker.
- Type of surgery; thoracic and abdominal surgery increase the risk of postoperative respiratory complications.

References

1. Hatfield A and Tronson M (2008). *The Complete Recovery Room Book* (4th edn). Oxford University Press: Oxford.

2. Sewell A and Young P (2003). Recovery & post-anaesthetic care. *Anaesthesia & Intensive Care* **4**(10), 329–32.

3. Grover A and Canavan C (2007). Critical incidents: the respiratory system. *Anaesthesia & Intensive Care Medicine* **8**(9), 352–7.

4. Al-Rawi S and Nolan K (2003). Respiratory Complications in the Postoperative Period. *Anaesthesia & Intensive Care Medicine* **4**(10), 332–4.

5. Westhorpe RN, Ludbrook GL, and Helps SC (2005). Crisis management during anaesthesia: bronchospasm. *Quality and Safety in Health Care* **14**(7),1–6.

Cardiovascular disorders

CV disorders of the body can be classified as either complications or events. CV complications describe minor-major conditions which are caused by homeostatic imbalance, such as hypotension and tachycardia. CV Events are conditions, which arise as a result of these complications.

Cardiovascular complications

- ↑ or ↓BP.
- Arrhythmias.
- ↑ or ↓HR.
- Chest pain.

Cardiovascular events

- Hypovolaemia.
- MI.
- Cardiac tamponade.
- Cardiac ischaemia.
- Cardiogenic shock.
- Cardiac arrest.

Cardiac arrest is very rare in the recovery room and is always precipitated by one or more of the complications and /or events described here.

Risk factors[1,2]

The predominant risk factors for the development of cardiovascular complications/events postoperatively are:

- History of CV disease—ischaemic heart disease, ↑ or ↓BP, arrhythmias.
- ↑ age
- Diabetes mellitus.
- Smoking.
- Altered electrolyte physiology preoperatively—emergency surgery.
- Renal impairment/history of renal disease.
- Regional anaesthetic technique.
- Type of surgery—cardiothoracic/major trauma.

Arrhythmias

Arrhythmias are common in the recovery room as many patients undergoing surgical intervention have altered cardiac function and status. Recognising them is not always easy and is dependent upon electrode position. A 12-lead ECG should always be performed in any patient with an altered 3-lead trace.

Remember, patients who have a cardiac history of surgery, infarction, and ischaemia will have an altered electrocardiogram wave. Such patients will never have 'textbook' rhythms.[3]

- *Hyper/hypokalaemia and metabolic disorders:* a ↑ or ↓K^+ is the most common metabolic cause of cardiac arrest. However, severe electrolyte disturbance can also cause arrest. Notable examples are hypoglycaemia, hypocalcaemia, and acidaemia. Correction of the abnormal value is the principal aim in such arrests.
- *Hypovolaemia:* severe intra/postoperative haemorrhage can result in arrest due to ↓ circulatory blood volume. GI bleeding, dehiscence,

and disseminated intravascular coagulation are notable causes (📖 see Hypovolaemia, p.566).

- *Thromboembolic/mechanical obstruction*: PE and MI are the most common causes of thromboembolic arrests. Surgical specialty can furthermore impact upon the risk of infarction; vascular and cardiac surgery being principal examples. Treatment of such arrests can be complicated and most are preventable if the signs of cardiac ischaemia (cardiac chest pain and radiation, ECG changes, SOB) are recognised.
- *Tension pneumothorax:* the progressive deterioration of a simple pneumothorax can lead to a tension pneumothorax. In such cases, the gradual build-up of escaped air/pressure ↑ mediastinal pressure, which leads to tracheal deviation and cardiac compression. Upon diagnosis of such an arrest, a needle thoracocentesis and insertion of a chest drain can quickly alleviate the compression.
- *Cardiac tamponade:* tamponade acts in a similar manner to tension pneumothorax. It is caused by a large pericardial effusion (build-up of fluid in the pericardium) and causes arrest via excessive myocardial compression. Tamponade is largely caused by penetrating chest injuries, cardiac surgery, infarct, and sepsis (pericarditis). The immediate management of such an arrest is a pericardiocentesis. Further surgery is often required at a later stage once the patient has been stabilised, to repair the rupture.
- *Toxic/therapeutic disturbances:* arrests due to toxicity and therapeutic disturbances can either be attributed to septic shock, poisoning, or drug overdose. In the recovery room, opiate overdosage is always a plausible cause for arrest if the patient's respiratory depression is ineffectively managed.[4]
- *Defibrillation:* defibrillation is only indicated in VF and pulseless VT arrests. This can be achieved via the use of a manual defibrillator or AED.

References

1. Beamer JER, Warwick J (2004). Critical incidents: The cardiovascular system. *Anaesthesia and Intensive Care Medicine* **5**(12), 426–9.

3. Hatfield A and Tronson M (2008). *The Complete Recovery Room Book* (4th edn). Oxford University Press: Oxford.

2. Kluger MT and Bullock MFM. (2002). Recovery room incidents: A review of 419 reports from the Anaesthetic Incident Monitoring Study (AIMS). *Anaesthesia* **57**, 1060–6.

4. Resuscitation Council UK (2006). *Advanced Life Support* (5th edn). Resuscitation Council (UK): London.

Further reading

Longmore M, Wilkinson I, and Torok E (2007). *Oxford Handbook of Clinical Medicine* (7th edn). Oxford University Press: Oxford.

Neurological disorders

Seizures and convulsions

A seizure can be defined as a sudden and uncontrollable discharge of electricity in the brain. A convulsion is the abnormal motor response that occurs during a seizure.[1]

Seizures can occur as a result of epilepsy or as a result of an underlying pathology, such as CNS imbalance. Irrespective of their cause, seizures should always be managed similarly—the maintenance of the airway taking precedence.

Types of seizure

There are several types of seizure that a patient can endure. These can be broadly categorised as: generalised, partial, and complex partial seizures.

- Generalised seizures summarise the traditional 'fit'. These describe tonic/clonic (grand mal) convulsions, myoclonic (brief arm contractions), and clonic seizures (rhythmic symmetrical movements of the arms, neck and face)
- Partial seizures (also known as focal seizures) are usually non-motor and involve sensory, autonomic, and/or higher conscious impairment.
- Complex partial seizures involve loss of consciousness, spatial awareness and memory.

Seizures can progress from one type to another. For example, complex partial seizures commonly develop into generalised seizures.[1]

Causes

These are the predominant causes of seizures in the recovery room:

- An epileptic who has not taken his/her medication or is undiagnosed.
- Adverse reaction to anaesthetic agents.
- Neurosurgery.   Most Common
- Hyperpyrexia and sepsis.
- Hypoglycaemia.
- Hypoxia.
- Fluid overload.
- Hypocalcaemia.
- Norpethidine toxicity (pethidine overdose).   Least Common

Adverse reaction to anaesthetic agents

With the exception of epilepsy, this is one of the most common reasons for postoperative seizures. Methohexitone, propofol, enflurane, and local anaesthetics are agents, which can directly stimulate convulsions. Abrupt withdrawal of alcohol (in alcoholics), benzodiazepines, and antiparkinsonians can also indirectly stimulate seizures.

Neurosurgery

All neurosurgical patients are at an increased risk of postoperative seizure, this may attributed to the surgery or the patient's medical history (which indicates the need for surgery).

Hyperpyrexia, sepsis, and febrile convulsions

Hyperpyrexia (high fever) refers to a core temperature >40°C. As the body's temperature begins to exceed this, its thermoregulatory cooling mechanisms begin to fail. A core temperature of 41°C+ can stimulate seizures and cellular decay in the brain. The body's consumption for O_2 will increase by 15% for every degree Celsius above 37°C therefore hyperpyrexic patients should always be administered high-flow O2. This can prevent and delay the onset of hyperpyrexic seizures.[2]

In children aged up to 6 years, seizures can occur once their core temperature reaches 39°C. In such instances, these seizures are referred to as febrile convulsions and are characterised by a rapid increase in core temperature. Febrile convulsions should be therapeutically managed by the administration of rectal diazepam (whilst the child is convulsing) and an antipyretic, such as paracetamol (if not administered prior to convulsion).[3]

In adults, sepsis is the most common cause of hyperpyrexia and the nature and type of operation can influence the risk of its development e.g. ruptured appendixes, external trauma, surgery involving the meninges.

Hypoglycaemia

A blood glucose level of <2mmol/l can result in a hypoglycaemic seizure. This type of seizure should be managed accordingly (☐ see Hypoglycemia, p.412) alongside an infusion of 50% glucose until the blood glucose level reaches between 5.5–11mmol/L.[2]

Norpethidine toxicity

Pethidine is metabolised by the body into norpethidine, which is a byproduct. Toxicity of norpethidine stimulates CNS activity and convulsions. Seizures can occur once the body's norpethidine levels exceed 1g and a maximum daily dosage of 25mg/kg (24 hour) is recommended.[4]

References

1. Denison D (2007).Degenerative Neurological Dysfunction: Nursing Management. In: Daniels R., Nosek. Nicoll L. (Eds). *Contemporary Medical-Surgical Nursing*. New York: Thomson Delmar Learning.

2. Hatfield A and Tronson M (2008). *The Complete Recovery Room Book* (4th edn). Oxford University Press: Oxford.

3. Wong V, Ho MHK, Rosman HP, et al. (2002). Clinical guidance on the management of febrile convulsion. *Hong Kong Journal of Paediatrics* **7**, 153–71.

4. Stone PA, MacIntyre, PE, and Jarvis DA (1993). Norpethidine toxicity and patient controlled analgesia. *British Journal of Anaesthesia* **71**, 738–40.

Seizure/convulsion management

The prevention of seizure is always the best form of management. A proactive approach, such as ensuring the epileptic patient is administered his/her anti-convulsant, maintenance of blood glucose level via sliding scale of insulin, and cooling of a patient before he/she becomes hyperpyrexic, can prevent a potential crisis from occurring.

When managing a convulsing patient reactively, a systematic approach should be adopted:

- Immediately check the pulse—if pulse absent, treat as cardiac arrest.
- Call for assistance and request the emergency trolley.
- Open the airway and support using jaw thrust/chin lift.
- Have suction available.
- Administer high-flow O_2 via non-rebreather mask, monitor breathing
- Protect the patient, raise cot sides on bed/trolley and support with padding or pillows.
- Monitor the seizure, note the time of onset and record the duration of convulsion.
- Ascertain cause of seizure: check blood sugar level, SpO_2, temperature, and medical/drug history.
- Lay the patient on their side and place into the recovery position until consciousness is regained.

Pharmacological management

- Most seizures will last no more than 3–5 minutes. Pharmacological management should be considered if the seizure exceeds this duration.
- The first-line treatment of postoperative seizures is benzodiazepines. IV lorazepam (0.1mg/kg, administered over 2 minutes) or diazepam (0.15–0.2mg/kg, administered over 5 minutes) should be used if the patient has IV access. PR diazepam can be administered (0.5mg/kg) if the patient does not have IV access. Alternatively, intranasal midazolam can be administered (0.2mg/kg).
- Second-line treatments (if the seizure has not resolved following administration of first-line agents) include phenobarbital sodium, clonazepam, fosphenytoin and most commonly, phenytoin. Phenytoin (15mg/kg dosage) and other second-line treatments should only be administered if the patient has been convulsing for ≥30 minutes.
- In worst case scenarios, propofol and thiopental can be used. In such instances, the patient should be re-intubated, ventilated, and transferred to intensive care.[1,2]

References

1. Allman KG, McIndoe AK, and Wilson IH (eds) (2005). *Emergencies in Anaesthesia.* Oxford University Press: Oxford.

2. Idrees U and Londner M (2005). Pharmacotherapy overview of seizure management in the adult emergency department. *Journal of Pharmacy Practice* **18**, 394–411.

Index

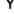